T0276559

Encyclopedia of Mesotheliomas

Encyclopedia of Mesotheliomas

Edited by **Aiden Logan**

New Jersey

Published by Foster Academics,
61 Van Reypen Street,
Jersey City, NJ 07306, USA
www.fosteracademics.com

Encyclopedia of Mesotheliomas
Edited by Aiden Logan

Printed in the United States of America.

Contents

Preface   VII

Chapter 1   **Molecular Pathogenesis of Malignant**
             Pleural Mesothelioma   1
             Philip A. Rascoe, Xiaobo X. Cao and W. Roy Smythe

Chapter 2   **Primary Malignant Pericardial Mesothelioma**   17
             Jesus Montesinos, Sílvia Catot,
             Francesc Sant and Montserrat Domenech

Chapter 3   **Para- and Intratesticular Aspects of**
             Malignant Mesothelioma   27
             Zachary Klaassen, Kristopher R. Carlson, Jeffrey R. Lee,
             Sravan Kuvari and Martha K. Terris

Chapter 4   **Testicular Mesothelioma**   43
             Alexander N. Zubritsky

Chapter 5   **Stem Cells and Mesothelioma**   65
             Bonnie W. Lau

Chapter 6   **Radiologic Evaluation of Malignant Pleural**
             and Peritoneal Mesothelioma   75
             Elif Aktas, Kemal Arda, Bora Aktas, Sahin Coban,
             Nazan Çiledağ and Bilgin Kadri Aribas

Chapter 7   **Mesothelioma in Domestic Animals:**
             Cytological and Anatomopathological Aspects   87
             Winnie A. Merlo and Adriana S. Rosciani

Chapter 8   **Immuno-Oncology and Immunotherapy**   97
             R. Cornelissen, J.G.J.V. Aerts and J.P.J.J. Hegmans

Chapter 9   **Connexin 43 Enhances the Cisplatin-Induced Cytotoxicity**
             in Mesothelioma Cells   121
             Hiromi Sato and Koichi Ueno

Chapter 10   **The Role of Immunotherapy in
the Treatment of Mesothelioma**   **137**
Saly Al-Taei, Jason F. Lester and Zsuzsanna Tabi

Chapter 11   **Cisplatin Resistance in Malignant Pleural Mesothelioma**   **169**
Parviz Behnam-Motlagh, Andreas Tyler, Thomas Brännström,
Terese Karlsson, Anders Johansson and Kjell Grankvist

Chapter 12   **The Central Role of Survivin in Proliferation and
Apoptosis of Malignant Pleural Mesothelioma**   **187**
Julija Hmeljak and Andrej Cör

Chapter 13   **The Impact of Extracellular Low pH on the Anti-Tumor
Efficacy Against Mesothelioma**   **201**
T. Fukamachi, H. Saito, M. Tagawa and H. Kobayashi

Chapter 14   **Why Anti-Energetic Agents Such as Citrate or
3-Bromopyruvate Should be Tested as Anti-Cancer
Agents: Experimental In *Vitro* and In *Vivo* Studies**   **225**
Philippe Icard, Xiao-Dong Zhang, Emilie Varin,
Stéphane Allouche, Antoine Coquerel,
Maria Paciencia, Luc Joyeux, Pascal Gauduchon,
Hubert Lincet and Laurent Poulain

Permissions

List of Contributors

Preface

The main aim of this book is to educate learners and enhance their research focus by presenting diverse topics covering this vast field. This is an advanced book which compiles significant studies by distinguished experts in the area of analysis. This book addresses successive solutions to the challenges arising in the area of application, along with it; the book provides scope for future developments.

Mesotheliomas are mysterious mesothelial tumors, in that they are relatively exceptional, hard to diagnose, and the etiology and pathogenesis of the disease are not yet completely revealed. Every year, this difficulty captures the attention of many specialists in the field of medicine and biology. An increase in growth of mesothelioma morbidity in many countries of the world has been observed because of additional industrialization of society in the last few years. Keeping that in mind, this book has been published with the involvement of an international group of experts with extensive experience. Intended for biologists, this book discusses the recent progressive achievements of all forms of the distinct categories of mesotheliomas, in humans as well as in domestic animals, at a great methodological level. The book would be beneficial for health care employees, oncologists and also the students of medical institutions working in the field of mesotheliomas.

It was a great honour to edit this book, though there were challenges, as it involved a lot of communication and networking between me and the editorial team. However, the end result was this all-inclusive book covering diverse themes in the field.

Finally, it is important to acknowledge the efforts of the contributors for their excellent chapters, through which a wide variety of issues have been addressed. I would also like to thank my colleagues for their valuable feedback during the making of this book.

Editor

Molecular Pathogenesis of Malignant Pleural Mesothelioma

Philip A. Rascoe, Xiaobo X. Cao and W. Roy Smythe
Texas A&M Health Science Center College of Medicine,
Scott & White Memorial Hospital & Clinic,
Olin E. Teague Veterans' Medical Center
USA

1. Introduction

Malignant mesothelioma is a rare, highly aggressive cancer which arises from the mesothelial cells which form the lining of the pleural, and less frequently the peritoneal cavities. Malignant pleural mesothelioma (MPM) is an emergent neoplasm, as it was rarely diagnosed prior to the middle of the 20th century. The incidence has risen steadily since 1970, and there are currently an estimated 3000 new cases per year in the United States. The peak incidence of mesothelioma may have occurred in the United States during the past decade, and the peak incidence in much of the developed world is expected to occur in the next 10-20 years. These data are thought to reflect the widespread occupational asbestos exposure in the Western world from the 1940s to the 1970s, as well as the inherent latency period of approximately 30 years between asbestos exposure and disease manifestation which is typical of MPM. Approximately 80% of mesothelioma cases can be directly attributed to asbestos fiber exposure. Additional suspected causes or co-carcinogens include other mineral fibers such as erionite, simian virus 40 (SV40), and radiation (Robinson and Lake 2005). Moreover, a mesothelioma epidemic in Turkey has demonstrated a likely genetic predisposition to mineral fiber carcinogenesis (Carbone, Emri et al. 2007).

Mesothelioma arises from multipotential mesothelial cells which are capable of differentiating into epithelial, sarcomatoid, or biphasic (mixed) neoplasms. There is lack of consensus on a staging system for MPM, however, most patients present with advanced disease. Advanced age, poor performance status, male sex, and sarcomatoid histologic subtype are all poor prognostic factors. Despite modest advances in clinical treatment, the mean overall survival for patients with MPM is approximately 12 months (Ducko and Sugarbaker 2008). There is also lack of consensus regarding treatment of MPM. Suitable surgical candidates with disease limited to one hemithorax may undergo surgical resection via extrapleural pneumonectomy (EPP) or pleurectomy/decortication (P/D) as part of a multimodality treatment approach. Radiation therapy alone is generally ineffective due to the large volume of primary tumor and its proximity to vital mediastinal structures. However, radiation therapy, particularly intensity-modulated radiation therapy (IMRT), has been demonstrated to reduce local recurrence following resection by EPP (Rice, Stevens et al. 2007). Historically, chemotherapy response rates have been less than 20%. However, improved response rates of 41% have been demonstrated with the addition of the folate antimetabolite pemetrexed (Vogelzang 2003). Highly selected patients appear to benefit from trimodality therapy consisting of aggressive surgical debulking followed by adjuvant radiation and chemotherapy (Sugarbaker, Flores et al. 1999). Failure of conventional therapies has led to interest in novel treatment approaches including intrapleural administration of immunotherapy and gene therapy, as well as intraoperative adjuncts such as intrapleural chemotherapy and photodynamic therapy (Friedberg, Mick et al. 2011; Vachani, Moon et al. 2011).

Studies of human cell lines and tissues as well as animal models of MPM have demonstrated genetic and epigenetic events which contribute to the multistep process of mineral fiber carcinogenesis. These events include inactivation of tumor suppressor genes, modulation of signal transduction pathways including receptor tyrosine kinases (RTKs), avoidance of apoptosis, and inhibition of the ubiquitin-proteosome degradation pathway. This chapter will focus on the molecular pathogenesis of malignant mesothelioma. Preclinical and clinical trials of targeted therapies such as tyrosine kinase, histone deacetylase, and proteosome inhibitors will be included in the discussion.

2. Etiology of mesothelioma

2.1 Asbestos

The vast majority of cases of mesothelioma can be linked in some fashion to asbestos exposure. Materials utilizing asbestos fibers have been present since ancient times. In fact, the word asbestos is derived from a Greek term meaning inextinguishable or unquenchable, a reference to its fire-resistant properties. It was these heat-resistant and insulating properties which made asbestos a valuable commodity, particularly as the industrial revolution began. In the United States, mining and subsequent use of asbestos increased steadily during the first half of the twentieth century, escalated rapidly following World War II, and peaked in 1973, after which it precipitously declined (Figure 1). Asbestos refers to a group of crystalline-hydrated silicate minerals which occur in one of two forms: serpentine and amphibole. Chrysotile is the only serpentine asbestos, and exists as a long, curly, and pliable fiber most suitable for making fabrics. Amphibole fibers are short, straight, and stiff, and have been used to make pipes and tiles. The major commercial amphiboles are amosite, crocidolite, and anthophyllite. Mixtures of chrysotile and amphiboles were used to produce an array of roofing, insulation, and fire-proofing materials. Evidence exists that all asbestos fiber types may demonstrate pulmonary toxicity in a dose-dependent fashion. Moreover, all fiber types possess carcinogenic potential, however, exposure to amphibole fibers is more likely to cause mesothelioma than chrysotile fibers (Cugell and Kamp 2004).

The pulmonary hazards of asbestos exposure, including asbestosis and bronchogenic carcinoma, were recognized and published by physicians in the early twentieth century. However, the link between asbestos exposure and mesothelioma was not established until 1960, when Wagner reported 33 cases of pleural mesothelioma occurring in a relatively short time period in an area of South Africa where crocidolite was mined (Wagner, Sleggs et al. 1960). In 1964, Selikoff and colleagues reported on the link between asbestos exposure and thoracic neoplasia (bronchogenic carcinoma and mesothelioma) in New York-area insulation workers in a variety of industries, including shipbuilding (Selikoff, Churg et al. 1964). Subsequently, this group reported mesothelioma as the cause of 10 of 307 consecutive deaths among these same workers, concluding that mesothelioma was indeed a complication of relatively light and intermittent (occupational) exposure to asbestos, including chrysotile, which was the dominant fiber in American industry at the time (Selikoff, Churg et al. 1965).

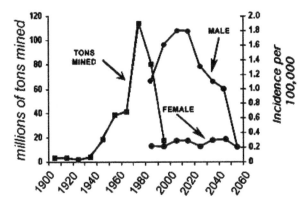

Fig. 1. Asbestos production and mesothelioma incidence: asbestos production in the United States in the last century and mesothelioma incidence from 1980 projected to 2055.
Reprinted from Cugell, D. W. and D. W. Kamp (2004). "Asbestos and the pleura: a review." Chest **125**(3): 1103-1117, with permission.

While smoking cigarettes has been proven to increase the likelihood of developing bronchogenic carcinoma in individuals exposed to asbestos, mesothelioma is not associated with smoking. It is also interesting that while most cases of mesothelioma are associated with asbestos exposure, only a small minority (approximately 5%) of exposed individuals develop mesothelioma (Gazdar and Carbone 2003). Asbestos exposure induces benign manifestations such as pleural effusion or plaques in some individuals, while causing malignant mesothelioma in others. Obviously, other etiologic factors, including genetics, play a role in mesothelioma pathogenesis.

2.2 SV40

SV40 is a polyoma virus of monkey origin which has been identified in a number of human tumors. SV40 contributes to the transformation of human cells by perturbing several intracellular pathways, including disabling the p53 and retinoblastoma (Rb) tumor suppressor pathways. In the 1960s, SV40 was found to be a contaminant in poliovirus vaccines which were prepared in primary cultures of rhesus monkey kidney cells. Contaminated vaccines were administered to children and adults in many countries including the United States. In fact, in the U.S. prior to 1963, approximately 90% of children and 60% of adults received at least one contaminated vaccination. The prevalence of SV40 infections in humans is not known. However, indirect evidence of widespread distribution of SV40 throughout the human population exists in that SV40-positive tumors have been detected throughout the world except in countries that reportedly did not use SV40-contaminated vaccine (Gazdar, Butel et al. 2002).

The human tumors most frequently found to have SV40 sequences are brain and bone tumors, lymphoma, and malignant mesothelioma. SV40 is also a potent oncogenic virus in rodents, and a similar spectrum of tumors is induced in hamsters following viral inoculation. In fact, the incidence of mesothelioma is 100% in hamsters following intrapleural inoculation. Human mesothelial cells contain high endogenous levels of p53 and are unusually susceptible to SV40-mediated transformation, with asbestos acting as a co-carcinogen. Despite powerful evidence regarding the biologic effects of SV40 in mesothelial cells, considerable skepticism exists within the scientific community regarding a causal relationship between the presence of SV40 viral sequences and development of mesothelioma (Gazdar and Carbone 2003).

2.3 Genetic predisposition: The cappadocia epidemic

In 1978, an unprecedented epidemic of mesothelioma was discovered in three villages located in Cappadocia, Turkey. Mesothelioma accounts for >50% of all deaths in these villages. Mineralogic studies of the volcanic rock in these villages demonstrated the presence of a fibrous mineral called erionite which shares some physical properties with crocodolite. Curiously, large erionite deposits are present in other parts of the world, including the western United States, but had never been associated with development of mesothelioma in these regions. The mesothelioma epidemic in Cappadocia was initially linked solely to exposure to erionite contained in the stones used to build houses in the region. However, construction and examination of careful pedigrees demonstrated that mesothelioma occurred in certain families but not in others. Studies have confirmed that the cause of the mesothelioma epidemic in Cappadocia is genetic predisposition to erionite-induced carcinogenesis which is transmitted in an autosomal dominant fashion (Carbone, Emri et al. 2007).

3. Molecular pathogenesis of mesothelioma

The mechanisms whereby inhaled asbestos fibers induce pleural disease, including mesothelioma, are diverse and likely multifactorial. The traditional explanation includes migration of fibers from the airway, through the visceral pleura, and eventual uptake from the parietal pleura. Alternative routes of fiber translocation to the parietal pleura include lymphatic and hematogenous dissemination (Cugell and Kamp 2004). There are several features of asbestos fibers which contribute to their carcinogenicity, including chemical composition, fiber length and form, and their biopersistence. Local responses to these characteristics include frustrated phagocytosis of fibers, generation of reactive oxygen and nitrogen species which may be genotoxic, initiation of inflammatory mechanisms, stimulation of growth factors and their receptors, and initiation of signal transduction pathways which stimulate proliferation and avoidance of apoptosis (Godleski 2004).

3.1 Chromosomal alterations

Allele loss, with subsequent loss of heterozygosity (LOH) at tumor suppressor loci, is a common occurrence in oncogenesis. Mutations and deletions of the p53 and pRb tumor suppressor pathways are prominent features in many human malignancies; however, p53 and pRb remain genetically intact in most mesotheliomas (Lee, Raz et al. 2007). Gene copy number alterations are present in mesothelioma. Common chromosomal regions of allele loss include 1p, 3p21, 6q, 9p21, 15q11-15, and 22q (Zucali, Ceresoli et al. 2011). Homozygous deletion of the 9p21 region is frequently present in mesothelioma cell lines and tumor specimens. Loss of 9p21 results in loss of the INK4a/ARF locus, which encodes two distinct proteins, p16INK4a and p14ARF, translated from alternatively spliced mRNA. p16INK4a inhibits the cyclin-dependent kinase (CDK)-mediated inactivation of pRb. p14ARF stabilizes p53 through its actions on Mdm2. As the INK4a/ARF locus plays an important role in the activity of both the p53 and pRb tumor suppressor pathways (Figure 2), a single mutational event may lead to the functional loss of both of these two key regulatory pathways (Lee, Raz et al. 2007).

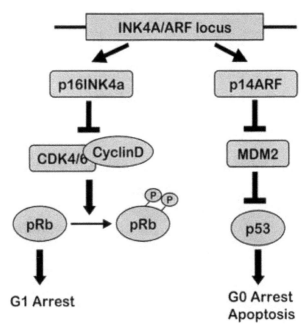

Fig. 2. The role of the INK4A/ARF locus in the regulation of the pRb and p53 tumor suppressor pathways. Reprinted from Lee, A. Y., D. J. Raz, et al. (2007). "Update on the molecular biology of malignant mesothelioma." Cancer **109**(8): 1454-1461, with permission.

3.2 Bcl-XL and resistance to apoptosis

Conventional chemotherapeutic agents and radiation therapy have been shown to exert their cytotoxic effects by inducing apoptosis via the mitochondrial (intrinsic) pathway (Figure 3). Alterations in expression levels of genes and proteins that regulate this pathway of programmed cell death occur frequently in tumor cells. These alterations favor inappropriate cell survival via increased expression of anti-apoptotic proteins. This in turn may lead to resistance to chemotherapeutics and radiation, as these therapies utilize apoptosis as a final common death pathway (Mow, Blajeski et al. 2001). Apoptotic resistance is therefore not only a hallmark of cancer but also a key mechanism of treatment failure (Hanahan and Weinberg 2011).

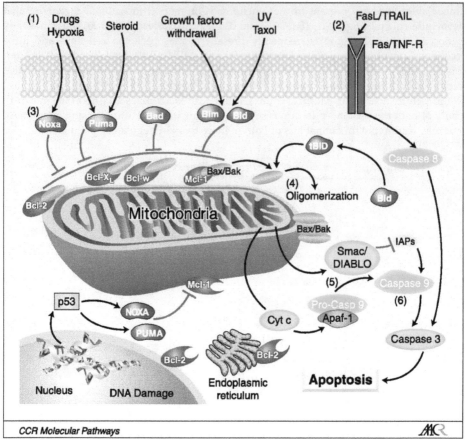

CCR Molecular Pathways

Fig. 3. The apoptotic pathway to cell death from the perspective of the Bcl-2 family of proteins. 1, The intrinsic pathway is initiated by various signals, principally extracellular stimuli. 2, The extrinsic pathway is activated by Fas ligand or TRAIL, subsequently activating caspase-8. Caspase-8 transforms Bid into truncated Bid. In addition, caspase-8 initiates a cascade of caspase activation. 3, BH3-only proteins (Bim, Bid, Bad, Noxa, Puma) engage with anti-apoptotic Bcl-2 family proteins to relieve their inhibition of Bax and Bak to activate them. 4, Next, Bax and Bak are oligomerized and activated, leading to mitochondrial outer membrane permeabilization. 5, Once mitochondrial membranes are permeabilized, cytochrome c and/or Smac/DIABLO is released into the cytoplasm, wherein they combine with an adaptor molecule, apoptosis protease-activating factor 1, and an inactive initiator caspase, procaspase-9, within a multiprotein complex called the apoptosome. Smac/DIABLO inhibits inhibitors of apoptosis proteins to activate caspase-9. 6, Caspase-9 activates caspase-3, which is the initiation step for the cascade of caspase activation. Intrinsic and extrinsic pathways converge on caspase-3. Bcl-2 family proteins are also found on the endoplasmic reticulum and the perinuclear membrane in hematopoietic cells, but they are predominantly localized to mitochondria. Reprinted from Kang M H , Reynolds C P Clin Cancer Res 2009;15:1126-1132, with permission.

The Bcl-2 family consists of 23-25 genes coding for proteins that, in conjunction with other constituents of programmed cell death pathways, regulate apoptotic homeostasis. The longer splice product of the *bcl-x* gene (located on the short arm of chromosome 20, 20pter-p12.1), Bcl-XL, is an important anti-apoptotic member of the family and is over-expressed in several solid tumors including malignant mesothelioma (Cao, Littlejohn et al. 2009). The physiological role of anti-apoptotic proteins is to prevent apoptosis by inhibiting release of soluble mitochondrial intermembrane proteins such as cytochrome c and DIABLO into the cytoplasm. The release of these proteins leads to caspase activation. Interactions of the various members of the Bcl-2 family have been revealed to be more complex than originally thought, but the role of BAX/BAK as effectors of mitochondrial membrane permeability remains central. The exact mechanism by which BAX/BAK affects membrane permeability is not completely understood, but it is known to involve membrane incorporation of these proteins, as well as autodimerization and interaction with VDAC proteins(Kim, Rafiuddin-Shah et al. 2006; Youle and Strasser 2008). Anti-apoptotic proteins such as BCL-XL act by sequestration of BAX/BAK "activator" proteins tBID, BIM and PUMA. This activity is antagonized by the interaction of "inactivator" proteins such as BIK, NOXA, and BAD with Bcl-XL. When challenged with pro-apoptotic stimuli in a wide variety of human tumor cell lines, Bcl-XL is at least as potent as Bcl-2 in prevention of apoptosis. In systems where Bcl-2 and Bcl-XL have been alternatively and co-over-expressed, Bcl-XL is more important to prevention of apoptosis.(Huang, Cory et al. 1997). Although there is significant homology between Bcl-2 and Bcl-XL, Bcl-XL has proved to be uniquely important in human disease, and has been the focus of our studies in mesothelioma, in which Bcl-2 is not typically overexpressed. Our laboratory has demonstrated the therapeutic potential of Bcl-XL down-regulation and functional inhibition both in vitro and in pre-clinical models of mesothelioma. In combination therapies, these models have proven successful in helping to overcome resistance to conventional chemotherapy.

Increased expression of pro-apoptotic members of the Bcl-2 family should favor programmed cell death in the presence of an appropriate stimulus. In fact, transduction of mesothelioma cell lines with an adenoviral vector containing the pro-apoptotic protein BAK induces decreased cellular viability and increased apoptosis in vitro (Pataer, Smythe et al. 2001). Antisense oligonucleotide (ASO) therapy directed at Bcl-XL mRNA has been shown to chemosensitize a number of tumor cell types, including mesothelioma. ASOs directed at Bcl-XL mRNA were utilized in vitro to down-regulate Bcl-XL protein expression, decrease viability, and engender apoptosis in human mesothelioma cell lines (Smythe, Mohuiddin et al. 2002). Furthermore, exposure of human mesothelioma cells to Bcl-XL ASOs in vitro was demonstrated to sensitize them to the conventional chemotherapeutic agent cisplatin in a synergistic manner (Ozvaran, Cao et al. 2004). Finally, the combination of Bcl-XL ASO and cisplatin was demonstrated to reduce the growth of established flank tumor xenografts in mice as well as extend survival in an orthotopic xenograft mouse model of mesothelioma (Littlejohn, Cao et al. 2008). Similar results have been obtained utilizing small interfering RNA (siRNA)-induced inhibition of Bcl-XL rather than antisense oligonucleotides.

Pharmacological agents that neutralize the functions of anti-apoptotic Bcl-2 family proteins have emerged as a promising new class of anti-cancer agents. These direct inhibitors of Bcl-XL function have a number of theoretical advantages over ASO and siRNA-based approaches, including facilitation of systemic delivery and cross reactivity with other anti-apoptotic members. 2-methoxy antimycin A3 is a small molecular ligand which inhibits binding of pro-apoptotic family members such as BAK by occupying the binding cleft of Bcl-XL and Bcl-2. Treatment of mesothelioma cell lines with 2-methoxy antimycin A3 results in apoptotic cell death without altering Bcl-2 family protein expression. Furthermore, co-adminstration of 2-methoxy antimycin A3 and cisplatin results in synergistic inhibition of tumor growth in an *in vivo* mesothelioma tumor model (Cao, Rodarte et al. 2007). Pharmacologic inhibitors of antiapoptotic Bcl-2 family members continue to undergo further refinement and have shown promise in a number of tumor types, including mesothelioma.

3.3 Histone Deacetylase Inhibitors (HDACi)

Histones are a family of proteins that serve as structural and regulatory components of chromatin. The fundamental complex of chromatin is the nucleosome, which consists of 146 base pairs of DNA wrapped around an octamer of histone subunits (Marks, Miller et al. 2003). Histone acetylation, regulated by histone acetyltransferases (HAT) and histone deacetylases (HDAC), affects the relative condensation of chromatin. In short, when histones are acetylated, chromatin is decondensed, and DNA is available for transcription. Histone deacetylases facilitate chromatin condensation, preventing transcription of genes which include tumor suppressors (Zucali, Ceresoli et al. 2011). In addition to effects on histone proteins and the structure of chromatin, histone deacetylase inhibitors (HDACi) also modulate the acetylation of nonhistone proteins such as transcription factors. This ultimately leads to a number of biologic effects such as promotion of apoptosis, cell cycle inhibition, and inhibition of angiogenesis (Paik and Krug 2010).

Sodium butyrate is a histone deacetylase inhibitor known to alter Bcl-2 family gene expression in a variety of tumor types. Exposure of mesothelioma cell lines to sodium butyrate leads to decreased mRNA transcription and protein expression of Bcl-XL as well as induction of apoptosis (Cao, Mohuiddin et al. 2001) In a subsequent study, cellular death and apoptosis of mesothelioma cell lines were augmented by the combination of sodium butyrate with proapoptotic gene therapy, namely adenoviral transfer of the proapoptotic Bcl-2 family members BAX and BAK (Mohiuddin, Cao et al. 2001). Similar *in vitro* effects have been demonstrated in mesothelioma utilizing the HDACi suberoylanilide hydroxamic acid (SAHA, Vorinostat). Others have demonstrated a synergistic response between HDACi and combination chemotherapy in mesothelioma. Treatment with valproic acid, another known HDACi, in combination with pemetrexed and cisplatin led to complete suppression of epithelioid mesothelioma growth in a mouse xenograft model (Vandermeers, Hubert et al. 2009).

An increasing amount of preclinical data demonstrating the utility of histone deacetylase inhibition *in vitro* and in mouse xenograft models has led to early phase clinical trials in patients with mesothelioma. Based on compelling evidence from two phase I trials involving mesothelioma patients who received Vorinostat, a multicenter, randomized, placebo-controlled phase III trial of Vorinostat in patients with advanced mesothelioma has been initiated. Patients who have progressed or relapsed following treatment with pemetrexed and platinum therapy are randomized 1:1 to receive Vorinostat or placebo. This study is ongoing (Paik and Krug 2010).

3.4 Receptor Tyrosine Kinases (RTKs)

Peptide growth factors are important in maintaining tumor cell viability, particularly in the face of apoptotic stimuli. These growth factors are well known to induce intracellular signal transduction pathways such as the phosphoinositide-3 (PI-3) kinase and mitogen-activated protein (MAP) kinase pathways through their interaction with specific cell surface transmembrane receptor tyrosine kinases (RTKs). Several growth factors and their receptors have been shown to play a significant role in the oncogenesis, progression, and resistance to therapy of malignant mesothelioma. Among them, Epidermal Growth Factor (EGF), Hepatocyte Growth Factor (HGF), Vascular Endothelial Growth Factor (VEGF), and Insulin-like Growth Factor (IGF) have been shown to be targets for therapy based on promising preclinical data (Villanova, Procopio et al. 2008).

3.4.1 Epidermal Growth Factor (EGF)

One of the most thoroughly studied targets in cancer therapeutics is the epidermal growth factor receptor (EGFR) and its ligand, EGF. EGFR is well known to be overexpressed in many human cancers, among them colon, breast, lung, and upper aerodigestive tract malignancies. In 1990, Dazzi and colleagues found that 68% of mesothelioma specimens stained positively for EGFR by means of immunohistochemistry and that EGFR positivity was more common in the epithelial subtype (Dazzi, Hasleton et al. 1990). In studying the immunohistochemical expression of EGFR and its ligand, transforming growth factor-alpha (TGF-α), Cai and associates found that 76% of mesotheliomas expressed TGF-α, whereas 45% expressed EGFR, indicating the possibility of an EGFR autocrine loop (Cai, Roggli et al. 2004). EGFR expression has also been linked to asbestos exposure in tissue culture. SV40-transformed human mesothelial cells exposed to asbestos fibers in vitro overexpress EGFR compared with control cells and EGFR expression is related to increasing fiber length of crocidolite asbestos (Pache, Janssen et al. 1998). Similar results have been obtained in vivo in rat pleural mesothelial cells (Faux, Houghton et al. 2001). A preclinical study using gefitinib (Iressa), an orally-bioavailable EGFR kinase inhibitor, demonstrated growth inhibition and G1 cell-cycle arrest in four mesothelioma cell lines (Janne, Taffaro et al. 2002). EGFR kinase inhibition led to apoptotic cell death via downregulation of PI-3 kinase/Akt signaling in mesothelioma in vitro (Rascoe, Cao et al. 2005). Finally, gefitinib was noted to potentiate the radiation response of mesothelioma xenografts in nude mice, with many animals demonstating complete regression with no tumor regrowth (She, Lee et al. 2003).

Based on the aforementioned preclinical data, pharmacologic inhibition of EGFR was thought to be a promising strategy in mesothelioma therapy. Moreover, the identification of activating mutations in the kinase domain of EGFR as a biomarker of response to tyrosine kinase inhibitor therapy in non-small cell lung cancer (NSCLC) patients was equally promising (Lynch, Bell et al. 2004) (Paez, Janne et al. 2004). While activating mutations of EGFR have been reported in patients with malignant peritoneal mesothelioma (Foster, Gatalica et al. 2008; Foster, Radhakrishna et al. 2010), no such activating mutations of EGFR have been discovered in patients with pleural mesothelioma, and the results of EGFR inhibitors in phase II clinical trials have been disappointing (Velcheti, Kasai et al. 2009). The Cancer and Leukemia Group B (CALGB) 30101 phase II trial enrolled 43 chemotherapy-naïve patients to receive 500 mg gefitinib (Iressa) daily. 3-month progression free survival was 40%, which was not different than historical controls, and the authors concluded that single-agent gefitinib was not active in malignant mesothelioma. 97% of the patients in CALGB 30101 who had EGFR expression scored by immunohistochemistry were found to have high expression (Govindan, Kratzke et al. 2005). A Southwest Oncology Group (SWOG) phase II trial enrolled 63 chemotherapy-naïve patients to receive erlotinib (Tarceva). Despite high EGFR expression in 75% of participants, only 42% of patients had stable measurable disease, and the median progression-free survival of 2 months was significantly lower than that observed with standard first-line chemotherapy (Garland, Rankin et al. 2007).

Phosphatase and tensin analog (PTEN) is a tumor suppressor gene which has been localized to chromosome 10q23. Loss of heterozygosity at 10q23 has been demonstrated in a number of tumor types, including mesothelioma. In a large tissue array study of clinical mesothelioma samples, 62% demonstrated absent PTEN expression while 14% demonstrated weak expression. Examination of clinical data from this cohort revealed that loss of PTEN expression was an independent predictor of poor survival in mesothelioma patients (Opitz, Soltermann et al. 2008). Our laboratory has previously demonstrated that adenoviral gene transfer and forced overexpression of PTEN engenders apoptosis in mesothelioma by Akt hypophosphorylation and decreased Akt kinase activity (Mohiuddin, Cao et al. 2002). It has been hypothesized that loss of PTEN and resultant constitutive Akt activation may explain the resistance seen with EGFR tyrosine kinase inhibitors, as they act upstream of PTEN (Agarwal, Lind et al. 2011).

3.4.2 Hepatocyte Growth Factor (HGF)

Hepatocyte Growth Factor (HGF) is a multifunctional growth factor known to induce cellular growth and proliferation, motility, and morphogenesis. HGF induces these biological functions through binding to its transmembrane tyrosine kinase receptor, c-Met (Zucali, Ceresoli et al. 2011). c-Met is overexpressed and activated in a majority of cases of mesothelioma when compared to normal tissues. In addition, the circulating serum levels of HGF are two-fold greater in mesothelioma patients as compared with healthy control patients. Upon HGF stimulation and c-Met phosphorylation, the PI-3 kinase and MAP kinase signal transduction pathways are activated in mesothelioma cell lines. Moreover, c-Met small interfering RNA (siRNA) and a pharmacologic c-Met inhibitor (SU11274) are effective in inhibiting cell growth and migration of these same cell lines (Jagadeeswaran, Ma et al. 2006).

An association between c-Met and Bcl-XL levels in malignant tissues has been established. In mesothelioma, the HGF/cMet axis appears to upregulate Bcl-XL expression at the transcriptional level. Specifically, via activation of MAP kinases, members of the ETS family of transcription factors are phosphorylated. This leads to nuclear importation of the factors ETS-2 and PU.1, both of which increase Bcl-XL promoter activity in mesothelioma. Conversely, the transcriptional repressor, Tel, is phosphorylated and exported from the nucleus to the cytoplasm (Cao, Littlejohn et al. 2009).

3.4.3 Vascular Endothelial Growth Factor (VEGF)

Vascular endothelial growth factor is an essential regulatory component of physiologic angiogenesis. Furthermore, its role in tumor pathogenesis, growth, and metastasis are well documented, and VEGF is overexpressed in most human malignancies. The effects of VEGF are mediated through binding to two tyrosine kinase receptors: VEGFR-1, or Flt-1 (fms-like tyrosine kinase-1), and VEGFR-2, or KDR/Flk-1 (kinase-insert domain receptor/fetal liver kinase-1) (Villanova, Procopio et al. 2008).

Mesothelioma patients have higher serum levels of VEGF than normal controls and, in fact, have higher VEGF levels than other solid tumor patients (Linder, Linder et al. 1998). VEGF and its two receptors are expressed in mesothelioma cell lines, biopsy specimens, and pleural effusions. VEGF levels in the pleural effusions of mesothelioma patients were 7-fold higher than levels in effusions in patients with non-malignant disease. Moreover, linear regression analysis has demonstrated an inverse correlation between serum VEGF levels and survival in mesothelioma patients (Strizzi, Catalano et al. 2001).

A number of angiogenesis inhibitors directed at VEGF and its receptors have been developed. The anti-VEGF monoclonal antibody bevacizumab (Avastin) has demonstrated modest survival benefit and is approved for use in metastatic colorectal carcinoma and non-small cell lung cancer. Unfortunately, despite the aforementioned promising preclinical data, a phase II trial combining cisplatin and gemcitabine with and without bevacizumab in unresectable, chemotherapy-naïve mesothelioma patients yielded no differences in progression-free or overall survival (Karrison, Kindler et al. 2007). A similar trial comparing bevacizumab and placebo in patients receiving current first-line chemotherapy (cisplatin/pemetrexed) is ongoing. Studies investigating several small molecule pharmacologic inhibitors of VEGF receptor tyrosine kinases have demonstrated only modest activity to date (Kelly, Sharon et al. 2011).

3.4.4 Insulin-like Growth Factors (IGF)

Insulin-like growth factors represent a family of peptides produced by various tissues throughout the body. IGFs possess growth stimulatory activities similar to insulin and may work in an autocrine, paracrine, or endocrine fashion. As such, IGF has been reported to be an important growth factor in many tumor types. Both normal mesothelial and mesothelioma cell lines express IGF-1 and IGF-1R mRNA, indicating the possibility of an autocrine loop (Lee, Raz et al. 2007). An IGF-1 receptor antisense expression vector led to a decrease in proliferation and tumorigenicity in a hamster mesothelioma cell line (Pass, Mew et al. 1996). We observed increased IGF-1R expression in mesothelioma cell lines relative to a transformed mesothelial line as well as decreased cellular viability and apoptosis in a sarcomatous-type mesothelioma line following IGF-1R inhibition (Rascoe, Cao et al. 2005). Others have demonstrated dose-dependent growth repression, inhibition of IGF-1R phosphorylation, and decreased activity of downstream PI-3 kinase/Akt and MAP kinase signal transduction pathways following treatment with an orally bioavailable IGFR inhibitor, NVP-AEW541 (Whitson, Jacobson et al. 2006).

3.5 Proteosome inhibitors

Investigation has revealed that the ubiquitin-proteosome pathway plays a key role in regulating homeostasis of cellular proteins that involve cell cycle, survival, and apoptosis. Therapeutically, targeting the proteosome with a specific inhibitor, bortezomib (Velcade), has been successful in selectively inducing apoptosis in a variety of human cancer cells including mesothelioma. Bortezomib is a selective inhibitor of the 20S proteosome. Its actions are pleiotropic and include inhibition of NF-kB activation by preventing degradation of its inhibitor IkB (Zucali, Ceresoli et al. 2011). Inhibition of constitutively activated NF-kB by bortezomib resulted in cytotoxicity and apoptosis in vitro and regression of mesothelioma xenografts in mice (Sartore-Bianchi, Gasparri et al. 2007). Furthermore, bortezomib potentiated the activity of pemetrexed and cisplatin in mesothelioma cell lines (Gordon, Mani et al. 2008). Bortezomib is currently under investigation in a number of mesothelioma trials, both as a single agent and in combination with chemotherapy. While bortezomib is approved for the treatment of multiple myeloma, cellular resistance to boretezomib-induced apoptosis may limit its successful application as a therapeutic agent in this context (Richardson, Sonneveld et al. 2007). In vitro development of a bortezomib-resistant mesothelioma cell line has demonstrated that evasion of the unfolded protein response (UPR) and concomitant reduction in pro-apoptotic gene induction accounts for resistance in bortezomib-adapted mesothelioma cells (Zhang, Littlejohn et al. 2010).

4. Conclusions and future directions

Despite modest advances in clinical treatment over the past decade, malignant pleural mesothelioma remains a vexing clinical problem. The mean overall survival for patients with MPM is approximately 12 months. Highly selected patients appear to benefit from aggressive surgical debulking followed by intensity-modulated radiation therapy (IMRT) to achieve local control of disease followed by systemic chemotherapy. Modest improvements in the treatment of unresectable mesothelioma have been made utilizing combination chemotherapy with cisplatin and pemetrexed. This combination is the current standard of care in the adjuvant setting as well.

Studies of human cell lines and tissues as well as animal models of MPM have demonstrated genetic and epigenetic events which contribute to the multistep process of mineral fiber carcinogenesis. These events include inactivation of tumor suppressor genes, modulation of signal transduction pathways including receptor tyrosine kinases (RTKs), avoidance of apoptosis, and inhibition of the ubiquitin-proteosome degradation pathway. Preclinical investigations of targeted therapies such as tyrosine kinase, histone deacetylase, and proteosome inhibitors have been promising. However, randomized clinical trials utilizing many of these same agents have been disappointing to date. Pharmacologic inhibitors of anti-apoptotic Bcl-2 family members continue to undergo refinement, and there is hope that they will emerge as a promising new class of anticancer agent. Preclinical data suggests they could demonstrate therapeutic effect in a number of tumor types, including mesothelioma.

Autophagy, a concerted process of intra-cellular breakdown within specialized double membrane vesicles, occurs in response to events such as metabolic stress. It is an evolutionarily conserved pro-survival mechanism, regulated downstream of MTOR in the PI-3kinase/Akt cell-survival pathway. While generally cytoprotective, excessive autophagy results in a type of programmed cell death that is morphologically distinct from apoptosis (Sinha and Levine 2008). It has been noted that, depending on context, autophagy can augment either cellular demise or protection. Apoptosis and autophagy are not mutually exclusive programmed cell death pathways, as evidenced by a specific physical interaction between regulators of the two pathways: Beclin-1 (autophagy) and Bcl-XL (apoptosis). Bcl-

XL has recently been determined to inhibit autophagy via a direct functional and physical interaction with Beclin-1, a protein essential for the initiation of autophagy (Maiuri, Le Toumelin et al. 2007). Beclin-1, characterized as a haploinsufficient tumor suppressor, is a known cytosolic mediator of autophagy, and a recent addition to the BH3-only members of the Bcl-family of proteins. These proteins govern intrinsic apoptosis, via selective interaction with the BH3 binding pocket of Bcl-XL (Oberstein, Jeffrey et al. 2007). Autophagy is likely important in response to toxic insults such as chemotherapy or irradiation, but its exact role in the context of a growing solid tumor remains unclear (Degenhardt, Mathew et al. 2006). Beclin-1 is known to promote cell survival in solid tumors via facilitation of autophagy, yet has also been shown to suppress tumorogenicity (Degenhardt, Mathew et al. 2006; Oberstein, Jeffrey et al. 2007). In malignant glioma cells, it has been shown that the anti-tumor effect of temozolomide can be suppressed by inhibiting early autophagy, but that inhibition of late autophagy enhances cytotoxicity (Kanzawa T 2008). Inhibition of autophagy in radiation resistant cell lines of breast, lung, pharyngeal, and cervical cancers resensitized them to radiation treatment (Apel, Herr et al. 2008). Thus, it is becoming clear that a greater understanding of autophagy in the context of chemotherapy-induced apoptosis within a growing solid tumor could add to our understanding of chemotherapeutic response and development of resistance.

Ongoing studies in our laboratory have demonstrated that both apoptosis and autophagy occur in malignant mesothelioma following histone deacetylase inhibition through mutually exclusive processes. Autophagy appears to occur much earlier than apoptosis, suggesting that autophagy may play a cytoprotective role in mesothelioma cells following cytotoxic therapy, thus subverting their entry into the apoptotic pathway.

5. References

Agarwal, V., M. J. Lind, et al. (2011). "Targeted epidermal growth factor receptor therapy in malignant pleural mesothelioma: Where do we stand?" *Cancer Treat Rev* 37(7): 533-542.

Apel, A., I. Herr, et al. (2008). "Blocked autophagy sensitizes resistant carcinoma cells to radiation therapy." *Cancer Research* 68(5): 1485-1494.

Cai, Y. C., V. Roggli, et al. (2004). "Transforming growth factor alpha and epidermal growth factor recpetor in reactive and malignant mesothelial proliferations." *Arch Pathol Lab Med* 128: 68-70.

Cao, X., J. Littlejohn, et al. (2009). "Up-regulation of Bcl-xl by hepatocyte growth factor in human mesothelioma cells involves ETS transcription factors." *Am J Pathol* 175(5): 2207-2216.

Cao, X., C. Rodarte, et al. (2007). "Bcl2/bcl-xL inhibitor engenders apoptosis and increases chemosensitivity in mesothelioma." *Cancer Biol Ther* 6(2): 246-252.

Cao, X. X., I. Mohuiddin, et al. (2001). "Histone deacetylase inhibitor downregulation of bcl-xl gene expression leads to apoptotic cell death in mesothelioma." *Am J Respir Cell Mol Biol* 25(5): 562-568.

Carbone, M., S. Emri, et al. (2007). "A mesothelioma epidemic in Cappadocia: scientific developments and unexpected social outcomes." *Nat Rev Cancer* 7(2): 147-154.

Cugell, D. W. and D. W. Kamp (2004). "Asbestos and the pleura: a review." *Chest* 125(3): 1103-1117.

Dazzi, H., P. S. Hasleton, et al. (1990). "Malignant pleural mesothelioma and epidermal growth factor receptor (EGF-R). Relationship of EGF-R with histology and survival using paraffin embedded tissue and the F4, monoclonal antibody." *Br J Cancer* 61: 924-926.

Degenhardt, K., R. Mathew, et al. (2006). "Autophagy promotes tumor cell survival and restricts necrosis, inflammation, and tumorigenesis." *Cancer Cell* 10(1): 51-64.

Ducko, C. T. and D. J. Sugarbaker (2008). Pleural Tumors. *Pearson's Thoracic & Esophageal Surgery.* J. D. C. G. Alexander Patterson, Jean Deslauriers, Antoon E.M.R. Lerut, James D. Luketich, Thomas W. Rice. Philadelphia, PA, Churchill Livingstone: 1121-1136.

Faux, S. P., C. E. Houghton, et al. (2001). "Increased expression of epidermal growth factor receptor in rat pleural mesothelial cells correlates with carcinogenicity of mineral fibres." *Carcinogenesis* 12: 2275-2280.

Foster, J. M., Z. Gatalica, et al. (2008). "Novel and Existing Mutations in the Tyrosine Kinase Domain of the Epidermal Growth Factor Receptor are Predictors of Optimal Resectability in Malignant Peritoneal Mesothelioma." *Annals of Surgical Oncology* 16(1): 152-158.

Foster, J. M., U. Radhakrishna, et al. (2010). "Clinical implications of novel activating EGFR mutations in malignant peritoneal mesothelioma." *World Journal of Surgical Oncology* 8(1): 88.

Friedberg, J. S., R. Mick, et al. (2011). "Photodynamic therapy and the evolution of a lung-sparing surgical treatment for mesothelioma." *Ann Thorac Surg* 91(6): 1738-1745.

Garland, L. L., C. Rankin, et al. (2007). "Phase II study of erlotinib in patients with malignant pleural mesothelioma: a Southwest Oncology Group Study." *J Clin Oncol* 25(17): 2406-2413.

Gazdar, A. F., J. S. Butel, et al. (2002). "SV40 and human tumours: myth, association or causality?" *Nat Rev Cancer* 2(12): 957-964.

Gazdar, A. F. and M. Carbone (2003). "Molecular pathogenesis of malignant mesothelioma and its relationship to simian virus 40." *Clin Lung Cancer* 5(3): 177-181.

Godleski, J. J. (2004). "Role of asbestos in etiology of malignant pleural mesothelioma." *Thorac Surg Clin* 14: 479-487.

Gordon, G. J., M. Mani, et al. (2008). "Preclinical studies of the proteasome inhibitor bortezomib in malignant pleural mesothelioma." *Cancer Chemother Pharmacol* 61(4): 549-558.

Govindan, R., R. A. Kratzke, et al. (2005). "Gefitinib in patients with malignant mesothelioma: a phase II study by the Cancer and Leukemia Group B." *Clin Cancer Res* 11(6): 2300-2304.

Hanahan, D. and R. A. Weinberg (2011). "Hallmarks of Cancer: The Next Generation." *Cell* 144: 646-674.

Huang, D. C. S., S. Cory, et al. (1997). "Bcl-2, Bcl-x(L) and adenovirus protein E1B19kD are functionally equivalent in their ability to inhibit cell death." *Oncogene* 14(4): 405-414.

Jagadeeswaran, R., P. C. Ma, et al. (2006). "Functional analysis of c-Met/hepatocyte growth factor pathway in malignant pleural mesothelioma." *Cancer Res* 66(1): 352-361.

Janne, P. A., M. L. Taffaro, et al. (2002). "Inhibition of epidermal growth factor receptor signaling in malignant pleural mesothelioma." *Cancer Res* 62: 5242-5247.

Kanzawa T, G. I., Komata T, Ito H, Kondo Y, Kondo S (2008). "Role of autophagy in temozolomide-induced cytotoxicity for malignant glioma cells. ." *Cell death and differentiation*(11): 448-457.

Karrison, T., H. L. Kindler, et al. (2007). "Final analysis of a multi-center, double-blind, placebo-controlled, randomized phase II trial of gemcitabine/cisplatin (GC) plus bevacizumab (B) or placebo (P) in patients (pts) with malignant mesothlioma (MM)." *J Clin Oncol* 25(18S): 7526.

Kelly, R. J., E. Sharon, et al. (2011). "Chemotherapy and targeted therapies for unresectable malignant mesothelioma." *Lung Cancer* 73(3): 256-263.

Kim, H., M. Rafiuddin-Shah, et al. (2006). "Hierarchical regulation of mitochondrion-dependent apoptosis by BCL-2 subfamilies." *Nature Cell Biology* 8(12): 1348-U1319.

Lee, A. Y., D. J. Raz, et al. (2007). "Update on the molecular biology of malignant mesothelioma." *Cancer* 109(8): 1454-1461.

Linder, C., S. Linder, et al. (1998). "Independent expression of serum vascular endothelial growth factor (VEGF) and basic fibroblast growth factor (bFGF) in patients with carcinoma and sarcoma." *Anticancer Res* 18(3B): 2063-2068.

Littlejohn, J. E., X. Cao, et al. (2008). "Bcl-xL antisense oligonucleotide and cisplatin combination therapy extends survival in SCID mice with established mesothelioma xenografts." *Int J Cancer* 123(1): 202-208.

Lynch, T. J., D. W. Bell, et al. (2004). "Activating mutations in the epidermal growth factor receptor underlying responsiveness of non-small-cell lung cancer to gefitinib." *N Engl J Med* 350(21): 2129-2139.

Maiuri, M. C., G. Le Toumelin, et al. (2007). "Functional and physical interaction between Bcl-X-L and a BH3-like domain in Beclin-1." *Embo Journal* 26(10): 2527-2539.

Marks, P. A., T. Miller, et al. (2003). "Histone Deacetylases." *Curr Opin Pharmacol* 3: 344-351.

Mohiuddin, I., X. Cao, et al. (2001). "Significant augmentation of pro-apoptotic gene therapy by pharmacologic bcl-xl down-regulation in mesothelioma." *Cancer Gene Ther* 8(8): 547-554.

Mohiuddin, I., X. Cao, et al. (2002). "Phosphatase and tensin analog gene overexpression engenders cellular death in human malignant mesothelioma cells via inhibition of AKT phosphorylation." *Ann Surg Oncol* 9(3): 310-316.

Mow, B. M., A. L. Blajeski, et al. (2001). "Apoptosis and the response to anticancer therapy." *Curr Opin Oncol* 13(6): 453-462.

Oberstein, A., P. D. Jeffrey, et al. (2007). "Crystal structure of the Bcl-X-L-beclin 1 peptide complex - Beclin 1 is a novel BH3-only protein." *Journal of Biological Chemistry* 282(17): 13123-13132.

Opitz, I., A. Soltermann, et al. (2008). "PTEN expression is a strong predictor of survival in mesothelioma patients." *Eur J Cardiothorac Surg* 33(3): 502-506.

Ozvaran, M. K., X. X. Cao, et al. (2004). "Antisense oligonucleotides directed at the bcl-xl gene product augment chemotherapy response in mesothelioma." *Mol Cancer Ther* 3(5): 545-550.

Pache, J. C., Y. Janssen, et al. (1998). "Increased epidermal growth factor-receptor protein in a human mesothelial cell line in response to long asbestos fibers." *Am J Pathol* 152: 333-340.

Paez, J. G., P. A. Janne, et al. (2004). "EGFR mutations in lung cancer: correlation with clinical response to gefitinib therapy." *Science* 304(5676): 1497-1500.

Paik, P. K. and L. M. Krug (2010). "Histone Deacetylase Inhibitors in Malignant Pleural Mesothelioma." *J Thorac Oncol* 5: 275-279.

Pass, H. I., D. J. Mew, et al. (1996). "Inhibition of hamster mesothelioma tumorigenesis by an antisense expression plasmid to the insluin-like growth factor-1 receptor." *Cancer Res* 56: 4044-4048.

Pataer, A., W. R. Smythe, et al. (2001). "Adenovirus-mediated Bak Gene Transfer Induces Apoptosis in Mesothelioma Cell Lines." *J Thorac Cardiovasc Surg* 121: 61-67.

Rascoe, P. A., X. Cao, et al. (2005). "Receptor tyrosine kinase and phosphoinositide-3 kinase signaling in malignant mesothelioma." *J Thorac Cardiovasc Surg* 130(2): 393-400.

Rice, D. C., C. W. Stevens, et al. (2007). "Outcomes after extrapleural pneumonectomy and intensity-modulated radiation therapy for malignant pleural mesothelioma." *Ann Thorac Surg* 84(5): 1685-1692; discussion 1692-1683.

Richardson, P. G., P. Sonneveld, et al. (2007). "Extended follow-up of a phase 3 trial in relapsed multiple myeloma: final time-to-event results of the APEX trial." *Blood* 110(10): 3557-3560.

Robinson, B. W. and R. A. Lake (2005). "Advances in malignant mesothelioma." *N Engl J Med* 353(15): 1591-1603.

Sartore-Bianchi, A., F. Gasparri, et al. (2007). "Bortezomib inhibits nuclear factor-kappaB dependent survival and has potent in vivo activity in mesothelioma." *Clin Cancer Res* 13(19): 5942-5951.

Selikoff, I. J., J. Churg, et al. (1964). "Asbestos Exposure and Neoplasia." *JAMA* 188: 22-26.

Selikoff, I. J., J. Churg, et al. (1965). "Relation Between Exposure to Asbestos and Mesothelioma." *N Engl J Med* 272(11): 560-565.

She, Y., F. Lee, et al. (2003). "The epidermal growth factor receptor tyrosine kinase inhibitor ZD1839 selectively potentiates radiation response of human tumor in nude mice, with a marked improvement of therapeutic index." *Clin Cancer Res* 9: 3773-3778.

Sinha, S. and B. Levine (2008). "The autophagy effector Beclin 1: a novel BH3-only protein." *Oncogene* 27 Suppl 1: S137-148.

Smythe, W. R., I. Mohuiddin, et al. (2002). "Antisense therapy for malignant mesothelioma with oligonucleotides targeting the bcl-xl gene product." *J Thorac Cardiovasc Surg* 123(6): 1191-1198.

Strizzi, L., A. Catalano, et al. (2001). "Vascular endothelial growth factor is an autocrine growth factor in human malignant mesothelioma." *J Pathol* 193(4): 468-475.

Sugarbaker, D. J., R. M. Flores, et al. (1999). "Resection margins, extrapleural nodal status, and cell type determine postoperative long-term survival in trimodality therapy of malignant pleural mesothelioma: results in 183 patients." *J Thorac Cardiovasc Surg* 117(1): 54-63.

Vachani, A., E. Moon, et al. (2011). "Gene Therapy for Mesothelioma." *Current Treatment Options in Oncology* 12(2): 173-180.

Vandermeers, F., P. Hubert, et al. (2009). "Valproate, in Combination with Pemetrexed and Cisplatin, Provides Additional Efficacy to the Treatment of Malignant Mesothelioma." *Clin Cancer Res* 15: 2818-2828.

Velcheti, V., Y. Kasai, et al. (2009). "Absence of mutations in the epidermal growth factor receptor (EGFR) kinase domain in patients with mesothelioma." *J Thorac Oncol* 4(4): 559.

Villanova, F., A. Procopio, et al. (2008). "Malignant Mesothelioma Resistance to Apoptosis: Recent Discoveries and their Implication for Effective Therapeutic Strategies." *Curr Med Chem* 15: 631-641.

Vogelzang, N. J. (2003). "Phase III Study of Pemetrexed in Combination With Cisplatin Versus Cisplatin Alone in Patients With Malignant Pleural Mesothelioma." *Journal of Clinical Oncology* 21(14): 2636-2644.

Wagner, J. C., C. A. Sleggs, et al. (1960). "Diffuse pleural mesothelioma and asbestos exposure in North Western Cape Province." *Brit J Indust Med* 17: 260-271.

Whitson, B. A., B. A. Jacobson, et al. (2006). "Effects of insulin-like growth factor-1 receptor inhibition in mesothelioma. Thoracic Surgery Directors Association Resident Research Award." *Ann Thorac Surg* 82(3): 996-1001; discussion 1001-1002.

Youle, R. J. and A. Strasser (2008). "The BCL-2 protein family: opposing activities that mediate cell death." *Nature Reviews Molecular Cell Biology* 9(1): 47-59.

Zhang, L., J. E. Littlejohn, et al. (2010). "Characterization of bortezomib-adapted I-45 mesothelioma cells." *Mol Cancer* 9: 110.

Zucali, P. A., G. L. Ceresoli, et al. (2011). "Advances in the biology of malignant pleural mesothelioma." *Cancer Treatment Reviews*.

2

Primary Malignant Pericardial Mesothelioma

Jesus Montesinos, Sílvia Catot, Francesc Sant and Montserrat Domenech
Althaia, Xarxa Assistencial de Manresa, Fundació Privada, Barcelona
Spain

1. Introduction

1.1 Epidemiology

Primary malignant pericardial mesothelioma is an extremely rare tumour. One of the largest autopsy series including about 500,000 cases gave an incidence of primary pericardial tumours of <0.0022% (Gossinger et al., 1998). However, it accounts for approximately 2-3% of all cardiac and pericardial primary tumours being the third tumour after angiosarcoma and rhabdomiosarcoma (Karadzic et al., 2005; Papi et al., 2005).

Mesothelioma arises from the serous epithelial cell of the mesothelium. The most common sites for this malignancy include the pleura (60-70%) and the peritoneum (30-35%). Primary pericardial mesothelioma accounts for only about 1% of all mesotheliomas (Karadzic et al., 2005; Papi et al., 2005).

Approximately 200 cases have been described in literature, of which most have been reported as case studies. The majority of diagnoses occur in the fourth to seventh decades of life with a median age of 46 years (Nilsson & Rasmuson, 2009) and on average, tends to develop in fairly young people compared to pleural or peritoneal mesothelioma. The male-to-female ratio is nearly 2:1, lower than the ratio of approximately 3.5:1 for mesotheliomas of the pleura.

The higher proportion of women suggests that the link with asbestos exposure is weaker for pericardial than for pleural mesothelioma, or that some pericardial mesotheliomas are pathogenetically distinct from their pleural counterparts (Burke et al., 1995). The etiology of malignant pericardial mesothelioma is not completely known. No obvious relationship between asbestos exposure and the development of pericardial mesothelioma has been established due, in part, to the very small number of cases reported (Kaul et al., 1994). An example of this is a recent article published by Nilsson et al., 2009, where they presented a case report and review of 29 primary pericardial mesotheliomas in English literature from 1993 through to 2008. They found that most of the reviewed articles contained no information about asbestos exposure and that only three cases were reported with known exposure to asbestos and 11 were reported with no known exposure (Nilsson et al., 2009), Table 1.

Furthermore, pericardial malignant mesothelioma has been described in patients with a prior history of irradiation showing pericardial effusion (Bendek et al., 2010; Yildirim et al., 2010). A rare association with pericardial mesothelioma and tuberculosis has also been reported (Narayanan et al., 1972).

Exposure to asbestos	n	%
Exposure	3/14	21
No known exposure	11/14	79
Not mentioned	16/30	53

Table 1. Asbestos exposure and primary pericardial mesothelioma

2. Clinical presentation

Symptoms arising from primary pericardial mesothelioma usually result from constriction of the heart or compression of surrounding structures, ranging from dyspnoea, cough, dysphagia, orthopnoea and chest pain (Aggarwal et al.,1991). The onset of symptoms is usually insidious. Common clinical manifestations of pericardial mesothelioma are constrictive pericarditis, pericardial effusion, cardiac tamponade and heart failure caused by myocardial infiltration (Suman et al., 2004). Compression of coronary arteries and local spread of the disease to surrounding large vessels can result in additional symptoms.

As with symptoms, the majority of physical findings are nonspecific. Tachycardia (a heart rate of more than 90 beats per minute) is usually present. Heart sounds may be attenuated if pericardial fluid is present. Clinically significant tamponade produces jugular venous distension, hypotension or even shock. A key diagnostic finding for tamponade is pulsus paradoxus, defined as an exaggeration (more than 10 mmHg) of the normal variation during the inspiratory phase of respiration, in which the blood pressure declines as one inhales and increases as one exhales, and is often palpable in muscular arteries. Sometimes, pulsus paradoxus can be caused by other pathologies, such as asthma, COPD, superior vena cava obstruction, pulmonary embolism or anaphylactic shock.

Additionally, distant metastasis, conduction blockade due to myocardial infiltration and tumour embolism causing neurological deficits have also been reported (Szczechowski et al., 1992). Metastases are present in about 25-45% of the patients and involve regional lymph nodes, lung and kidney (Karadzic et al., 2005; Lagrotteria et al., 2005).

3. Diagnosis

Diagnosis of the disease can be challenging because of nonspecific symptoms and therefore usually only detected at an advanced stage. Usually, tumour presentation consists of coalescent irregular lobular masses that obliterate the pericardial space and tend to constrict the heart. Although a mild infiltration into the subepicardial muscle may occur, the underlying myocardium is frequently not affected. The malignant involvement of pericardium may lead to the development of pericardial effusion, which results from blockage of venous and lymphatic circulation of pericardial fluid.

Often, a multimodal imaging approach, including echocardiography, computed tomography (CT), magnetic resonance imaging (MRI) and FDG-PET scans, is required. Chest radiography of patients reveals cardiomegaly, an irregular cardiac silhouette or diffuse mediastinal enlargement. Transthoracic echocardiography is the mainstay imaging technique for cardiac tumour detection. Although generally robust, it carries several well-described limitations, including operator dependence, restricted field of view and occasional limited imaging of the right heart chambers. Transesophageal echocardiography improves image quality considerably, but is more invasive and carries a restricted field of view. CT scan can demonstrate the extent of the cardiac tumour, the extent of pericardial thickening, the mediastinal lymph node and the extracardiac lesions, Figure 1. These can be useful in distinguishing primary pericardial tumours from other causes of constrictive pericarditis. Cardiovascular magnetic resonance imaging is the reference non-invasive imaging technique for assessment and characterization of a suspected cardiac mass. It allows accurate confirmation of the presence of a space occupying lesion, localization and assessment of the extent of involvement, evaluation of the functional impact of the lesions, as well as tissue characterization, Figure 2. Such information is important not only for diagnosis, but also determination of prognosis and in planning of therapy (Randhawa et al., 2011). Integrated positron-emission tomography (PET)/Computed tomography (CT) imaging has not established itself in routine evaluation, probably due to their low frequency. However, in a recent report, PET-CT was useful in the staging and preoperative evaluation of pleural or pericardial mesothelioma, detection of unsuspected nodal and occult distant metastases (Ost et al., 2008).

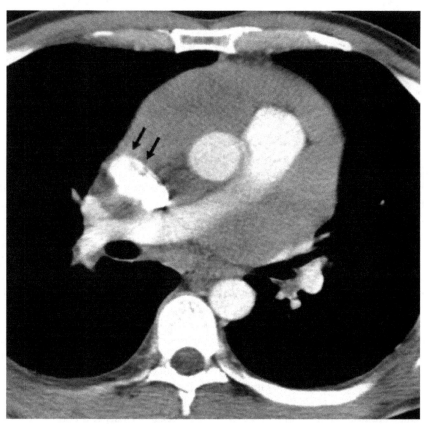

Fig. 1. Axial contrast-enhanced chest CT scan (mediastinal window) shows a soft-tissue mass with homogenous enhancement that encases the ascending aorta and right pulmonary artery. The mass is compressing the right atrium (arrows).

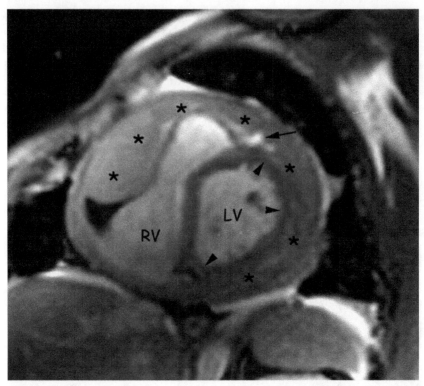

Fig. 2. Contrast-enhanced short-axis steady-state free precession MR image, demonstrates extensive pericardial involvement of the tumour that encases the ventricles and also compresses the right ventricle. It is possible to differentiate the myocardium (arrowheads) from the mass (asterisks). In this sequence, liquids show high attenuation and only minimal pericardial fluid is seen (arrow). RV: right ventricle; LV: left ventricle.

The diagnosis of the disease is made as a result of the pathologic assessment of pericardial fluid or tissue generally obtained with the guidance of echocardiogram, ultrasonography or CT scans. Moreover, cytological examination, immunohistochemistry and the high pericardial hialuronic acid content of the pericardial aspirate can be diagnostic. As with any tumour, reliable diagnosis of mesothelioma depends on obtaining adequate and representative tissue samples. Antemortem diagnosis is notoriously difficult because the clinical presentation is nonspecific, the radiological findings are sometimes non-contributory and the cytological analysis of pericardial fluid is often inconclusive. In only 10-20% of cases can the diagnosis be made before the death of the patient (Papi et al., 2005). It is important to differentiate between malignancy and mesothelial reactive hyperplasia associated with inflammatory disease. In biopsy specimens, features that indicate the presence of a malignancy are infiltration of deep tissues, atypical cells, necrosis and confluent forms. In these cases it is useful to obtain additional anamnesis, clinical and radiological information. Immunohistochemistry has a limited role and the more useful antibodies have diagnostic sensitivity and specificity < 90% (table 2).

Antibody	Sensitivity (%)	Specificity (%)
Epithelial membrane antigen	74	89
p53	58	91
Desmin	83	83

Table 2. Antibodies distinguishing between malignant mesothelioma and reactive mesothelial hyperplasia (Addis B & Roche H, 2009).

On microscopy, malignant mesotheliomas of the pericardium resemble pleural mesotheliomas. Mesotheliomas are divided into epithelial, mixed (biphasic) and sarcomatous types on the basis of histologic growth patterns, Figure 3,4. The less common mixed and sarcomatous variants show poorer survival. Immunohistochemically, almost 100% of pleural mesotheliomas express cytokeratin in epitheloid areas. Sarcomatoid cells express cytokeratin in about 75% of cases, vimentin is preferentially expressed in the spindle cell areas and epithelioid membrane antigen (EMA) is frequently present in the epitheloid areas. With pericardial mesotheliomas, EMA and vimentin are present in fewer than 50% of pericardial cases. As with pleural mesothelioma, a panel of antibodies should be used for differential diagnosis with metastatic pericardial tumours, so much frequent than mesothelioma. For adenocarcinoma, the most common metastatic pericardial tumour, a panel of positive (CK5/6, calretinina) and negative (CEA, ber-EP4 y CD15) antibodies allow the diagnosis of mesothelioma in the context of the morphologic findings. In this case, antibodies usually positive in epithelial mesothelioma are presented in Table 3 (Addis & Roche, 2009).

Antibody	Sensitivity (%)	Specificity (%)
CK5/6	83	85
Calretinin	82	85
HBME 1	85	43
Thrombomodulin	61	80
N-cadherin	78	84
Wilms tumour product-1	77	96

Table 3. Antibodies usually positive in epithelial mesothelioma.

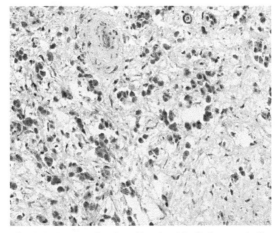

Fig. 3. Positivity for calretinin in neoplastic cells of epithelial mesothelioma.

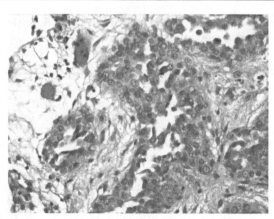

Fig. 4. Epithelial mesothelioma in invasive pattern. Hematoxylin-eosin x 200.

4. Treatment and prognosis

Pericardial mesothelioma is a highly aggressive tumour with global survival of less than 6-12 months, depending on histological type, tumour stage, performance status and treatment, and other factors, such as gender and age (Papi et al., 2005; Suman et al., 2004). Its molecular profile indicates that most of the known genes for radio- and chemoresistance are overexpressed (Roe et al., 2009). Treatment tends to be mainly palliative rather than radical and based on surgery, chemotherapy and radiotherapy. However, despite best efforts, no significant difference has been achieved in regards to prognosis.

Surgery plays a limited role as the disease is often locally advanced when diagnosis is reached. Its main role is therefore to control symptoms, as in the case of partial pericardiectomy in cardiac tamponade (Vigneswaran et al., 2000).

Treatment options for the control of malignant pericardial effusions or tamponade should be individualized to maximize symptom relief and minimal impact in quality of life. Several techniques have been used, percutaneous pericardiocentesis, pericardial sclerosis, subxiphoid pericardial window, pericardiectomy or pericardiectomy by thoracotomy or video-assisted thoracoscopy. However, a retrospective comparison of cases published in 1998 by Girardi, showed that periocardiocentesis with intrapericardial sclerotherapy was as effective as open surgical drainage for the management of malignant pericardial effusions and also showed similar rates of complications (Girardi et al., 1997). Surgical drainage is desirable in patients with intrapericardial bleeding and in those with clotted hemopericardium or thoracic conditions that make needle drainage difficult or ineffective. If treatment is indicated for management of tamponade, percutaneous subxiphoid pericardiocentesis is the treatment of choice in the acute setting, guided by echocardiography. Recurrent pericardial effusion occurs in approximately 21-50% of cases (Anderson et al., 2001; Tsang et al., 2000). Limited cases suggest rates of pericardial fluid reaccumulation at 30 days ranging 5-33% after periocardiocentesis and intrapericardial treatment with sclerosing drugs versus more than 50% in cases treated with pericardial drainage alone (Anderson et al., 2001). Several sclerosing agents have been used, tetracycline, bleomycin, thiotepa, mitoxantrone, docetaxel, among others. Some cases may required three or more treatments to achieve adequate sclerosis. A prospective comparison study of doxycicline versus bleomycin showed a similar rate of success, but less morbidity in cases treated with bleomycin, especially in severe retroesternal chest pain, 70% of patients treated with tetracyclines versus 0% with bleomycin (Liu et al., 1996).

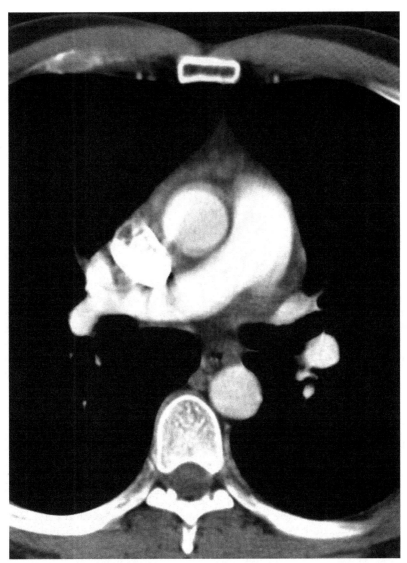

Fig. 5. Chest CT scan performed after three cycles of chemotherapy. Axial contrast enhanced CT scan (mediastinal window) at the same level as Figure 1 shows marked improvement in the mass (Santos et al., 2008).

Scheme of bleomycin chemical sclerosis: after catheter is correctly placed and drainage is effective, bleomycin 10 to 20mg dissolved in 10 to 20 mL of normal saline is inserted through the catheter into the pericardial sac. The catheter is clamped for 1 to 2 hours and then reopened and allowed to drain. Special positioning of the patient is not required. Procedure could be repeated every 24-48h until volume of drainage was less than 25 mL per 24 hours. Maximum number of procedures is 3 or 4. Catheter is definitively removed when the echocardiogram confirms that the effusion is resolved.

Radiation therapy has been used as adjuvant treatment in patients with incomplete tumour resection with or without chemotherapy (Papi et al., 2005; Suman et al., 2004) but pericardial mesothelioma responds poorly to radiotherapy and we have to be cautious with the side effects of such radiation that can cause primarily pericarditis or myocarditis.

The use of new drugs offers further treatment options. The therapeutic schemes generally used are the same as those used in pleural mesothelioma, mainly a combination of platin-infusion plus gemcitabine or paclitaxel with and objective response rates of 16-48% and median survivals of 9.6-11.2 months. Recently, pemetrexed, a multitargeted antifolate, has demonstrated modest activity against malignant pleural mesothelioma in combination with cisplatin (Volgenzang et al., 2003) or carboplatin (Ceresoli et al., 2006). Some cases report excellent tumour response with a combination of carboplatin and pemetrexed unusual in this type of tumours with progression-free survival and overall survival of 10 and 18 months, respectively (Doval et al., 2007; Fujimoto et al., 2009; Santos et al., 2008), Figure 5.

5. Conclusion

Malignant pericardial mesothelioma is a rare malignancy with a poor prognosis. Diagnosis procedures are sometimes difficult and a multidisciplinary approach, including pathologists, clinicians and radiologist, is often required. Due to few cases being described, management is based on knowledge obtained from usual presentations of malignant mesothelioma, such as pleural or peritoneal. Systemic treatments can be used and tumoural responses have been described, especially with new antineoplastic agents. With respect to the treatment of local complications as pericardial effusions with tamponade, options include pericardiocentesis with or without chemical sclerosis as an initial procedure. Other more aggressive surgical approaches may be recommended in selected cases.

6. References

Addis, B. & Roche, H. Problems in mesothelioma diagnosis. *Histopathology* Vol.54, (2009), pp.55-68, ISSN 1365-2559

Aggarwal, P.; Wali, JP. & Agarwal,J. Pericardial mesothelioma presenting as a mediastinal mass. *Singapore Medical Journal* , Vol.32, No.3, (June 1991), pp.185-6 ISSN 0037-5675

Anderson, TM.; Ray, CW.; Nwogu, CE.; Bottiggi, AJ.; Lenox, JM.; Driscoll, DL. & Urschel, JD. Pericardial catheter sclerosis versus surgical procedures for pericardial effusions in cancer patients. *Journal of Cardiovascular Surgery (Torino)* Vol.42, No.3, (June 2001), pp.415-9 ISSN 0021-9509

Bendek, M.; Ferenc, M. & Freudenberg, N. Post-irradiation pericardial malignant mesothelioma: an autopsy case and review of the literature. *Cardiovascular Pathology* Vol.19,(2010), pp.377-379 ISSN 1054-8807

Burke, A. & Virmani R. Malignant mesothelioma of the pericardium. Tumors of the Heart and Great Vessels. Wahington DC: *Atlas of Tumor Pathology* (1995), pp.181-94 ISSN 1532-2114

Ceresoli, G.; Zucali, PA.; Favaretto, AG; Grossi, F.; Bidoli, P.; Del Conte, G.; Ceribelli, A.; Bearz, A. & Morenghi, E. Phase II study of pemetrexed plus carboplatin in malignant pleural mesothelioma. *Journal of Clinical Oncology* Vol.24, No.9, (Mar 2006), pp.1443-1448 ISSN 1527-7755

Doval, DC.; Shripad, B.; Pande, MD.; Sharma, J.; Rao, S.; Neeraj Prakasj & Vaid, A. Report of a case of pericardial mesothelioma with liver metastases responding well to pemetrexed and platinum-based chemotherapy. *Journal of Thoracic Oncology* Vol.2, No.8, (August 2007), pp.780-1 ISSN 1556-0864

Fujimoto, N.; Gemba, K.; Wada, S.; Ono, K., Fujii, Y.; Ozaki, S.; Ikeda, T.; Taguchi, K.; Junitomo, T. & Kishimoto, T. Malignant pericardial mesothelioma with response to chemotherapy. *Journal of Thoracic Oncology* Vol.4, No.11, (November 2009), pp. 1440-41. ISSN 1556-0864.

Girardi, LN.; Ginsberg, RJ. & Burt, M. Periocardiocentesis and intrapericardial sclerosis: effective therapy for malignant pericardial effusions. *The Annals of Thoracic Surgery* Vol.64, No.5, (November 1997), pp.1422-1428 ISSN 1552-6259

Gossinger, H.; Siostrzonek, P.; Zangeneh, M.; Neuhold, A.; Herold, C.; Schmoliner, R.; Laczkovics, A.; Tscholakoff, D. & Mösslacher, H. Magnetic resonance imaging findings in a patient with pericardial mesothelioma. *American Heart Journal Vol. 115, No.6, (June 1988)*, pp.1321-2 ISSN 0002-8703

Grebenc, ML.; Rosado de Christenson, ML.; Burke, AP.; Green, CE. & Galvin, JR. Primary cardiac and pericardial neoplasms: radiologic-pathologic correlations. *Radiographics Vol.20*, No.4, (Jul-August 2000), pp.1073-103 ISSN 1527-1323

Karadzic, R.; Kostic-Banovic, L. & Antovic, A. Primary pericardial mesothelioma presenting as constrictive pericarditis. *Archive of Oncology* Vol.13, issue 3-4, (2005), pp.150-152 ISSN 0354-7310

Kaul, TK.; Fields, BL. & Kahn, DR. Primary malignant pericardial mesothelioma: a case report and review. The *Journal of Cardiovascular Surgery (Torino)* Vol.35, No.3, (June1994), pp.261-7 ISSN 0021-9509

Lagrotteria, DD., Tsang, B., Elevathil, LJ. & Tomlinson, CW. A case of primary malignant pericardial mesothelioma. *The Canadian Journal of Cardiology* Vol.21, No.2, (February 2005), pp.185-7 ISSN 1753-4313

Liu, G.; Crump, M.; Goss, PE.; Dancey, J. & Shepherd, FA. Prospective comparison of the sclerosing agents doxicycline and bleomycin for the primary management of malignant pericardial effusion and cardiac tamponade. *Journal of Clinical Oncology* Vol.14, No.12, (December 1996), pp.3141-3147 ISSN 1527-7755

Narayanan, PS.; Chandrasekar, S. & Madhavan, M. Intrathoracic mesotheliomas associated with tuberculosis. *Indian Journal of Medical Sciences* Vol.26, No.7, (July 1972), pp.432-6

Nilsson, A. & Rasmuson, T. (2009). Primary pericardial mesothelioma: report of a patient and literature review. *Case Reports in Oncology* Vol.2, (July 2009), pp.125-132. ISSN 1662-6575

Ost, P.; Rottey, S.; Boterberg, T.; Stragier, B. & Goethals, I. (2008). F-18 fluorodeoxyglucose PET/CT scanning in the diagnostic work-up of a primary pericardial mesothelioma. *Journal of Thoracic Imaging* Vol.23, (2008), pp.35-8 ISSN 0883-5993

Papi, M.; Genestreti, G.; Tassinari, D.; Lorenzini, P.; Serra, S.; Ricci, M.; Pasquini, E.; Nicolini, M.; Pasini, G.; Tamburini, E.; Fattori, PP. & Ravaioli, A. Malignant pericardial mesothelioma. Report of two cases, review of the literature and differential diagnosis. *Tumori* Vol.91, No.3, (May-june 2005), pp. 276-9 ISSN 2038-2529

Roe, OD.; Anderssen, E.; Helge, E.; Pettersen, CH.; Olsen, KS.; Sandeck, H.; Haaverstad, R.; Lundgren, S. & Larsson, E. (2009). Genome-wide profile of pleural mesothelioma versus parietal and visceral pleura: the emerging gene portrait of the mesothelioma phenotype. *PLoS ONE* 2009, ISSN 1932-6203

Santos, C.; Montesinos, J.; Castañer, E.; Sole, JM. & Baga, R. Primary pericardial mesothelioma. *Lung Cancer* Vol.60, (2008) , pp. 291-293, ISSN 0169-5002

Suman, S.; Schofield, P. & Large, S. Primary pericardial mesothelioma presenting as pericardial constriction: a case report. *Heart* Vol.90, (2004), e4. ISSN 1532-4427

Szczechowski, L. & Janiec, K. Pericardial mesothelioma as a very rare cause of recurrent cerebral emboli. *Wiad Lek* Vol.45, No.21-22, (November 1992), pp.857-61 ISSN 0043-5147

Tsang, TS.; Seward, JB.; Barnes, ME.; Bailey, KR.; Sinak, LJ.; Urban, LH. & Hayes, SN. Outcomes of primary and secondary treatment of pericardial effusion in patients with malignancy. *Mayo Clinic Proceedings* Vol.75, No.3, (March 2000), pp.248-53 ISSN 0025-6196

Vigneswaran, WT. & Stefanacci, PR. Pericardial mesothelioma. *Current Treatment Options in Oncology* Vol.1, No.4, (October 2000), pp.299-302 ISSN 1527-2729

Vogelzang, NJ.; Rusthoven, JJ.; Symanowski, J.; Denham, C.; Kaukel, E.; Ruffie, P.; Gatzemeier, U.; Boyer, M.; Emri, S.; Manegold, C.; Niyikiza, C. & Paoletti, P. Phase III study of pemetrexed in combination with cisplatin versus cisplatin alone in patients with malignant pleural mesothelioma. *Journal of Clinical Oncology* Vol.21, No.14, (July 2003), pp.2636-2644 ISSN 1527-7755

Yildirim, H.; Metintas, M. & Ak, G. (2010). Malignant pericardial mesothelioma following thoracical radiotherapy: dissemination from pericardium to pleura. *Tüberküloz ve Toraks Dergisi* Vol.58, No.3, (2010), pp.301-305 ISSN 0494-1373

3

Para- and Intratesticular Aspects of Malignant Mesothelioma

Zachary Klaassen[1], Kristopher R. Carlson[1],
Jeffrey R. Lee[2], Sravan Kuvari[2] and Martha K. Terris[1]
[1]*Department of Urology*
[2]*Department of Pathology*
Georgia Health Sciences University,
United States of America

1. Introduction

While the pleural and pericardial forms of malignant mesothelioma account for the majority of cases, this tumor has important and often overlooked urological implications. Embryologically, the vaginal process is an evagination of the peritoneum and indents the scrotal swelling to form the inguinal canal. During migration from the abdomen, the testes are covered by reflected folds of the vaginal process and subsequently form the visceral and parietal layers of the tunica vaginalis. Given this continual lining of epithelial cells of endodermal origin, the potential for transformation into malignant mesothelioma is possible from the peritoneal cavity to the tunica vaginalis covering the testis (Lane, 2001). Although the majority of literature is dedicated to malignant mesothelioma of the tunica vaginalis, relationships between other genitourinary organs and this disease have been described and will be discussed. This chapter will focus on the epidemiology, physical examination findings, diagnostic modalities, histopathologic analysis, treatment, recurrence rates, follow-up guidelines and prognostic factors for male patients with genitourinary malignant mesothelioma.

2. Malignant mesothelioma by genitourinary anatomic location

2.1 Tunica vaginalis testis

The most common urologic site of mesothelioma is the tunica vaginalis testis, accounting for ~1% of all mesothelioma cases (Attanoos & Gibbs, 2000) and the majority of urologic cases (Plas et al., 1998). The tunica vaginalis is an embryonic evagination of the abdominal peritoneum residing in the scrotum, and similar to thoracic mesothelioma, risk factors for malignant mesothelioma include a history of asbestos exposure or a family member with a history of asbestos exposure (may be present in up to 1/3 of patients) (Plas et al., 1998; Vianna & Polan, 1978). Other possible etiological factors that have been suggested for malignant disease include previous testicular trauma and hernia repair; however these factors have not been corroborated (Amin, 1995; Antman et al., 1984). In the few cases reported in patients in the first three decades of life, no history of asbestos exposure was reported in the patient or family and the etiological factor in these cases remains unclear (Antman et al., 1984; Johnson et al., 1973; Jones et al., 1995; Linn et al., 1988; McDonald et al., 1983; Plas et al., 1998; Stein and Henkes, 1986).

In their report of 74 patients, Plas et al. (1998) reported that the highest incidence of disease is noted in the 6th and 7th decades of life, although 1/3 of cases have been reported in patients less than 44 years of age. Among 16 patients identified in The National Cancer Institute's Surveillance, Epidemiology, and End Results (SEER) Program (2009) with disease of the tunica vaginalis the mean age was 68 ± 12 years with a range of 44 to 88 years. Furthermore, 15 of these 16 patients were Caucasian, suggesting a possible race predilection. No predilection for the right or left tunica vaginalis has been elucidated to date (Plas et al., 1998), however two cases of malignant bilateral disease have been reported (McDonald et al., 1983; Menut et al., 1996).

2.2 Spermatic cord

Malignant mesothelioma of the spermatic cord is an extremely rare tumor with less than 10 cases reported in the literature (Arlen et al., 1969; Leiber et al., 2000; Pizzolato & Lamberty, 1976; Silberblatt & Gellman, 1974; Tobioka et al., 1995; Torbati et al., 2005; Tuttle Jr et al., 1977; Vyas et al., 1990) including 4 patients identified in the SEER database (National Cancer Institute, 2009). Tuttle et al. (1977) have suggested that a mesothelial histogenesis of the spermatic cord should not be surprising as the testis descend to the scrotum giving the opportunity for nests of mesothelial cells from the urogenital ridge to implant along this route. Furthermore the spermatic cord is in immediate contact with tunica vaginalis.

Men of all ages may be affected as cases from the literature have a median age of 46 years of age (range: 37-60 years), while patients from the SEER Program have identified young (one patient 11 years of age) and elderly patients (three patients >60 years of age). In all studies reviewed from the literature and 3 of 4 patients identified in the SEER database presented with right-sided disease, however due to the paucity of cases, any causal anatomic relationship would be speculative.

2.3 Epididymis/testis

Although the literature does not explicitly report cases of malignant mesothelioma confined to the true testis or epididymis (perhaps diagnosed and/or conglomerated with malignant mesothelioma of the tunica vaginalis), the SEER database identified three patients with disease of the epididymis and 12 patients with testicular disease between 1973 and 2007 (National Cancer Institute, 2009). Comparable to other urologic anatomic sites, elderly patients are more susceptible (mean age – 59 ± 21 years of age; median 65 years of age), however younger patients are not without risk (one patient 24 years of age). Among 13 of 15 patients the database reported laterality of the lesion, 7 (54%) patients had right sided and 6 (46%) patients had left sided lesions. Furthermore, 9 patients had a reported tumor size, ranging from 0.9 to 11.2 cm (mean ± SD, 3.9 ± 3.2). Comparable to disease of the tunica vaginalis testis, 14 of 15 (94%) patients with disease of the epididymis or testis were Caucasian, further suggesting a race predilection for malignant mesothelioma.

3. Physical examination and diagnostic modalities

The majority of patients present to their primary care physician or urologist with a scrotum that has been enlarging over the course of several months and patients typically receive a preoperative diagnosis of hydrocele or testicular tumor (Figure 1) (Spiess et al., 2005). Patients with spermatic cord disease commonly present with scrotal or inguinal swelling or mass that may be assumed to be inguinal hernia and go undiagnosed for years (Leiber et al., 2000).

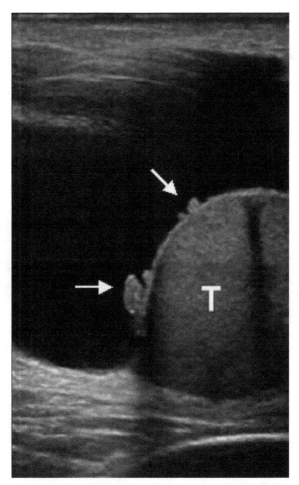

Fig. 1. Preoperative ultrasonography demonstrating the testicle (T) and a paratesticular mass (arrows - mesothelioma of the tunica vaginalis testis).

One of the most significant issues with managing patients with malignant disease is accurate preoperative diagnosis [less than 3% of cases of malignant mesothelioma of the tunica vaginalis (Plas et al., 1998)]. Although relatively nonspecific, typical sonographic appearance of malignant mesothelioma is a paratesticular papillary excrescence or nodularity that is often associated with hydrocele (Boyum & Wasserman, 2008). Recently, color Doppler sonography has emerged as a possible imaging modality for preoperative diagnosis. Initial studies (Mak et al., 2004; Wang et al., 2005; Wolanske & Nino-Murcia, 2001) documented an intratesticular mass that was hypovascular in comparison to surrounding testicular tissue, and 2 recent cases (Aggarwal et al., 2010; Boyum and Wasserman, 2008) report hypervascularity within a paratesticular nodule or stalk arising from the tunica vaginalis. Thus, discrepancies in color Doppler sonography, whether hypovascularity or hypervascularity of paratesticular nodules, may increase preoperative diagnosis of malignant mesotheliomas (Klaassen & Lehrhoff, 2010).

4. Histopathology

Malignant mesothelioma of the tunica vaginalis comprise the histopathological reports to date and are generally subclassified into epithelial type and biphasic or mixed type (Figure 2). Sarcomatous type is generally found in the pleural cavity however there has been one

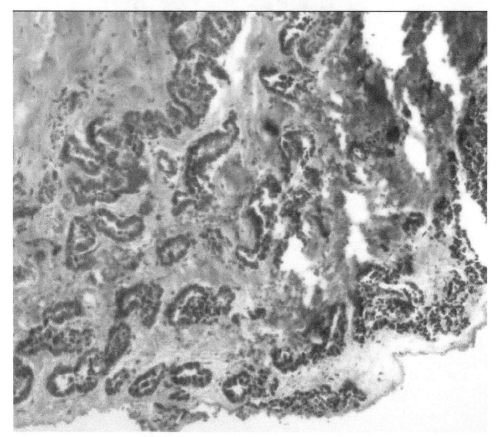

Fig. 2. Malignant mesothelioma of the tunica vaginalis testis (Hematoxylin and Eosin stain 100x). The tumor is predominantly epitheliod, which is the most common histological type.

reported case of this histological subtype for the tunica vaginalis (Eimoto and Inoue, 1977). A large immunohistochemical profile by Winstanley et al. (2006) reported 18 cases of malignant mesothelioma specific to the tunica vaginalis from the UK between 1959 and 2004. They found that all cases were positive for calretinin (Figure 3) and EMA, 16 cases were positive for thrombomodulin, 15 cases were positive for CK7, 13 cases were positive for CK5-CK6, and all cases were negative for CK20 and carcinoembryonic antigen (CEA). Furthermore, tumors are characteristically vimentin positive (Figure 4) and MOC 31 negative (Figure 5). On gross examination, the tumor is usually poorly demarcated, with intermittent firm and friable whitish and yellowish regions (Richie & Steele, 2007).

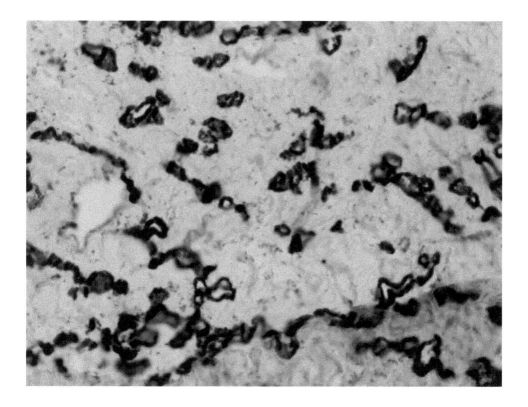

Fig. 3. Malignant mesothelioma of the tunica vaginalis testis staining positive for calretinin (100x).

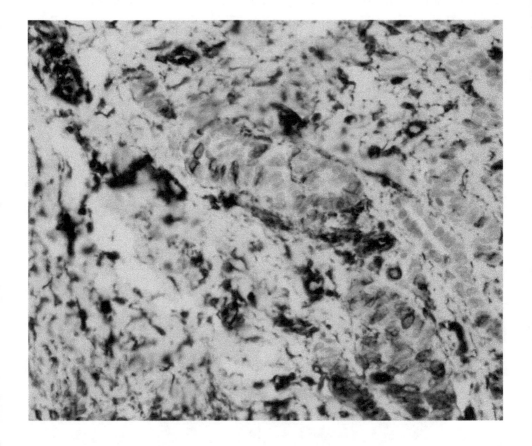

Fig. 4. Malignant mesothelioma of the tunica vaginalis testis staining positive for vimentin (100x).

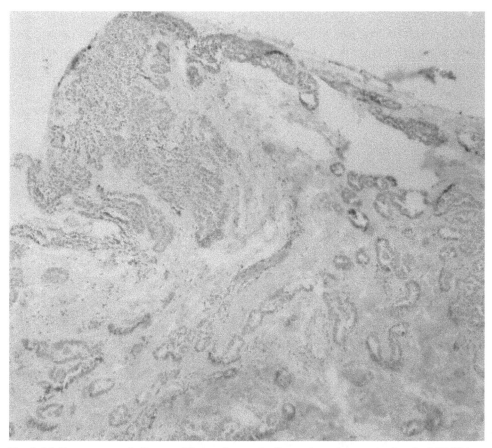

Fig. 5. Malignant mesothelioma of the tunica vaginalis testis staining negative for MOC 31 (40x).

5. Treatment

Intraoperative or postoperative diagnosis of malignant mesothelioma most commonly results in inguinal orchiectomy, orchiectomy, or hydrocele wall excision of the tumor (Figure 6).

In their review of 74 cases of malignant mesothelioma of the tunica vaginalis, Plas et al. (1998) reported first-line surgical approach (available for 62 patients) as inguinal orchiectomy in 26 patients, orchiectomy in 19 patients, resection of hydrocele wall in 15 cases and individual cases of hemiscrotectomy and local excision of the tumor. Following histologically proven malignant mesothelioma inguinal orchiectomy was performed as a second procedure for 14 patients and hemiscrotectomy in 12 patients (Plas et al., 1998). Furthermore, lymphadenectomy was performed in 17 patients (N=8 retroperitoneal, N=5 inguinal, N=4 iliac) with evidence of metastasis in 11 of these patients (Plas et al., 1998). Fifty of 51 patients identified in the SEER database (National Cancer Institute, 2009) underwent surgical excision of the tumor. Black et al. (2003) advocate early aggressive local resection for palliation in patients who have significant symptoms, as they described a patient who underwent multiple aggressive resections and experienced a remarkable, albeit transient, improvement in symptoms following each resection.

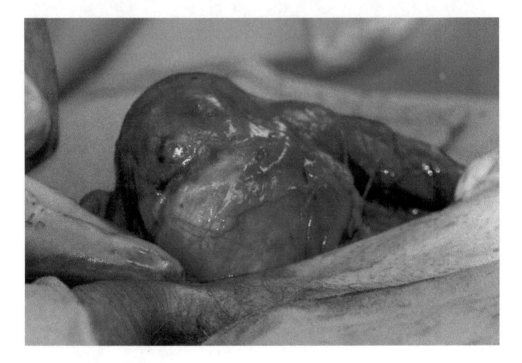

Fig. 6. An intraoperative image demonstrating a paratesticular mass during orchiectomy (mesothelioma of the tunica vaginalis testis).

Adjuvant treatment strategies include chemotherapy, radiotherapy or a combination of chemotherapy and radiotherapy, with heterogenous regimens and outcomes reported (Plas et al., 1998). Plas et al. (1998) identified 10 patients who underwent chemotherapy (most commonly doxorubicin and cyclophosphamide) 2 of which had partial remission and 6 of which had no improvement in symptoms. Plas et al. (1998) also identified 10 patient who underwent radiotherapy (40-60 gray; varying duration of therapy), reporting complete remission with 12 months of follow up in 5 patients, partial remission in 1 patient and no change in tumor size in 2 patients. Among 6 patients who underwent chemotherapy and radiotherapy, Plas et al. (1998) reported no cases of complete remission however 3 patients had partial remission. At the present time, adjuvant treatment of malignant mesothelioma remains experimental and physician dependent with no set guidelines or appropriate follow-up analysis available.

6. Recurrence, follow-up guidelines and prognosis

6.1 Recurrence

To date, Plas et al. (1998) have reported the only comprehensive study identifying factors that may influence local recurrence. In their report, patients with a positive histology of asbestos exposure (N=2) had a significantly shorter interval before tumor recurrence than patients with no history of exposure (N=7) (p < 0.05). Furthermore, Plas et al. (1998) reported an increased incidence of local recurrence after resection of the hydrocele wall alone compared to scrotal excision and inguinal orchiectomy, however there was no survival advantage when more radical excision was performed.

6.2 Follow-up guidelines

Presently, there are no established follow-up guidelines for malignant mesothelioma. We agree with Plas et al. (1998) who have suggested clinical examinations and CT scan or retroperitoneal ultrasound every 3 months for the first 2 years, followed by yearly observation for the subsequent 3 years. Since malignant mesothelioma of the genitourinary tract may be diagnosed at any age, the fact that there are no established tumor markers to use during the follow-up period, and due to the possibility of recurrence up to 15 years after primary therapy (Jones et al., 1995), there is an argument that surveillance should continue for up to 10 years and perhaps for the rest of the patient's life.

6.3 Prognosis (Table 1)

The SEER database (National Cancer Institute, 2009) and Plas et al. (1998) provide the largest sample size and provide the most significant analyses for determining prognosis of genitourinary malignant mesothelioma.

	Age			
	≤ 40	41-69	≥ 70	p-value
Patients, N=(%)	7 (14)	24 (47)	20 (39)	<0.0001
Age (mean ± SD)	23.3 ± 7.6	59.2 ± 7.7	76.1 ± 5.2	
Location, N=(%)	Testis - 3 (43) Penis - 1 (14) Scrotum - 1 (14) Spermatic Cord - 1 (14) Overlapping Lesion - 1 (14)	Tunica vaginalis - 8 (33) Overlapping Lesion - 8 (33) Testis - 3 (13) Spermatic Cord - 2 (8) Epididymis - 2 (8) Scrotum - 1 (4)	Tunica vaginalis - 8 (40) Testis - 6 (30) Overlapping Lesion - 2 (10) Scrotum - 2 (10) Spermatic Cord - 1 (5) Epididymis - 1 (5)	
Mean Survival, years (95% CI)	16.1 (8.0-24.2)	12.3 (6.2-18.4)	5.0 (3.0-7.0)	0.06
Median Survival, years (95% CI)	14.7 (4.2-25.3)	7.0 (1.2-12.8)	3.3 (2.7-3.9)	

	Stage[a]			
	Localized	Regional	Distant	p-value
Patients, N=(%)	23 (47)	18 (37)	8 (16)	<0.0001
Age (mean ± SD)	61.9 ± 14.0	62.8 ± 17.6	63.6 ± 23.5	
Location, N=(%)	Tunica vaginalis - 6 (26) Overlapping Lesion - 5 (22) Testis - 5 (22) Scrotum - 3 (13) Spermatic Cord - 2 (9) Epididymis - 2 (9)	Tunica vaginalis - 7 (39) Testis - 5 (28) Overlapping Lesion - 4 (22) Spermatic Cord - 1 (6) Epididymis - 1 (6)	Tunica vaginalis - 3 (38) Overlapping Lesion - 2 (25) Scrotum - 1 (13) Spermatic Cord - 1 (13) Testis - 1 (13)	
Mean Survival, years (95% CI)	16.7 (10.4-23.0)	7.7 (3.5-11.9)	2.4 (0.7-4.1)	0.02
Median Survival, years (95% CI)	8.0 (NR)	3.4 (2.3-4.5)	1.3 (0-3.2)	

Abbreviations: SD, standard deviation; CI, confidence interval; NR, not reported
[a] Two patients unstaged (one penile and one testis mesothelioma)

Table 1. Clinical outcomes of male patients with malignant mesothelioma stratified by age and stage of disease, from the Surveillance, Epidemiology, and End Results (SEER) database (2009).

6.3.1 Age (Figure 7)

Among the 51 patients identified in the SEER database (National Cancer Institute, 2009), 7 (14%) were ≤40, 24 (47%) were 41-69 and 20 (39%) were ≥70 years of age (p < 0.0001). Mean survival was progressively worse for older patients, with mean survival rates of 16.1 (95% CI 8.0-24.2), 12.3 (95% CI 6.2-18.4) and 5.0 years (95% CI 3.0-7.0), respectively (p = 0.06). The 3- and 5-year survival rate for patients ≤40 years of age was 100% and 80%, for patients 41-69 was 56% and 38%, and for >70 was 29% and 23%, respectively. In their meta-analysis patients with malignant mesothelioma of the tunica vaginalis, Plas et al. (1998) reported that univariate analysis revealed a significant correlation of age with survival (p < 0.01), emphasizing longer survival for younger patients (N=29, <60 years of age) compared to older patients (N=29, ≥60 years of age). Among these two sample populations, it is evident that elderly patients have a survival disadvantage compared to younger patients with genitourinary malignant mesothelioma.

6.3.2 Extent of disease (Figure 8)

Among the 51 patients in the SEER database (National Cancer Institute, 2009), 49 patients were categorized as having localized (N=23, 47%), regional (N=18, 37%) or distant (N=8, 16%) disease (p < 0.0001). Mean survival was significantly worse for patients with non-localized disease, with mean survival rates of 16.7 (95% CI 10.4-23.0), 7.7 (95% CI 3.5-11.9) and 2.4 years (95% CI 0.7-4.1), respectively (p = 0.02). The 3- and 5-year survival rate for patients with localized disease was 65% and 48%, for patients with regional disease was 40%

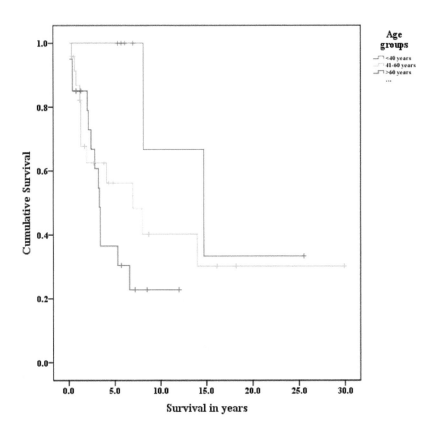

Fig. 7. Kaplan-Meier survival analysis of male patients with urologic malignant mesothelioma stratified by patients <40, 41-60 and >60 years of age from the Surveillance, Epidemiology, and End Results (SEER) database (2009) ($p = 0.06$).

and 35% and for patients with distant disease was 29% and 29%, respectively. Comparatively, Plas et al. (1998) also found a significant correlation between the presence of primary metastatic disease and survival (p < 0.05, N=11 metastatic disease; N=46 organ confined disease). Not surprisingly, patients with advanced malignant mesothelioma have significantly poorer outcomes compared to patients with locoregional controlled disease.

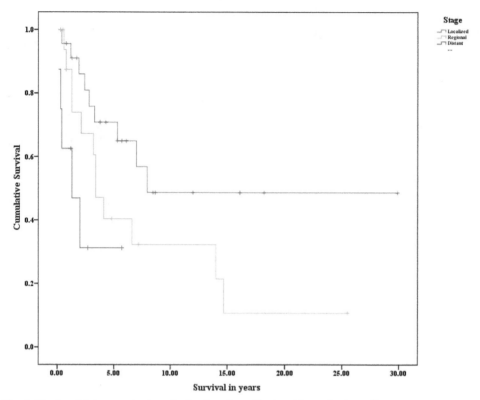

Fig. 8. Kaplan-Meier survival analysis of male patients with urologic malignant mesothelioma stratified by localized, regional and distant disease from the Surveillance, Epidemiology, and End Results (SEER) database (2009) (p = 0.02).

6.3.3 Other variables

Since there are no tumor markers available for patients with malignant mesothelioma, other factors have been tested for prognostic significance. Competing-risks regression analyses performed for the 51 patients in the SEER database (National Cancer Institute, 2009) did not identify a significant prognostic correlation for disease of the tunica vaginalis, patients of non-Caucasian race, year of diagnosis before 2001 and tumor size. Plas et al. (1998) reported that a history of asbestos exposure, tumor histology or primary therapy did not correlate with survival.

7. Conclusions

Malignant mesotheliomas with urologic connotations need to be considered as these tumors have been termed "well described pathologies at unusual sites" (Lane, 2001). At this point in time, analysis suggests a predilection for Caucasian males (however, without a survival disadvantage) and poorer prognosis for elderly patients and patients without locoregional control. The advent of color Doppler sonography will potentially increase the rate of correct preoperative diagnosis and allow for the appropriate primary surgical approach to be performed (Boyum & Wasserman, 2008; Wolanske & Nino-Murcia, 2001; Mak et al., 2004; Wang et al., 2005) (Figure 9). Surgical therapy remains the cornerstone of initial treatment with a need for further analysis and resources directed toward identifying appropriate adjuvant treatment regimens. This disease is rare but has the potential for aggressive and deadly behavior necessitating a correct preoperative diagnosis, aggressive surgical management and likely lifelong surveillance.

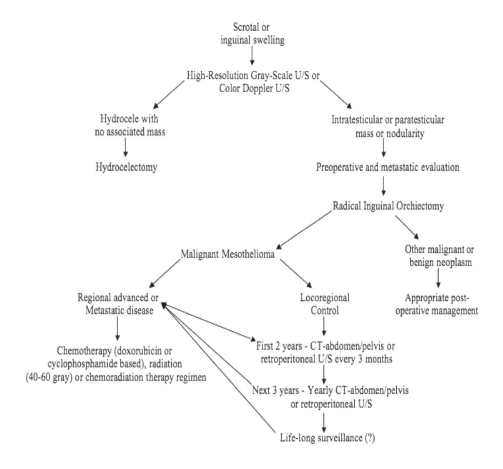

Fig. 9. An evidence-based algorithm for the diagnosis, treatment and follow-up of malignant mesothelioma of the male genitourinary tract (U/S – ultrasonography; CT – computed tomography

8. Acknowledgment

Sachin Patil, MD – for statistical analysis

9. References

Aggarwal P, Sidana A, Mustafa S & Rodriguez R. (2010). Preoperative diagnosis of malignant mesothelioma of the tunica vaginalis using Doppler ultrasound. *Urology*, Vol. 75, No. 2, (Feb 2010), pp. (251-252), 0090-4295.

Amin R. (1995). Case report: Malignant mesothelioma of the tunica vaginalis: an indolent course. *Br J Radiol*, Vol. 68, No. 813, (Sept 1995), pp. (1025-1027), 0007-1285.

Antman K, Cohen S, Dimitrov NV, Green M & Muggia F. (1984). Malignant mesothelioma of the tunica vaginalis testis. *J Clin Oncol*, Vol. 2, No. 5, (May 1984), pp. (447-451), 0732-183X.

Arlen M, Grabstald H & Whitmore Jr WF. (1969). Malignant tumors of the spermatic cord. *Cancer*, Vol. 23, No. 3, (Mar 1969), pp. (525-532), 1097-0142.

Attanoos RL & Gibbs AR. (2000). Primary malignant gonadal mesotheliomas and asbestos. *Histopathology*, Vol. 37, No. 2, (Aug 2000), pp. (150-159), 1365-2559.

Black PC, Lange PH & Takayama TK. (2003). Extensive palliative surgery for advanced mesothelioma of the tunica vaginalis. *Urology*, Vol. 62, No. 4, (Oct 2003), pp. (748vii-748ix), 0090-4295.

Boyum J & Wasserman NF. (2008). Malignant mesothelioma of the tunica vaginalis testis: a case illustrating Doppler color flow imaging and its potential for preoperative diagnosis. *J Ultrasound Med*, Vol. 27, No. 8, (Aug 2008), pp. (1249-1255), 1550-9613.

Eimoto T & Inoue I. (1977). Malignant fibrous mesothelioma of the tunica vaginalis. *Cancer*, Vol. 39, No. 5, (May 1977), pp. (2059-2066), 1097-0142.

Johnson DE, Fuerst DE & Gallager HS. (1973). Mesothelioma of the tunica vaginalis. *South Med J*, Vol. 66, No. 11, (Nov 1973), pp. (1295-1297), 0038-4348.

Jones MA, Young RH & Schully RE. (1995). Malignant mesothelioma of the tunica vaginalis: a clinicopathologic analysis of 11 cases with review of the literature. *Am J Surg Pathol*, Vol. 19, No. 7, (July 1995), pp. (815-825), 0002-9440.

Klaassen Z & Lehrhoff BJ. (2010). Malignant Mesothelioma of the Tunica Vaginalis Testis: A Rare, Enigmatic Tumor. *UroToday Int J*, Vol. 3, No. 6, (December 2010), 1944-5784.

Lane T. (2001). Tumor of the spermatic cord: an unusual primary manifestation of an epithelial mesothelioma of the peritoneum with patent processus vaginalis. *BJU Int*, Vol. 87, No. 4, (March 2001), pp. (415), 1464-410X.

Leiber C, Katzenwadel A, Popken G, Kersten A & Schultze-Seemann W. (2000). Tumor of the spermatic cord: An unusual primary manifestation of an epithelial mesothelioma of the peritoneum with patent processus vaginalis. *BJU Int*, Vol. 86, No. 1, (July 2000), pp. (142), 1464-410X.

Linn R, Moskovitz B, Bolkier M, Munchoir M & Levin DR. (1988). Paratesticular papillary mesothelioma. *Urol Int*, Vol. 43, No. 1, (1988), pp. (60-61), 1464-410X.

Mak CW, Cheng TC, Chuang SS, Wu RH, Chou CK & Chang JM. (2004). Malignant mesothelioma of the tunica vaginalis testis. *Br J Radiol*, Vol. 77, No. 921, (Sept 2004), pp. (780-781), 0007-1285.

McDonald RE, Sago AL, Novicki DE & Bagnall JW. (1983). Paratesticular mesotheliomas. *J Urol*, Vol. 130, No. 2, (Aug 1983), pp. (360-361), 0022-5347.

Menut P, Herve JM, Barbagelata M & Botto H. (1996). Bilateral malignant mesothelioma of the tunica vaginals: apropos of a case. *Prog Urol*, Vol. 6, No. 4, (Aug-Sept 1996), pp. (587-589), 1166-7087.

National Cancer Institute, Division of Cancer Control and Population Sciences, Surveillance Research Program, Cancer Statistics Branch. Surveillance, Epidemiology, and End Results (SEER) Program. Limited-use data (1973-2007), released April 2010, based on November 2009 submission. Accessed May 31, 2011.

Pizzolato P & Lamberty J. (1976). Mesothelioma of Spermatic Cord: Electron Microscopic and Histochemical Characteristics of Its Mucopolysaccharides. *Urology*, Vol. 8, No. 4, (Oct 1976), pp. (403), 0090-4295.

Plas E, Riedl CR & Pfluger H. (1998). Malignant mesothelioma of the tunica vaginalis testis: Review of the literature and assessment of prognostic parameters. *Cancer*, Vol. 83, No. 12, (December 1998), pp. (2437-2446), 1097-0142.

Richie JP & Steele GS. (2007). Chapter 29: Neoplasms of the Testis, In: *Campbell-Walsh Urology, Ninth Edition*, Wein AJ, Kavoussi LR, Novick AC, Partin AW, Peters CA, pp. (893-935), Saunders Elsevier, 978-0-7216-0798-6, Philadelphia, USA.

Silberblatt JM & Gellman SZ. (1974). Mesotheliomas of spermatic cord, epididymis, and tunica vaginalis. *Urology*, Vol. 3, No. 2, (February 1974), pp. (235-237), 0090-4295.

Spiess PE, Tuziak T, Kassouf W, Grossman HB & Czerniak B. (2005). Malignant mesothelioma of the tunica vaginalis. *Urology*, Vol. 66, No. 2, (August 2005), pp. (397-401), 0090-4295.

Stein N & Henkes D. (1986). Mesothelioma of the testicle in a child. *J Urol*, Vol. 135, No. 4, (Apr 1986), pp. (794), 0022-5347.

Tobioka H, Manabe K, Matsuoka S, Sano F & Mori M. (1995). Multicystic mesothelioma of the spermatic cord. *Histopathology*, Vol. 27, No. 5, (November 1995), pp. (479-481), 1365-2559.

Torbati PM, Parvin M & Ziaee SA. (2005). Malignant Mesothelioma of the Spermatic Cord: Case Report and Review of the Literature. *Urol J*, Vol. 2, No. 2, (Spring 2005), pp. (115-117), 1735-1308.

Tuttle Jr JP, Rous SN & Harrold MW. (1977). Mesotheliomas of spermatic cord. *Urology*, Vol. 10, No. 5, (November 1977), pp. (466-468), 0090-4295.

Vianna NJ & Polan AK. (1978). Non-occupational exposure to asbestos and malignant mesothelioma in females. *Lancet*, Vol. 1, No. 8073, (May 1978), pp. (1061-1063), 0140-6736.

Vyas KC, Khamesara HL, Gupta AS & Sarupariya A. (1990). Adenomatoid tumor of the spermatic cord. *J Indian Med Assoc*, Vol. 88, No. 1, (Jan 1990), pp. (15-16), 0019-5847.

Wang MT, Mak CW, Tzeng WS, Chen JC, Chang JM & Lin CN. (2005). Malignant mesothelioma of the tunica vaginalis testis: unusual sonographic appearance. *J Clin Ultrasound*, Vol. 33, No. 8, (Oct 2005), pp. (418-420), 1097-0096.

Winstanley AM, Landon G, Berney D, Minhas S, Fisher C & Parkinson MC. (2006). The immunohistochemical profile of malignant mesotheliomas of the tunica vaginalis: a study of 20 cases. *Am J Surg Pathol*, Vol. 30, No. 1, (Jan 2006), pp. (1-6), 0147-5185.

Wolanske K & Nino-Murcia M. (2001). Malignant mesothelioma of the tunica vaginalis
    testis: atypical sonographic appearance. *J Ultrasound Med,* Vol. 20, No. 1, (Jan 2001),
    pp. (69-72), 1550-9613.

4

Testicular Mesothelioma

Alexander N. Zubritsky
Moscow
Russian Federation

1. Introduction

The testicular mesothelioma is one of the rare tumor from other types of mesotheliomas (less than 1%)[9, 43, 81, 104]. In light of this are clear of the difficulties encountered by some clinicians, radiologists, pathologists and cytologists in differential diagnosis. In addition, they are so rare that there is no more the researcher, which would focus in his hands a sufficient number of his own observations to make serious conclusions. That is why, apparently, the question of the tumor so far in the literature are not systematically developed. The lack of sufficient information on the morphology of mesothelioma are often a cause of incorrect diagnosis. It should also be recognized that a lack of sufficient morphological data about testicular mesothelioma considerably narrows the diagnostic possibilities for dissector and thereby restricts the advice assistant to clinic in establishing the correct diagnosis. In this regard, it seems appropriate to offer for the attention of specialists is one of the literary reviews, focusing on the pathological anatomy of this enigmatic tumor, thereby making an attempt to systematize to some extent, knowledge of mesothelial tumors. We hope that the proposed work will be useful and necessary in the daily work of professionals and will be of interest for researchers studying and developing one of the important problems in oncology - the problem of testicular mesothelioma.

2. Synonyms and definition

Testicular mesothelioma is one of the testis-specific and aggressive form of cancer that develops from the mesothelium covering the tunica albuginea as well as parietal and visceral sheets of the tunica vaginalis of the testis, epididymis, and spermatic cord, and surrounding it, thereby providing protection and support of this body [68, 79]. Among the primary tumors of serous integument mesothelioma (synonyms: adenofibroma, adenofibromyoma, adenoma, adenoma of Müllerian moves, adenomatoid genital tract tumor, adenomatoid leiomyoma, adenomatoid tumor, adenomatous tumor, angiomatoid tumor, angiomatoid tumor of endothelium, cancerous endothelioma, carcinosarcoma, celomic cancer, celothelioma, cystadenoma, endothelial cancer, endothelioma, fibroadenoma, lymfangioendothelioma, lymphangioma, malignant epithelioma, malignant epithelioma of serosa, malignant tumor of the serous covering of cells, primary carcinoma, sarcomatous endothelioma) of the testis is a relatively rare [49, 96, 99].

3. Epidemiology: Frequency and age

Considered a type of cancer in this chapter is most common with a high socio-economic status, mainly in the elderly, but is in young and even in the children, and the incidence has two peaks: the first in 20-30 years, the second after 50 years [110]. Testicular tumors are about 1% of the total number of tumors in men [25]. They occur with a frequency of 20-25 per 1 million men, most aged 20-35 years (3, 40). Testicular tumors in 60% of the observations affect the boys up to 3 years of age, with 80% of them are malignant [5, 60, 67] . The high incidence of testicular tumors for 1998-2002 is registered in most countries of Western Europe: Denmark (9.2 per 100 000 population), Germany (8.1), Scotland (7.6), Italy (7.3), Switzerland (6.9), Czech Republic (6. 5), Netherlands (6.0), Russia, St. Petersburg (1.7); among the white U.S. population (6.0-6.8) [110]. Throughout the second half of the last century there has been an increase of morbidity by testicular cancer. In 2002 in Russia revealed 1189 testicular cancer, representing 1.8 per 100 000 population[64]. Most often, these tumors were observed in age from 0 to 4 years, 30 to 34 years and older than 75 years. The countries with high mortality (> 0.5) from testicular cancer are almost all represented by the WHO the countries of Eastern and Central Europe (Croatia, Czech Republic, Estonia, Hungary, Latvia, Lithuania, Poland, Romania, Slovakia, Slovenia, etc.) [44, 71]. In Western Europe and the U.S., that is, in regions with a high morbidity of testicular cancer, the mortality rate is low, which can be attributed to advances in the treatment of tumors of the body. Mortality, respectively, is low and in countries with low morbidity, namely in East Asia. In Russia, the mortality statistics from testicular cancer is not provided and there is still no national registry of mesothelioma.

However, Kashansky [51] in Russia for the period from 1881 to 2006 has conducted a time-consuming retrospective analysis of published by Russian-speaking authors of 872 papers containing descriptions of 3576 observations of mesotheliomas in different locations, including 29 (0.8%) - of testis, but without a clear representation of literary references proving the obtained data that undoubtedly reduces the quality of his work. The decrease of the reliability of this work also can be attributed to a lack of the Russian national mesothelioma registry. Currently, the epidemiology of the disease being studied in the Altai Territory and the Sverdlovsk region of Russia, and the mesothelioma monitoring was organized in St. Petersburg.

According to Butnor, et al [15] revealed 80 observations of paratesticular adenomatoid tumor, and Murai [78] reports only 6 (0.3%) cases of malignant mesothelioma from 1785 of mesotheliomas of various localizations during 1958-1996, arising from the tunica vaginalis of testes.

Testicular mesothelioma occurs at various ages, from newborns to 80 years. Over the past 50 years, have been documented about 100 cases of testicular mesothelioma [113]. About 80 cases of malignant testicular mesothelioma are reported in the literature, and the frequency of mesothelioma is 1: 1 000 000 [43]. Al-Qahtani, et al. [4] indicate that 73 surveillances of malignant mesothelioma arising from the testicular serous membranes, are published in the literature for the period 1966-1997. Mesothelioma varies in a wide range from 0.6 cases per 1 million inhabitants per year in Tunisia, and 35 in Australia [63]. The background morbidity is 1-2 cases per 1 million of population per year (39). According to forecasts Peto, et al. [84] the mortality from mesothelioma in Western European countries will grow from 5,000 cases in 1998 to 9,000 in 2018 and over the next 35 years from mesothelioma dies about 250 000 people.

According to the International Agency for Research on Cancer, in Europe there is a significant variation between the levels of mesothelioma morbidity in different countries [10, 110]. Thus, in 1993-1997 the largest number of cases of mesothelioma among men are registered in Scotland and the Netherlands - 34 cases per million, whereas in Estonia and Belarus - only 3 cases per million. The situation with the frequency of detection of mesothelioma in the USA and Canada is different from Australia, France and Great Britain, where the number of cases is much higher and continues to grow [85]. For example, in Australia in 1993-1997 were recorded an average of 23 cases with mesothelioma per million among men. In 2000, there were already 60 cases per million in men [45].

Among the economically developed countries of Western Europe, only in Sweden is a similar situation to the United States. In 1993-1997 the morbidity among Swedish men was at the level of the13 cases per million population, but in recent years, the downward trend of these indicators. Projected to peak IARC mesothelioma in Western Europe will be in the 2015-2030 years. According to the International Agency for Research on Cancer the peak of mesothelioma morbidity in Western Europe will be in the 2015-2030 [11, 110].

Thus, epidemiological data about this type of cancer are inconsistent and is explained by the fact that some authors consider the testicular tumors with the positions of germ cell tumors, not considering the mesothelioma of the paratesticular zone, other researchers lead only statistics of the mesotheliomas of other more frequent localizations, not focusing its attention on the testicular mesothelioma because of its great rarity, and numerous publications on the paratesticular mesothelioma are, unfortunately, mostly descriptive in nature. That is why out of the contradictory situation is advisable to establish national centers of pathology with the formation of these cytology, biopsy and autopsy banks, followed by an examination of questions of etiology, epidemiology, patho-and morphogenesis of tumor diseases and, in particular, testicular mesothelioma, as well as analysis of the intravital diagnosis of pathological processes in order to the timely treatment and prevention [116].

4. Etiology and pathogenesis

The exact cause of the testicular mesothelioma is not installed, but the known risk factors that may contribute to its development [20, 64]. Factors of the testicular tumors are as follows: 1. Age. The majority of cases of the testicular cancer are detected from 15 to 40 years. However, the tumor may occur at any age, including infants and the elderly. 2. Cryptorchidism, in which the possibility of the tumor defeat is growing at 40-60 times. 3. Professional career: the miners, firefighters, utility workers, leather, printing, oil and gas industry have an increased risk of testicular cancer. Rather, it involves the use of certain solvents and dyes. Therefore, the risk group usually consists of firefighters, miners, plumbers, builders and gasman. 4. AIDS. Men living with human immunodeficiency virus, there is an increased role in the development of the testicular cancer. 5. Race. The probability of occurrence of the testicular cancer among white Americans is 5-10 times higher than among African-American men. The risk of the testicular cancer in men of Asia and Africa is low. 6. Nutrition. The excessive consumption of animal fat is a risk factor for the testicular cancer. 7. A small increase in risk of the testicular cancer is associated with the trauma of the scrotum. 8. The risk of the testicular cancer raised among young people whose mothers used to maintain the pregnancy is estrogenic drugs, in particular, diethylstilbestrol, and who were, respectively, in vitro exposed to estrogens.

In recent years actively accumulates information indicating about polyetiology of the disease [83]. There is increasing works on mesothelial activity of chemical (salts of nickel, beryllium, silica, tobacco, iron oxide, manganese, carbon black, polyurethane, polysilicon, ethylene oxide, wollastonite, erionite, etc.), physical (microwave and ionizing radiation) and biological (fungi , mycobacterium tuberculosis, viruses of the avian leukemia (MS 29) and simian virus 40) agents [30, 37, 42, 77, 82, 111]. Presently, a considerable role in the development of mesothelioma is assigned to viral etiology, with the Simian virus 40 being isolated in 47-83% of human mesotheliomas, yet the currently available epidemiological evidence seems insufficient to duly evaluate the impact of this virus on the increased incidence of mesothelioma in the second half of the last century [17, 20]. Among the carcinogenic factors contributing to the emergence of mesothelioma, the asbestos is in the first place, especially the impact of asbestos and its derivatives (actinolite, zeolite, amosite, anthophyllite, chrysotile, crocidolite and tremolite), which are classified by the International Agency for Research on Cancer in Group 1 of the carcinogen risk to human where asbestos can be both a stimulant and an initiator of carcinogenesis, it has its own cancer-causing properties and, moreover, can enhance the carcinogenic effect of other factors [12, 33, 62, 90]. Like all other types of mesothelioma, testicular mesothelioma is believed to be caused by exposure to asbestos [7, 87]. In 40% of patients had contact with asbestos, and notes the synergy effects of smoking and asbestos at risk of developing mesothelioma [43]. Despite the fact that in some developed countries reduces production and use of asbestos, the morbidity and mortality from mesothelioma continues to rise. This can be explained to the delayed effect of asbestos. It is known that for development of malignant tumor the latency period is required, the duration of which depends from the carcinogenic factor could be 20 years or more. However, it is possible that increases in the morbidity of mesothelioma is related to other unknown factors [29, 32]. Since the beginning of 1970 in the XX century in Western countries, the development of mesothelioma were due solely to the inhalation of asbestos-containing dust, and, above all, amphibole asbestos, especially crocidolite, and tremolite asbestos, which currently have a crucial role in the etiology of the disease [22, 36]. Human exposure occurs through inhalation of asbestos fibers from the polluted air in the working environment, as well as from the ambient air near of the sources of such pollution, or in rooms that contain the fragile asbestos materials. Such exposure may occur during the installation and use of asbestos-containing materials, and of the vehicle maintenance. In 1977 in Germany, then in France, Japan, Finland, USA and other countries, and since 1996 in Russia the mesotheliomas through law were classified as occupational diseases associated with exposure to asbestos [51]. In a number of countries have established national cancer registers of mesothelioma and operate numerous government agencies and public associations, to examine various aspects of this pathology. The incidence of diseases caused by asbestos is related to fiber type, size of fibers, the dose and the industrial processing of asbestos [89].

The mechanisms of carcinogenicity of asbestos may be associated with the formation in target organs of the active forms of oxygen, which are known to be capable of damaging cell membranes, including the genetic structure of cells [91]. Under the influence of iron contained in large quantities in the amphibole asbestos minerals, oxygen is restored to superoxide with subsequent formation of hydrogen peroxide and later hydroxyl radical. In addition, the active forms of oxygen appear as a result of damage to the phagocytes by asbestos fibers longer than 10 μm (0. 01 mm — the so-called "long fibers") and the emergence of "oxidative stress" is directly into the phagocytes.). In the literature there are data that the short asbestos fibers (up to 10 μm - and thickness of elementary fiber in 26 nanometers) can directly damage the chromosomes and cell division apparatus (fragmentation of the chromosomes, micronuclei, mitotic spindle damage). The initial event in a row, leading to a malignant tumor is the emergence of cells with damaged hereditary structures, which is either removed from the body or remains and gives rise to a tumor. Recent results revealed that asbestos carcinogenesis in humans and in rodents is linked to the activation of the AP-1 pathway, which induces cell division, and to the secretion of TNF-alpha (and the expression of its receptor) by mesothelial cells and by nearby macrophages exposed to asbestos [18]. In mesothelial cells, TNF-alpha signaling through NF-kappaB activation prevents apoptosis and cell death, allowing mesothelial cells to survive the genetic damage induced by asbestos and divide. In addition, mutagenic oxygen radicals released mainly by lung macrophages may contribute to asbestos carcinogenesis. Very recent results indicate that mineral fiber carcinogenesis can be influenced by genetics and microbial infections [19]. Genetic susceptibility to the mineral fiber erionite has been demonstrated in some Turkish families and causes a malignant mesothelioma epidemic in Cappadocia, Turkey. In these mesothelioma families, exposure to minimal amounts of erionite or asbestos appears sufficient to cause mesothelioma. Recent results demonstrate that SV40 and crocidolite asbestos are cocarcinogens and that, in the presence of SV40, significantly lower amounts of asbestos suffice to induce malignant mesothelioma [55]. These findings indicate that the risk varies among asbestos- and erionite-exposed individuals because of their genetic background or because of exposure to other carcinogens. Moreover, these data provide a rationale for the observation that only a fraction of heavily exposed asbestos workers developed mesothelioma, and novel targets for prevention and therapy.

How the fibers reach the testicular area has yet to be determined, but it is understood that asbestos fibers can cause tumors to form in that region of the body. While there is currently no theory to explain why asbestos exposure might cause a primary tumor to develop in the testicles, it is understood that once the asbestos fibers are in the body, they can become lodged in organs and cause inflammation or infection that can result in the development of mesothelioma. The fibers cause cancerous cells to divide abnormally, causing build up of fluid and the development of tumors. Once cells have become cancerous, they are no longer able to regulate their own cycles of growth and division. A primary tumor that develops in the testicle is formed from cancerous cells that divide without restraint, which causes the thickening of the tunica vaginalis and can eventually lead to the formation of tumors.

Thus, the etiology and pathogenesis of testicular mesothelioma to date until the end are unknown, although there are various factors that may influence for the occurrence of the disease, and may play a significant role to asbestos and its derivatives, and these issues require careful further study on the modern level.

5. Pathological anatomy: The macroscopic and cyto-histopathological features

Serous membranes in general, and the testicular membranes, in particular, are difficult to built connective tissue membranes, which have a rich network of blood and lymph vessels, and their surface is covered by one layer of mesothelial cells - mesotheliocytes located on the basement membrane.

Like any cancer testicular mesothelioma can be categorized generally into two types according to the type of cancerous cells. These are benign mesothelioma and malignant mesothelioma. The former one is a non cancerous condition while the latter is the more dangerous one as it spreads to other body parts. The first is the so-called adenomatoid tumor of genitals (mesotheliomas of sex organs), as well as fibrous mesothelioma. All other types of mesotheliomas, including localized in the large serous cavities are malignant.

In International histological classification of tumors of the testis number 16, in section VII «"Tumors of the straight tubules, network testis, epididymis, spermatic cord, the capsule, supporting structures and vestigial structures" under the letters "A" and "B" are introduced such titles as "Adenomatoid tumor" and "Mesothelioma", respectively [48, 49]. According to the international histological classification of tumors of soft tissue № 3 distinguish predominantly epithelioid, predominantly fibrous (spindle) and a two-phase form of benign and malignant mesothelioma [46, 47]. In the modern classification of tumors of the urinary system and male reproductive organs and tumors of the lung, pleura, thymus and heart differentiate the: diffuse malignant mesothelioma and its types - epithelial, sarcomatoid, desmoplastic, biphasic (a combination of epithelial and sarcomatoid features) and localized (nodal) [106, 107]. It should be noted that macro-and microscopic pattern of testicular mesothelioma is usually no different from similar tumors of other localizations.

Adenomatoid tumor is often benign, usually unilateral tumor of the epididymis , sometimes of the testicular tunica albuginea, which is about 69% of all cancers of the epididymis, but they can meet as malignant analogues of neoplasms [56]. Macroscopically, it is represented by an encapsulated, rarely plaque-like node in diameter from a few millimeters to 5 cm, consisting of soft or compact tissue, ivory. The tumor is usually detected in the lower pole of the epididymis, most of the right testicle. The histological pattern is the same everywhere. It does not depend on the location, but depends on the phase of the tumor development. Golovin [35] distinguishes the epithelial, endothelial-like, and fibromatous stage. At the epithelial stage the tumor is represented a conglomerate of small tubules lined by mostly a cuboidal epithelium. The next stage is characterized by a unique, peculiar only to the tumor, changes in the epithelial cells that vacuolating, flatten and become similar to endothelial (or mesothelial) elements. The last stage is "strangling" of the parenchymatous elements by growing fibrous tissue with an admixture of smooth muscle fibers, the tumor becomes a so-called fibroma, in which only here and there is saved the remnants of the adenomatoid structures. The fibrous stroma may be by hyalinized, there is lymphoid infiltration. Often seen the smooth muscle elements, which should not be seen as a sign of invasion [34]. However, the confusion that reigns in the literature about its supposed histogenesis and, consequently, the classification provisions still exists. As potential sources of tissue called the endothelium, mesothelium and derivatives of mezonefron and müllerian remnants of moves (adenomatoid tumors in the fallopian tubes) [59]. Most of the authors believe the most likely the mesothelial origin. Hence the another name - a benign mesothelioma of genital tract. Thus adenomatoid tumor and testicular mesothelioma, as would put on an equal footing, that is totally unjustified and could only lead to confusion. These two tumors anything among themselves do not have any clinical behaviour, histological pattern or histogenesis. If true mesothelioma develops in the mesothelium covering the testicular membranes, then adenomatoid tumor because of its epithelial nature, it is obvious in the early stages of development - most likely from embryonic remnants or Wolf and Müllerian duct. Therefore, these tumors are confused and unite under one name can not be. Testicular mesotheliomas grow diffusely in the form papillae, causing dropsy, the cytoplasm of tumor cells is not vacuolated, tumors never exposed to total fibrosis. Adenomatoid tumors originating from the testicular membranes, do not grow diffusely, but as a node, the papillary structures do not form, the dropsy do not give, their cells have characteristic large vacuole; tumors over time are converted into fibroma, leiomyoma rarely [35].

Squamous cell carcinoma and adenocarcinoma in the area of testis epididymis and spermatic cord are extremely rare and do not have here any special clinical and morphological features that distinguish them from similar tumors at other sites [59].

In addition to the adenomatoid tumor which are viewed as a derivative of the mesothelium, is the tumor proliferation of mesothelium benign or malignant nature, but sometimes the differences between the two tumors is very difficult to establish [23]. The tumor must also distinguish between hyperplasia, often papillary, and desquamation of the mesothelium in inflammatory lesions [49]. From the testicular membranes may develop benign mesothelial tumors. In rare instances in the testes mesothelium can be a source of papillary tumors. The structure of these tumors resembles that of similar tumors originating from ovarian membrane[34].

The type of benign mesothelioma is the non cancerous form of the mesothelioma and is rare [108]. Recently it was referred to as the "solitary fibrous tumor." It is not a cancer itself but can develop into cancerous forms. The benign mesothelioma usually starts in the sub mesothelium layer that lies beneath the mesothelium of the testicular membranes.

The structure of benign mesotheliomas is rather monotonous [105]. On the connective tissue basis with small lymphoid cell clusters are highlighted a cellular bands of the solid structure or in the form of tubes, closely contacting each other, anastomosing and branching. In the interstitial tissue are sometimes found smooth muscle fibers. Careful examination of the tumor proves that solid cell bands and tubular structures are a continuation of the same cell formations. Tumor bands are surrounded by argyrophilic frame and formed large cells with acidophilic cytoplasm and large round nucleus with a centrally located nucleolus. Sometimes the tumor bands are soft and formed a single row of cells, sometimes bands are wider and consist of several rows. In this case there may be gaps that have irregular shape and are always formed between the tumor cells in tumor bands, rather than between them and argyrophilic frame. These gaps include the slightly mucikarminofil liquid. The gaps may expand and connect with each other, and the cells on the edge of the gap are first cube, and then acquire the endothelial form. The cellular bands turn into tubes. Some cells are separated and placed in the cavity gaps. Depending on the case and the location, as well as in different parts of the same tumor may dominate the solid cellular bands or tubular formation. In the latter case, the tumor resembles and is often mistakenly regarded as a lymphangioma. This similarity is enhanced by the presence in the interstitial tissue of the lymphoid clusters. Proof of their origin is the mesothelial brush fringe lining the cavity. A detailed study revealed that the apical surface of endothelial-like cells is not smooth, like endothelial cells, and is provided with a cuticular border and even ciliate formations. No similar formations in vascular endothelium and they are unique to the mesothelium. Can thus be considered reliable, such that tumor formation is not lymphangioma, and certainly not with cancer, and a benign mesothelioma. It still remains to clarify why only mesothelium of genital tract leads to such tumors [26, 27, 68, 69].

Fibrous mesothelioma is a slowly growing, well-delimited node (no more than 3 cm in diameter) has a conical shape, the apex is directed upwards along the spermatic cord, grow together at the base of the epididymis, a very dense, layered on the section, whitish or light brownish. Only in tissue culture can prove the mesothelial origin of the tumor cells. On histological pattern, it has the structure of fibroma, rich in cellular elements, so it is called fibrous mesothelioma [26, 27, 68, 69, 96]. The structure of malignant mesothelioma in its main features is everywhere the same and different only in its details of macroscopic pattern and clinical course associated with the anatomical features of each serous cavity [13, 75]. Macroscopically, the tumor is in the form of a dense infiltrate, causing a dramatic thickening (2-3 cm, and sometimes more) of the serous membranes in a limited area or extends to the entire parietal and visceral sheets of the tunica vaginalis surrounding the body in the form of the shell, sometimes has the form of the mild delimited node from 0.5 to 6 cm oval, or merging several nodes with the villous surface resembling moss, destroys the epididymis and causes the testicular atrophy. It is white, yellow or brownish color, granular, often crumbles easily, in its upper part can move in the spermatic cord, and lower - in the epididymis [26, 27, 79]. In the thicker of infiltrates and nodes is a lot of cracks and cystic cavities with serous, bloody or cloudy mucus content. In the serous cavity, if it is not obliterated, accumulated serous or hemorrhagic exudate, often in large quantities [96]. Mesothelioma is prone to rapid dissemination through the lymph vessels of the serous membrane, resulting in the latter occurs tumor 'lymphangitis' and formed the small nodular lesions. Typical regional and distant metastases in lymph nodes, namely, inguinal, iliac and para-aortic. Hematogenous metastases is usually not excessive, but it may metastasize to the lungs, liver, kidneys, heart, bone, brain, thyroid, adrenal gland, skin, soft tissue. The tumor may grow into other body, mainly on the connective tissue interlayers with the formation in it of small nodules and tumor brands, but the invasive growth is not typical for mesothelioma, it has the exophytic growth in the thickened serous membrane. In the presence of a large tumor node in the body is always an assumption to metastatic lesion of serous membrane.

Microscopic pattern is expressed in the appearance of papillary, solid, alveolar, glandular (tubular), cystic, myxomatous, fibrous, perithelial, sarcomatoid and angioma-like structures, which in some cases may dominate [74, 80, 101, 115]. All this creates considerable polymorphism of the microstructure of the tumor [96]. The types of malignant tumor or cancer cells involved in the development of mesothelioma are of three main types namely epithelioid, sarcomatoid and mixed or biphasic cells [46, 106]. Among the most frequent histological variants of mesothelioma is epithelioid (50-70%) as a set of buds with delicate gripping growths covered with prismatic, cubic or polygonal cells with pale vacuolated cytoplasm and with evidence of cellular polymorphism, hyperchromatosis of the nuclei, the presence of pathological mitoses and giant cells, as if spun from each other, that is, in our opinion, the pathognomonic morphological sign of mesothelioma, and for which can not be wrong [115]. The other type is sarcomatoid which is much more serious than the epithelioid, and it affects the secondary tissues including the bone, muscles, cartilage or fat [94]. This type of cancer cell is a much more rare type that occurs in 7-20% of the cases. Mixed (biphasic) refers to both types of cancers that occurs simultaneously, and making up the rest of the 20-35% of the mesothelioma cases that are reported. A feature of the tumor is large variety of morphological structure, as well as the ability to form structures characteristic of both epithelial and connective tissue for growth. Connective tissue differentiation is less common than epithelial. It is expressed in the transformation of mesothelial cells into elongated elements, such as fibroblasts, which are formed into bundles, severed in various directions. Between the tumor cells are elongated in one way or another including argyrophilic and collagenous fibers. Tumor cells were clearly involved in their formation. These special morphogenetic potency are disclosed already in conditions of inflammation and tissue culture [26, 27]. Histological structure of the epithelial type of mesothelioma is typical enough: they are not similar to any other epithelial tumors and are recognized easily [76]. Connective tissue options is more difficult to distinguish from fibrosarcoma. And they both consist of elongated cells that produce collagen fibers. But fibrosarcomas are small-spindle-cells tumors and relatively rich in mitoses, whereas fibroblasts of mesothelial origin differ by polymorphism and this polymorphism in a strange way contrasts with the paucity of mitoses. In general, cells of all types of mesotheliomas is rarely share by mitosis and is a valuable diagnostic feature.

In the study of tumors of this region has to overcome some difficulties to determine their exact location. Of course, when the tumor is small and not adherent to surrounding tissues, then we can easily establish that it is within the epididymis, spermatic cord, or testicular membranes. But often fall into the hands of a pathologist large tumors that were released outside the body in which they are evolved, and spliced to the surrounding tissues. In such cases, the localization can be expected speak only. This circumstance creates a condition where in each case it would be better to speak in favour of mesothelioma of paratesticular zone, but without precise localization. However, I would like to focus on those cases where the tumor location is beyond doubt.

According to Klimanova [54], the cellular composition of the exudate with mesothelioma in each case differs significantly by originality, but on aggregate the most of common cytomorphological features all cytograms can be summarized in three main groups. When cytograms having a picture of glandular cancer, tumor cell elements are arranged as a circular complexes, rosettes, and glandular-like and papilla-like structures, clusters and isolated. According to the degree of polymorphism and anaplasia of tumor cells in each case the cytograms are somewhat different. However, as a rule, the cell structure consists mainly of rounded cells, there are cubic and prismatic cells. Sometimes there is a sharply pronounced nuclear and cellular polymorphism, in the cytoplasm along with the large cells are small and giant cells, the latter are often multinucleated. Cell nuclei predominantly round and oval, of different sizes, coarse-grained chromatin pattern or small-grained, sometimes thin with non-uniform illumination. Sharply hypertrophied nucleoli are seen in the nuclei. With a low differentiation of cellular elements the cytogram looks more monomorphic, since the basic number of elements are rounded cells of medium size with a narrow zone of basophilic cytoplasm.

Among cytograms of mesothelioma, like cytograms for regenerative proliferative processes, can be identified two types. When one of these cellular elements are very similar to the lining of a serous cover under physiological conditions, and only the abundance of them in the exudate indicates a pathology. The cells are arranged as a vast, one-layer clusters, bands, and layers, are enlarged to the round, polygonal and elongated shape. Signs of atypia of the cellular elements are expressed mild. However, there are discomplexation of nuclei, their polymorphism, the uneven pattern of chromatin (granular or small-grained with broad achromatic zones). The hypertrophied nucleoli are visible in the nuclei. In part of the nuclei with large size have revealed signs of severe dystrophy. In the second form of mesothelioma cells cytograms by location is very similar to the elements of a well differentiated glandular cancer or of proliferating mesothelium. They are mostly round-shaped, medium sized, form a round, or similar to the papillae complexes, glandular-like structure, rows and clusters of other shapes. Enlarged cell nuclei are located centrally and eccentrically, the cytoplasm is colored differently intensively, smile-grained or fine-vacuolated.

In cytograms of mixed type are present both epithelial and connective tissue cells. Epithelial cells are arranged in the form of the layers, papilla-like, glandular-like structures, and clusters and isolated. They are the same type, mostly rounded, sometimes cubic, vary considerably in size. Cell nuclei are rounded or oval shape of various sizes, located centrally or eccentrically. The structure of chromatin in some nuclei are uniformly grained, in other small-grained. Many nuclei are hyperchromatic, some of them contain the hypertrophied nucleoli. The cytoplasm surrounds the nucleus in a narrow or wide rim, is stained unevenly. In some cells more intensely it is stained in the center around of the nucleus, the other reveals a bright ring in the middle of the cytoplasm. There are cells with the morphological characteristics of secretion (the signet ring cell is a cell type with a narrow intensively stained rim of the cytoplasm, which surrounds the vacuole filled with grainy masses of secretion). The cells form of connective tissue similar to the fibroblasts or fibrocytes, are arranged in bundles, bands, clusters and isolated. They are small in size, of the spindle or elongated shape, often with spines of different lengths. The cell nuclei are of round and oval shape, average sizes, sometimes large. Many nuclei are hyperchromatic stained, with irregular contours and uneven chromatin pattern. The cytoplasm of most cells are stained weakly basophilic, granular or has bands. Both types of cellular elements (epithelial and connective tissue) as is mixed in cytogram and often formed intimately the interrelated clusters. Cytologic differential diagnosis of mesothelioma in exudate is very difficult Most often, the cytogram has a pattern of the glandular cancer. Suspected mesothelioma, in this case can only be a careful examination of the entire cellular composition, when I find an abundance of cells and different cell groups, characteristic of epithelial tumors, some types of connective tissue cells and structural formation of them. It should be noted that the mesothelioma even with sharply expressed atypia cells has elements similar to proliferating or dystrophic mesothelium. Especially valuable if all three types of cellular elements (specific to cancer, similar to the mesothelium and the connective tissue nature) are in close contact, and often in direct connection. In the absence of pronounced signs of mesothelioma cells atypia have many similarities with their mesothelium in able of regenerative proliferation, diagnosis can be made only when taken into account the clinical data for this disease.

Cytological diagnosis of mesothelioma is set in the mixed cellular composition of cytograms if, in addition to the cells and structures of the epithelial type observed a large number of fibroblastic cells type and structures with the nature of the connective tissue growth.

Thus, in accordance with the macroscopic, histological and cytological study of tumor substrate of paratesticular zone are released the benign and malignant mesotheliomas, cyto-histological pattern which it is extremely polymorphic and not always pathologists, experiencing the considerable difficulties, can reliably determine their precise localization, namely, the testicular membranes, spermatic cord or its epididymis.

6. Clinical data: Signs and symptoms

Clinical picture is made up of symptoms caused by the presence of the primary paratesticular tumor and its metastases, or a combination thereof [92]. Mesothelioma originating from the serous membranes of the testis, epididymis or its spermatic cord, accompanied by increased and in most cases combined with a hydrocele [28, 83, 100]. Initially the testicular tumor is asymptomatic. The speed of its development is uncertain. However, most often asymptomatic tumor growth lasts no more than 1-2 months. The most frequent symptoms of primary paratesticular tumor are pain, increasing in size or swelling of the body with the appearance of palpable tumor in their formation. With the growth of tumor the testis increases, it becomes dense, lumpy due to the appearance of testicular lumps, which are pathognomonic diagnostic symptom of testicular mesothelioma, and later joins the adhesion process associated with the skin of scrotum [57, 95]. The increase of the testis as the main and only symptom noted in 54% of patients. The pain is the result of a significant increase of intratesticular pressure, germination of the tunica vaginalis of testis or elements of the spermatic cord and is often a sign of far-gone of the disease. Acute pain in the testicle and his the increasing simulate the clinical picture of acute epididimoorhit, the accession of hydrocele in 10% of the cases is typical for tumor lesion. The pain may radiate to the groin, thigh and lower back before the emergence of metastases. In 5% of cases the only symptom may be pain in the back. Often the symptoms associated with the presence of metastases predominate over local symptoms of the testicular lesion. Thus, severe pain in the back may indicate to an increase in the retroperitoneal lymph nodes, which squeeze the nerve rootlets, or to the involvement in the process of the psoas muscle. Often there are gastrointestinal symptoms (nausea or vomiting, diarrhea, abdominal pain), loss of weight, fatigue, muscle weakness, and sometimes in the abdominal cavity on palpation is revealed a tumor. The spread of the tumor above the diaphragm can lead to the discovery in the left supraclavicular area of the visible tumor masses and to the complaints of shortness of breath, chest pain, cough, hoarseness, and heart palpitations.

7. Diagnosis and differential diagnosis

The rarity of the testicular mesothelioma makes it extremely difficult to diagnose [61].The primary malignant neoplasm of the testis serous membranes, its epididymis and the spermatic cord is very difficult for intravital diagnosis, not only in earlier, but in the later stages of the disease. In addition, the diagnosis of mesothelioma is imperfect, usually heavily delayed and it is no accident that this tumor remains an enigma for the oncologist [53]. The cancer typically progresses to the later developmental stages before the patients learned of their diagnosis in the documented cases of the testicular mesothelioma.

Its an accurate diagnosis is obtained at best from pathologic study of resected tumor and at worst from postmortem examination [114]. A combination of clinical, X-ray, laboratory, and instrumental techniques is used to make the diagnosis. The diagnosis should be based primarily on the exclusion of the primary tumor in various internal organs, and first of all, lung, stomach, pancreas, gall bladder and others. The diagnosis is based on precise localization of the tumor and the availability in it of ciliated epithelial cells (primitive cells of the coelom), while using the testicle self-examination can be established an early diagnosis of the testicular cancer. Be that as it may be, any tumor in the testis should be considered as a possible his cancer, and every patient with suspected to a malignant tumor of the testicular region should be examined promptly by a surgeon-urologist, or oncologist. Diagnosis is made up of data history, physical examination, palpation, laboratory tests, radionuclide diagnostics, ultrasound, positron emission tomography, remote infrared thermography, magnetic resonance imaging for detection of metastases and a biopsy [39]. The palpation study is the first diagnosis stage of testicular mesothelioma. With continued examination the doctor should carefully to investigate the status of inguinal, abdominal, supraclavicular, and other lymph nodes accessible to research, to draw an attention to the breasts to detect a possible gynecomastia. Transillumination, which allows to distinguish a tumor that does not transmit light from a cyst filled with fluid, refers to an affordable and highly informative survey techniques [3]. In all patients with suspected to the testicular malignant tumor is necessary to conduct an ultrasound of the scrotum [70]. An ultrasound is a noninvasive and relatively inexpensive method, and accuracy of study in testicular tumors is very high and reaches 90% [14, 25]. Testicle ultrasound is used for differential diagnosis of testicular tumors and other diseases, such as epididymitis. However, basing a diagnosis solely on ultrasound imaging can not, because based on the results of the study can not clearly differentiate tumor from inflammation. Magnetic resonance imaging is more accurate method, but because of the high cost is not always used in routine practice. Nevertheless, in some observations the magnetic resonance imaging should be used to resolve disagreements arising between the ultrasound and physical examination [6]. Cytological examination of the tumor punctate has supporters and opponents. The puncture of the tumor is a danger of its dissemination. In addition, the puncture biopsy does not give the full picture of the morphological features of the tumor, but negative cytology does not exclude the existence of neoplasms. However, in recent years strengthened the view that the puncture in suspected testicular tumor is very valuable, simple and harmless study [1, 52]. Hydropic fluid from the testicular membranes should be subjected to compulsory cytology. Radiacal orchiectomy with subsequent histological examination of obtained material allows to diagnose a testicular tumor.

After identifying of the primary tumor is necessary to determine the stage of disease in the light of the lesion of lymph nodes and presence of distant metastases [73]. Computed tomography is the most accurate method of determining the lesion of the lymph nodes, mainly retroperitoneal. However, be aware that 25-30% of patients with testicular tumor and the absence of data computed tomography showing the lesion of the lymph nodes, and morphological study revealed the microscopic metastases in the last. Other frequently used methods of diagnosis of retroperitoneal lymph node metastases are cavography and lymphangiography. With a significant increase of retroperitoneal lymph nodes in the excretory urogram is possible to detect a displacement or compression of the ureter. The lungs are the most frequent localization of distant metastases of testicular tumor. To identify them it is need perform not only lung X-rays in two projections, but also computed tomography of the chest, allowing to detect metastases in diameter up to 3 mm [26]. Metastatic liver lesions can be detected by ultrasound and scintigraphy of the liver, and the presence of metastases in the brain of an informative role in the diagnosis is given of magnetic resonance imaging. Experts are reserved to the primary tumor biopsy, and with great enthusiasm to the removal of metastases for histological examination. So much activity can be explained by three reasons. First, the biopsy helps to determine the extent of distribution of the tumor process. Secondly, if you delete metastasis, in addition to histological examination, it is possible that he was single and, of course, the procedure would be of great benefit to the patient. Third, the histological study of metastasis, despite the fact that there is a conclusion of the primary tumor, can make a change in the morphological verification of diagnosis, and consequently in the nature of the treatment. The task of staging process is to determine the prevalence and nature of both the primary tumor and its metastases. The level of serum markers of human chorionic β-gonadotropin, α-fetoprotein and lactate dehydrogenase to be determined in pre-and postoperative period, and in the future - with weekly intervals. The situation in which after the operation the level of α-fetoprotein and human chorionic β-gonadotropin is not normal, indicates the prevalence of the disease, which makes justified those serological tests. In this case, shortly after radical orhiectomy should be performed computed tomography (an advantage of magnetic resonance imaging has not yet proved) of the chest, abdomen and pelvis. When using classification by the TNM system is required histological confirmation of the diagnosis [8]. Histological verification of both mature and immature mesotheliomas is very difficult. Histogenesis and morphology of testicular tumors can be reliably determined only by histotopographical, and sometimes even serial sections. Therefore, the best way to determine the diagnosis is to obtain a tissue sample from the area. The sample may then be biopsied and examined for the presence of cancerous cells. Once a diagnosis is confirmed, the patient will be referred to an oncologist to determine a course of treatment.

Differential diagnosis between mesothelioma and their simulating metastatic tumors is based on the combined of anatomical, histological and clinical data. On the basis of a microscopic examination of mesothelioma from adenocarcinoma is difficult to differentiate [2]. In the analysis of the microstructure is of great importance to the presence of polymorphism of the tumor areas resembling to the angioendothelioma, spindle-polymorphocellular sarcoma, etc., which is not characteristic of cancerous tumors. The structure of mesothelioma is also unlike to any the testicular disgerminoma. The latter has a pronounced solid-alveolar structure, and is too small glandular differentiation, to assume that it occurs in the epididymis or testicular tubules [26].

Recently, using different immunohistochemical markers for mesotheliomas, in particular, they are positive for cytokeratin, cytokeratin 7, γ-glutamylcysteine synthetase, vimentin, mesothelin, epithelial membrane antigen, thrombomodulin, calretinin, and mesothelial antibody, whereas mesotheliomas are negative for cytokeratin 20 and carcinoembryonic antigen [24, 50, 65, 112]. However, it is not always and not all the conventional tumor markers allow you to make a diagnosis [16, 97]. For example, the carcinoembryonic antigen, usually is determined at low concentrations, whereas, the tissue polypeptide specific antigen and the cytokeratin fragment 21-1 are identified only occasionally in high concentrations. Differential diagnosis of testicular tumor have to spend with specific and nonspecific inflammatory diseases of the testis, as well as with a hydrocele, hematocele, hematoma, hernia, and testicular torsion [66]. Tuberculous orchitis is confirmed by the tuberculous lesion of kidney, prostate, seminal vesicles. The gender history and Wasserman'reaction have an important role in cases of suspected syphilis in the testis. If you suspect a diagnosis of brucellosis orchitis is specified by the agglutination test, at Wright-Haddlson, complement fixation reaction with allergic intracutaneous test. In doubtful cases, for the differential diagnosis of chronic orchitis and testicular tumor is shown holding of an emergency open biopsy on the operating table. Accurate diagnosis can be made using the immunohistochemical typing with the use of monoclonal antibodies, as well as the method of tissue culture.

Thus, the difficulty of the diagnostic process in the diagnosis of testicular mesothelioma is obvious. Therefore, a breakthrough in improving its diagnosis should be sought in the widespread institutional arrangements, consisting in close collaboration of the various medical specialties in specialized medical centers a qualitatively of new level.

8. Treatment

Over the past two decades in the treatment of testicular cancer has been quite remarkable, resulting in 5-year survival rate in the U.S. and Europe has reached 90-95% [3, 31]. However, in many countries rates of 5-year survival rate is much lower. In Russia (St. Petersburg), 5-year survival rate for patients with testicular cancer is 73%. In the treatment of testicular mesothelioma distinguish 3 main methods: 1) the operation, 2) radiation therapy, and 3) chemotherapy. Often, depending on the tumor stage is used combined (multimodal) treatment with two or all three methods, which is recommended, particularly, for the treatment of diffuse mesothelioma [109]. Approaches to treatment are being developed for neoadjuvant therapy with cytokines only in the early stages. Operation is possible only in the early stages of the disease [102]. Treatment is surgical of adenomatoid tumors, usually with a good prognosis. Radiation therapy is used mainly with palliative purpose. Radiation may be used if the patient's health cannot withstand a major operation. The treatment of the testicular tumors depends on several factors including the histological structure of the tumor, stage of disease, the presence of contralateral testicular damage and general state of the patient and his opinion. The main problem is the timeliness of treatment and the sequence of preoperative radiation execution, the remove of the primary tumor, the diagnostic and therapeutic lymphadenectomy and the chemotherapy effects in the cancer institutions [21, 98]. Malignant mesothelioma is difficult to treat, because it is not a centralized tumor mass [72]. Mesothelioma tends to spread along nerves, blood vessels, and surfaces. Because of this tendency to spread, multiple methods of treatment must be employed to fight the cancer, and treatment is often unsuccessful if the cancer is in a later stage.

The most common treatment option available for testicular mesothelioma is the removal of the testicles, or a portion of it [40]. If the cancer has advanced very high, it may be necessary to remove the entire testicles. Surgery can be performed to remove the cancer in addition to radiation and chemotherapy. These methods are usually used to relieve symptoms related to mesothelioma. Other treatment options available are chemotherapy or radiation therapy [41]. Chemotherapy or radiation may also be suggested following surgery to kill any cancerous cells that may remain. Radiation therapy will attempt to kill any cancerous cells in the testicles via the help of a high beam razor that directly targets tumorous cells. As the successful schemes used chemotherapy for tumors of the testis recommend complex, involving the use of cisplatin, mitomycin, vinblastine, etoposide, doxorubicin, bleomycin, gemcitabine, and folic acid, which in combination are effective in 90% of cases [64].

If malignant mesothelioma is diagnosed in stage I of the disease, surgery is often used to remove tumor masses. If mesothelioma is diagnosed during the initial stage, surgery will usually be performed to remove the tumor. The use of chemotherapy and radiation after surgery is still being studied to determine a good course of action for mesothelioma treatment. In stages II and III, symptom relief is stressed because mesothelioma is often incurable at this level of development of the cancer. Surgery to remove as much of the cancer as possible is employed, as well as some chemotherapy and radiation. In stage IV, malignant mesothelioma spreads to organs distant from the original site of disease and becomes impossible to cure. A hospice or supportive care is usually the best option for this advanced form. The patient may also wish to try alternative methods of therapy for pain relief, including acupuncture. In addition, testicular mesothelioma tends to recur within a few years, even in cases where tumors are surgically removed [58]. It is also necessary to remember that 1-3% of patients with testicular cancer is the risk of cancer in the other testicle. Therefore, it is necessary to improve methods of treatment to reduce the frequency of relapses and worsening prognosis [88]. In this sense, periodic surveillance and screening are important in patients with testicular cancer. With a view to early detection of tumor recurrence must regularly determine the levels of tumor markers such as alpha-fetoprotein, human chorionic β-gonadotropin and lactate dehydrogenase. Moreover, it should be regularly assigned to X-rays of the chest and the appropriate methods of radiological investigations to detect recurrence, metastases or occurrence of multiple primary tumors.

It is always necessary to remember that in the course of treatment for testicular mesothelioma or after may occur the following complications [25]:

1. Practically in all patients with radio-and chemotherapy leads to oligospermia. Many observations of spermatogenesis recovered in 1-2 years and 2 years after chemotherapy with one testicle preserved the ability to fertilize are generally returned.
2. Chemo-and radiotherapy increase the risk of secondary leukemias. The greatest risk of leukemia (0.5% in 5 years) has been established for patients receiving etoposide.
3. Nephrotoxicity. During chemotherapy with platinum drugs may be a slight decrease in creatinine clearance - on average by 15%.
4. Ototoxicity. Decreases mainly the perception of sounds with a frequency of 4.8 kHz, ie not spoken frequency.
5. Retrograde ejaculation. Occurs as a complication of retroperitoneal lymphadenectomy due to standard intraoperative intersection of sympathetic pathways, providing a reflex contraction of the bladder neck during ejaculation.
6. The development of secondary tumors. Established higher incidence of stomach cancer, bladder and pancreas.

Thus, treatment in testicular tumors developed in some detail, but research in this area are continuing. The main areas of focus are to develop the optimal treatment strategy of residual retroperitoneal tumors after chemo- or radiation therapy, treatment of patients with bilateral tumors and cancer of the single testis, more efficient treatment of chemoresistant cancer. Given the rarity of the disease, it is advisable to carry out the treatment in the specialized cancer institutions that have experience in treating such patients. For each method of treatment are possible complications that may persist for several months. Knowledge of therapy complications may help to fight them. Currently, there is intensive development of promising new methods of treatments, like gene therapy, photodynamic therapy and immunotherapy, which are the subject of clinical studies and that really can qualitatively change the suffering of the patients with testicular mesothelioma in the near future.

9. Prognosis

Testicular malignant mesothelioma is considered to be a very clinically aggressive form of cancer, spreading quickly [86, 103]. Because of this, the prognosis for a patient with this form of mesothelioma is often poor [73, 93]. However, the prognosis depends on factors such as age, macro-microscopic version, stage of disease, intercurrent illness. Severe intercurrent diseases, stage 3 and 4, diffuse form and sarcomatoid or biphasic types of testicular mesothelioma and advanced age are associated with a poor prognosis [38]. The median survival after diagnosis of testicular mesothelioma is 1 year and five-year survival is 10%. Most patients die within 2 years after their diagnosis. In the U.S., a 5-year survival rate for mesothelioma patients is 28%. In Russia the figure is 23%. Out of all types of testicular cancers, the survival rate after ten years is around 98%.

Thus, the prognosis for testicular mesothelioma in the light of certain factors set forth above are generally unfavorable, and the determination of histological variants of tumors has important prognostic value in relation to anything other than light microscopy in the diagnosis of mesothelioma are commonly used methods of immunohistochemistry and electron microscopy.

10. Conclusion

From this analytical review of the world literature implies that the testicular mesothelioma is a mysterious and rare tumor originating from mesotheliocytes, covering the serous membranes of the testis, epididymis and spermatic cord with an unknown etiology and pathogenesis, a poor clinic and prognosis, and as a rule, of the late diagnosis, in spite of intensive development and application of new methods of diagnosis and treatment in recent years. The speed of the correct diagnosis establishing, prevention and treatment of the testicular mesothelioma depend on the attention to the health of the patient's cancer, oncological vigilance and art of a doctor, from the provision of modern medical equipment, from a qualitative immunohistochemical, immunophenotypical and cytogenetic studies with the use of modern medical and computer technologies and techniques, as well as on the creation in all highly developed countries of the united, up-to-date, organizational, methodical, consultative, and statistical centres on studying human pathology at a qualitatively new level – the national centres of pathology, in which multiple studies on the etiology, patho-and morphogenesis of tumors, and in particular, mesothelioma testis, and also analysis of the intravital diagnosis of the character of pathological processes according to data of cytologic, biopsy and autopsy banks with the help of modern computer and telecommunication technologies would be carried out.

11. References

[1] Ahmed M, Chari R, Mufi GR, Azzopardi A. Malignant mesothelioma of the tunica vaginalis testis diagnosed by aspiration cytology – A case report with review literature. Int Urol Nephrol 1996; 28 (6): 793–796.

[2] Akyildiz EU, Oz B., Schitoglu I, Demir H. The diagnostic utility of maspin in the distinction between malignant mesothelioma and pulmonary adenocarcinoma. J Int Med Res 2010; 38 (3): 1070–1076.

[3] Alexandrov VP, Mikhailichenko VV. Urology and andrology. The modern guide for physicians. In: Diseases and injuries of the scrotum. Chapter 12; 414–440. Moscow: "AST"; St. Petersburg: "Sova" 2005; 576 p (in Russian).

[4] Al-Qahtani M, Morris B, Dawood S, Okerheim R. Malignant mesothelioma of the tunica vaginalis. Can J Urol 2007; 14 (2): 3514–3517.

[5] Al-Shukri SKh, Tkachuk VN. Tumors of the genitourinary organs. Guide for physicians. In: Testicular tumors. Chapter 8; 159–181; Tumors of the testicular epididymis. Chapter 9; 182–183; Tumors of the spermatic cord. Chapter 10; 184–187. St. Petersburg: "Piter" 2000; 320 p (in Russian).

[6] Andipa E, Liberopoulos K, Asvestis C. Magnetic resonance imaging and ultrasound evaluation of penile and testicular masses. World J Urol 2004; 22: 382–391.

[7] Attanoos RL, Gibbs AR. Primary malignant gonadal mesotheliomas and asbestos. Histopathology 2000; 37: 150–159.

[8] Avtandilov GG. Fundamentals of pathoanatomical practice. Leadership. Moscow: "RMAPO" 1994; 512 p (in Russian).

[9] Benchekroun A, Jira H, Ghadouane M, Kasmaoui EH, Marzouk M, Faik M. Paratesticular malignant mesothelioma. Report of a new case. Ann Urol (Paris) 2001; 35 (5): 293–295.

[10] Bianchi C, Brollo A, Ramani L and Bianchi T. Malignant mesothelioma in Europe. Int J Med Biol Environ 2000; 28 (2): 103–107.

[11] Bianchi C, Brollo A, Ramani L and Bianchi T. Malignant mesothelioma in Central and Eastern Europe. Acta med Croat 2000; 53 (4–5): 161–164.

[12] Bianchi C, Bianchi T. Amianto un secolo di sperimentazione sull'uomo. Trieste: Hammerle Editori 2002; 102 p.

[13] Bisceglia M, Dor DB, Carosi I, Vairo M, Pasquinelli G. Paratesticular mesothelioma. Report of a case with comprehensive review of literature. Adv Anat Pathol 2010; 17: 53–70.

[14] Blaivas M, Brannam L. Testicular ultrasound. Emerg Med Clin North Amer 2004; 22: 723–748.

[15] Butnor KJ, Sporn TA, Hammnar SP, Roggli VL. Well-differentiated papillary mesothelioma. Am J Surg Pathol 2001; 25: 1304–1309.

[16] Cabay RJ, Siddiqui NH, Alam Sh. Paratesticular papillary mesothelioma: A case with borderline features. Arch Pathol Lab Med 2006; 130 (1): 90–92.

[17] Carbone M. Simian virus 40 and human tumors: It is time to study mechanisms. J Cell Biochem 1999; 76 (2): 189–193.

[18] Carbone M, Barbanti-Brodano G. Viral Carcinogenesis. Chapter 17; 214–232. In: Section Two. Translational Basic Science / Oncology. An Evidence-Based Approach Edited by Alfred E Chang, Patricia A Ganz, Daniel F Hayes, Timothy J Kinsellla, Harvey I Pass, Joan H Schiller, Richard M Stone, Victor J Strecher. New York: Springer 2006; 2022 p.

[19] Carbone M, Bedrossian CW. The pathogenesis of mesothelioma. Semin Diagn Pathol 2006; 23 (1): 56–60.

[20] Carbone M, Fisher S, Powers A, Pass HI, Rizzo P. New molecular and epidemiological issues in mesothelioma: Role of SV 40. J Cell Physiol 1999; 180(2): 167–172.

[21] Castillo OA, Alvarez JM, Vitagliano G, Ramirez D, Diaz M, Sanchez-Salas R. Limfadenectomia retroperitoneal laparoscopia en cancer de testiculo no seminoma estadio. Arch esp urol 2007; 60 (1): 59–66.

[22] Churg A. Chrysolite, trenolite, and malignant mesothelioma in man. Chest 1988; 93 (3): 621–628.

[23] Churg A, Colby TV, Cagle P, et al. The separation of benign and malignant mesothelial proliferations. Am J Surg Pathol. 2000; 24: 1183-2000.

[24] Ekman S, Eriksson P, Bergstrom S, Johansson P, Goike H, Gulleo J, Henriksson R, Larsson A, Berqovist M. Clinical value of using serological cytokeratins as therapeutic markers in thoracic malignancies. Anticancer Res 2007; 27 (5B): 3545–3554.

[25] Fedorov VD, Pikunov MYu, Shchegolev AI, Dubova EA, Kamalov AA, Nikushina AA. Tumors of testicle. Khirurgiya. Zhurnal imeni NI Pirogova 2007; (5): 68–74 (in Russian).

[26] Foot N. Identification of Tumors. Philadelphia, London, Montreal: J.B.Lippincott Co 1948; 397 p.

[27] Foot N. Identification of Tumors. Translated from English V.B.Freiman / Prof. Ya.L.Rapoport (Ed). Moscow: Foreign Literature Publishing House 1951; P.41–42; P.140 (in Russian).

[28] Fujii Y, Masuda M, Hirokawa M, Matsushita K, Asakura S. A case of benign mesothelioma of the tunica vaginalis testis. Hinyokika Kiyo 1993; 39 (1); 89–92.

[29] García de Jalón A, Gil P, Azúa-Romeo J, Borque A, Sancho C, Rioja LA. Malignant mesothelioma of the tunica vaginalis. Report of a case without risk factors and review of the literature. Int Urol Nephrol 2003; 35: 59–62.

[30] Gibbs GW, Berry G. Mesothelioma and asbestos. Regul Toxicol Pharmacol 2008; 52: S223–31.

[31] Gilligan T, Kantoff PW. Testis Cancer. Chapter 49; 844–873. In: Section Five. Solid Tumors / Oncology. An Evidence-Based Approach Edited by Alfred E Chang, Patricia A Ganz, Daniel F Hayes, Timothy J Kinsellla, Harvey I Pass, Joan H Schiller, Richard M Stone, Victor J Strecher. New York: Springer 2006; 2022 p.

[32] Goel A, Agrawal A, Gupta R, Hari S, Dey AB. Malignant mesothelioma of the tunica vaginalis of the testis without exposure to asbestos. Cases J 2008; 1:310.

[33] Goldberg S, Rey G, Luce D, Ilg AGS, Rolland P, Brochard P, Imbernon E, Goldberg M. Possible effect of environmental exposure to asbestos on geographical variation in mesothelioma rates. Occup Environ Med 2010; 67 (6): 417–421.

[34] Golovin DI. Atlas of human tumours. Leningrad: Publishing House "Meditsina" 1975; P.201–205 ; P.306–309 (in Russian).

[35] Golovin DI. Errors and difficulties in histological diagnosis of tumors: (a guide for physicians). Leningrad: «Meditsina» 1982; 304 p (in Russian).

[36] Gorini G, Pinelli M, Sforza V, Simi U, Rinnovati A, Zocchi G. Mesothelioma of the tunica vaginalis testis: reported of 2 cases with asbestos occupational exposure. Int J Surg Pathol 2005; 13 (2): 211–214.

[37] Grove A, Jensen ML, Donna A. Mesotheliomas of the tunica vaginalis testis and hernial sacs. Virchows Archiv 1989; 415: 283–292.

[38] Guney N, Basaran M, Karayigit E, Muslumanoglu A, Guney S, Kilicaslan I, Gulbarut S. Malignant mesothelioma of the tunica vaginalis testis: a case report and review of the literature. Med Oncol 2007; 24 (4): 449–452.

[39] Gupta NP, Agrawal AK, Sood S, Hemal AK, Nair M. Malignant mesothelioma of the tunica vaginalis testis: a report of two cases and review of literature. J Surg Oncol 1999; 70: 251-254.

[40] Gupta NP, Kumar R. Malignant gonadal mesothelioma. Curr Treat Opt Oncol 2002; 3 (5): 363–367.

[41] Hamm M, Rupp C, Rottger P, Rathert P. Malignant mesothelioma of the tunica vaginalis testis. Chirurg 1999; 70 (3): 302–305.

[42] Hassan R, Alexander R. Nonpleural mesotheliomas: mesothelioma of the peritoneum, tunica vaginalis, and pericardium. Hematol Oncol Clin North Am. 2005; 19: 1067–1087.

[43] Hatzinger M, Hacker A, Langbein S, Grobholz R, Alken P. Malignant mesothelioma of the testes. Aktualle Urol 2006; 37 (4): 281–283.

[44] Hodgson JT, McElvenny DM, Darnton AJ, Price MJ, Peto J. The expected burden of mesothelioma mortality in Great Britain from 2002 to 2050. Br J Cancer 2005; 92: 587–593.

[45] Hyland RA, Ware S, Johnson AR, Yates DH. Incidence trends and gender differences in malignant mesothelioma in New South Wales, Australia. Scand J Work Environ Health 2007; 33 (4): 286–292.

[46] International Histological Classification of Tumours N 3. Histological Typing of Soft Tissue Tumours / FM Enzinger, R Lattes, H Torloni (Eds). World Health Organization. Geneva, 1969.

[47] International Histological Classification of Tumors N 3. Histological Typing of Soft Tissue Tumors / FM Enzinger, R Lattes, H Torloni (Eds). World Health Organization. Geneva, 1974; P.23–24 (in Russian).

[48] International Histological Classification of Tumours N 16. Histological Typing of Testis Tumours / FK Mostofi, LH Sobin, et al (Eds). World Health Organization. Geneva, 1977.

[49] International Histological Classification of Tumours N 16. Histological Typing of Testis Tumours / FK Mostofi, LH Sobin, et al (Eds). World Health Organization. Geneva, 1981; P.16; P.36 (in Russian).

[50] Jones MA, Young RH, Scully RE. Malignant mesothelioma of the tunica vaginalis. A clinicopathologic analysis of 11 cases with review of the literature. Am J Surg Pathol 1995; 19: 815-825.

[51] Kashansky SV. Mesothelioma in Russia: systematic review of 3576 published cases from occupational medicine viewpoint. Occupational medicine and industrial ecology 2008; (3):15–21 (in Russian).

[52] Kimura N, Dota K, Araya Y, Ishidate T, Ishizaka M. Scoring system for differential diagnosis of malignant mesothelioma and reactive mesothelial cells on cytology specimens. Diagn Cytopathol 2009 ; 37 (12): 885–890.

[53] Klaassen Z, Lehrhoff BJ. Malignant Mesothelioma of the Tunica Vaginalis Testis: A Rare, Enigmatic Tumor. UroToday Int J 2010; 3(6).

[54] Klimanova Z F. Tumor processes of the serous membranes (for exudates of the serous cavities). In: A guide to the cytological diagnosis of human tumors / AS Petrova, MP Ptokhov (Eds). Moscow: Publishing House "Meditsina" 1976; 279–301 (in Russian).

[55] Kroczynska B, Cutrone R, Boccheta M, Yang H, Elmishad AG, Vacek P, Ramos-Nino M, Mossman BT, Pass HI, Carbone M. Crocidolite asbestos and SV40 are cocarcinogens in human mesothelial cells and in causing mesothelioma in hamsters. Proc Natl Acad Sci USA 2006; 103: 14128-14133.

[56] Kuzaka B, Biernacka-Wawrzonek D, Szymanska K, et al. Adenomatoid tumors of the testis and epididymis. Przegl Lek 2004 ; 61: 531–534.

[57] Lee SC, Lee JK. A case of primary malignant mesothelioma of tunica vaginalis testis. Korean J Urol. 1991; 32: 843–845.

[58] Liguori G, Garaffa G, Trombetta C, Bussani R, Bucci S, Belgrano E. Inguinal recurrence of malignant mesothelioma of the tunica vaginalis: one case report with delayed recurrence and review of the literature. Asian J Androl 2007; 9 (6): 859–860.

[59] Likhachev YuP, Shtern RD. Tumors of the testis, seminal vesicles and penis. In: A guide to the pathoanatomical diagnosis of human tumors /NA Kraevsky, A.V Smoliyannikov (Eds). Moscow: "Meditsina", 1971; 258–277 (in Russian).

[60] Livingstone RR, Sarembock LA. Testicular tumours in children. S Afr Med J 1986; 70 (3): 168–169.

[61] Mak CW, Cheng TC, Chuang SS, Wu RH, Chou CK, Chang JM. Malignant mesothelioma of the tunica vaginalis testis. Br J Radiol 2004; 77: 780–781.

[62] Malignant mesothelioma edited by Andrea Tannapfel. Springer-Verlag 2011 ; 193 p.

[63] Malignant mesothelioma: advances in pathogenesis, diagnosis, and translational therapies edited by Harvey I Pass, Nicholas J Vogelzang, and Michele Carbone. New York, NY: Springer 2005; 854 p.

[64] Manual of Urology: In three volumes. Vol. 3. In: Testicular tumors. Chapter 23; 317–348; Tumors of the testicular epididymis. Chapter 24; 349–350; Tumors of the spermatic cord. Chapter 25; 351–353 / Prof. NA.Lopatkin (Ed). Moscow: Publishing House "Meditsina" 1998; 672 p (in Russian).

[65] Marchevsky AM. Application of immunohistochemistry to the diagnosis of malignant mesothelioma. Arch Pathol Lab Med 2008; 132: 397–401.

[66] Marinbakh EB. Malignant tumors of the testis (clinic, diagnosis and treatment): Abstract of thesis. … Doctor of Medical Sciences. Moscow 1970; 25 p (in Russian).

[67] Marinbakh EB. Tumors of the testis and its epididymis. Moscow: Publishing House "Meditsina" 1972; 216 p (in Russian).

[68] Masson P. Tumeurs Humaines. Histologie Diagnostics et Techniques. Paris: Librairie Maloine 1956.

[69] Masson P. Tumeurs Humaines. Histologie Diagnostics et Techniques. Translated from the French Prof. SA Vinogradova / AI Strukov (Ed). Moscow: Publishing House "Meditsina" 1965; 108–110; 308 (in Russian).

[70] Matsuzaki K, Nakajima T, Katoh T, Kitoh H, Mizoguchi K, Akahara K, Inone T. Malignant mesothelioma of the tunica vaginalis : a case report. Hinyokika Kiyo 2008; 54 (9): 629–631.

[71] McElvenny DM, Darnton AJ, Price MJ, Hodgson JT. Mesothelioma mortality in Great Britain from 1968 to 2001. Occup Med (Lond) 2005; 55: 79–87.

[72] Melloni G, Puglisi A, Ferraroli GM, Carretta A, et al. Il trattamento del mesotelioma pleurico maligno. Minerva chir 2001; 56 (3):243–250.

[73] Mesothelioma edited by Bruce WS Robinson and A Philippe Chahinian. London: Martin Dunitz 2002; 366 p.

[74] Mikuz G, Hopfel-Kreiner I. Papillary mesothelioma of the tunica vaginalis propria testis. Virchows Archiv 1982; 396 (2): 231–238.

[75] Moore AJ, Parker RJ, Wiggins J. Malignant mesothelioma. Orphanet J Rare Dis. 2008; 3: 34.

[76] Morikawa Y, Ishihara Y, Yanase Y, et al. Malignant mesothelioma of tunica vaginalis with squamous differentiation. J Urol Pathol 1994; 2: 95–102.

[77] Mossman BT, Gruenert DC. SV 40, growth factors, and mesothelioma; another piece of the puzzle. Am J Respir Cell Mol Biol 2002 ; 26 (2): 167–170.

[78] Murai Y. Malignant mesothelioma in Japan : analysis of registered autopsy cases. Arch Environ Health 2001; 56: 84–88.

[79] Olkhovskaya IG. Tumors of the testis, seminal vesicles and penis. In: Pathoanatomical diagnosis of human tumors. Handbook / NA Kraevsky, AV Smoliyannikov, DS Sarkisov (Eds). - 3rd Edition. Moscow: "Meditsina" 1982; 296–312 (in Russian).

[80] Park HM, Kim JH, Bae SG, Kwon TK, Chung SK. A case of malignant mesothelioma of tunica vaginalis. Korean J Urol. 1997; 38: 1132–1134.

[81] Park YJ, Kong HJ, Jang HC, Shin HS, Oh HK, Park JS. Malignant mesothelioma of the spermatic cord. Kor J Urol 2011; 52 (3): 225–229.

[82] Pathology of malignant mesothelioma edited by Francoise Galateau-Salle. Springer-Verlag London 2010; 198 p.

[83] Perez-Ordonez B, Srigley JR. Mesothelial lesions of the paratesticular region. Semin Diagn Pathol 2000 ; 17: 294–306.

[84] Peto J, Decarli A, Vecchia CLa, Levi F, Negri E. The European mesothelioma epidemic. Br J Cancer 1999; 79 (3–4): 666–672.

[85] Peto J, Hodgson JT, Matthews FE, Jones JR. Continuing increase in mesothelioma mortality in Britain. Lancet 1995; 345: 535–539.

[86] Plas E, Riedl CR, Pflüger H. Malignant mesothelioma of the tunica vaginalis testis: review of the literature and assessment of prognostic parameters. Cancer. 1998;83:2437–2446.

[87] Reynards JM, Hasan N, Baithun SI, Neuman L, Lord MG. Malignant mesothelioma of the tunica vaginalis testis. Br J Urol 1994; 74: 389-390.

[88] Rekhi B, Pathuthara S, Ajit D, Kake SV. «Signet-ring» cells – A caveat in the diagnosis of a diffuse peritoneal mesothelioma occuring in a lady presenting with recurrent ascites: An unusual case report. Diagn Cytopathol 2010; 38 (6): 435–439.

[89] Roggli VL, Pratt PC, Brody AR. Asbestos fiber type in malignant mesothelioma : an analytical scanning electron microscopic study of 94 cases. Am J Ind Med 1993 ; 23 (4): 605–614.

[90] Roggli VL, Vollmer RT, Butnor KJ, Sporn TA. Tremolite and mesothelioma. Ann Occup Hyg 2002 ; 46 (5): 447–453.

[91] Sabo-Attwood T, Ramos-Nino M, Mossman BT. Environmental Carcinogenesis. Chapter 18; P.233-243 In: Section Two Translational Basic Science / Oncology. An Evidence-Based Approach Edited by Alfred E.Chang, Patricia A.Ganz, Daniel F.Hayes, Timothy J.Kinsellla, Harvey I.Pass, Joan H.Schiller, Richard M.Stone, Victor J.Strecher. New York: Springer, 2006; 2022 p.

[92] *Sawada K, Inoue K, Ishihara T, Kurabayashi A, Moriki T, Shuin T. Multicystic malignant mesothelioma of the tunica vaginalis with an unusually indolent clinical course. Hinyokika Kiyo 2004; 50 (7): 511–513.

[93] *Schure PJ, van Dalen KC, Ruitenberg HM, van Dalen T. Mesothelioma of the tunica vaginalis testis: a rare malignancy mimicking more common inguino-scrotal masses. J Surg Oncol 2006; 94 (2): 162–164.

[94] Shimada S, Ono K, Suzuki Y, Mori N. Malignant mesothelioma of the tunica vaginalis testis: a case with a predominant sarcomatous component. Pathol Int 2004; 54 (12): 930-934.

[95] Shin TK, Lee TY, Park MH. Mesothelioma of the tunica vaginalis of the spermatic cord with coincidental finding renal cell carcinoma. Korean J Urol. 1995; 36: 1142–1146.

[96] Smoliyannikov AV. Tumors of serous membranes. In: A guide to the pathoanatomical diagnosis of human tumors /NA Kraevsky, A.V Smoliyannikov (Eds). Moscow: "Meditsina" 1971; 77–79 (in Russian).

[97] Spiess PE, Tuziak T, Kassouf W, Grossman HB, Czerniak B. Malignant mesothelioma of the tunica vaginalis. Urology 2005; 66: 397–401.

[98] Stathopoulos J, Antoniou D, Stathopoulos GP, Rigatos SK, Dimitroulis J, Koutandos J, Michalopolou P, Athanasiades A, Veslemes M. Mesothelioma: Treatment and survival of a patient population and review of the literature. Anticancer Res 2005; 25 (5): 3671-3676.

[99] *Strukov AI, Serov VV. Pathological anatomy. Textbook. Moscow: Publishing House "Meditsina" 1979; 188-189 (in Russian).

[100] Thomas C, Hansen T, Thuroff JW. Malignant mesothelioma of the tunica vaginalis testis. Urologe A 2007; 46 (5): 538-540.

[101] Tolhurst SR, Lotan T, Rapp DE, Lyon MB, Orvieto MA, Gerber GS, Sokoloff MH. Well-differentiated papillary mesothelioma occurring in the tunica vaginalis of the testis with contralateral atypical mesothelial hyperplasia. Urol Oncol: Semin Orig Invest 2006; 24 (1): 36-39.

[102] Torbati PM, Parvin M, Ziaee SA. Malignant Mesothelioma of the Spermatic Cord: Case Report and Review of the Literature. Urol J 2005; 2: 115-117.

[103] Tuttle Jr JP, Rous SN, Harrold MW. Mesotheliomas of spermatic cord. Urology 1977; 10: 466-468.

[104] Urology: Textbook / Prof. NA Lopatkin (Ed). Fifth Edition, revised and enlarged. Moscow: GEOTAR-MED, 2002; 520 p (in Russian).

[105] van Poppel H, van Renterghem K, Claes H, et al. Benign Mesothelioma of the Epididymis: Case Report. Urol Int 1988; 43: 370-371.

[106] World Health Organization Classification of Tumours. Pathology and Genetics of Tumours of the Lung, Pleura, Thymus and Heart / WD Travis, E Brambilla, HK Muller-Hermelink, CC Harris (Eds). International Agency for Research on Cancer Press. Lyon, 2004 ; 344 p.

[107] World Health Organization Classification of Tumours. Pathology and Genetics of Tumours of the Urinary System and Male Genital Organs / John N Eble, Guido Sauter, Jonathan I Epstein, Isabell A Sesterhenn (Eds). International Agency for Research on Cancer Press. Lyon, 2004; 359 p.

[108] Xiao SY, Rizzo P, Carbone M. Benign papillary mesothelioma of the tunica vaginalis testis. Arch Pathol Lab Med 2000; 124: 143-147.

[109] Ya TD, Welch L, Black D, Sugarbaker PH. A systemic review on the efficacy of cytoreductive surgery combined with perioperative intraperitoneal chemotherapy for diffuse malignancy peritoneal mesothelioma. Ann Oncol 2007; 18 (5): 827-834.

[110] Zaridze DG. Cancer prevention. Guide for physicians. Moscow: IMA-PRESS 2009; 224 p.

[111] Zerbino DD, Dmitruk IM. Aetiology, pathogenesis and clinico- morphological peculiarities of mesothelioma: A review of the literature. Vrach Delo 1984; (10): 4-8 (in Russian).

[112] Zervos MD, Bizekis C, Pass HI. Malignant mesothelioma 2008. Curr Opin Pulm Med 2008; 14: 303-309.

[113] Zubritsky AN. Mesothelioma. Principal bibliographic index of Russian and foreign literature. Moscow: Meditsina Publishers, 2004; 64 p (in Russian).

[114] Zubritsky AN. Mesothelioma revisited. Acta Medica Bulgarica 2008; 35(2): 31-34.

[115] Zubritsky AN. Mesothelioma (a review of the literature). Present Interests of Pathological Anatomy: Proceedings. The 3rd Congress of Russian Society of Pathologists, Samara, May 26-30, 2009 / Phedorina TA (Ed). Samara, 2009; 2: 604-605 (in Russian).

[116] Zubritsky AN. Multiple primary tumours. Bibliographical index of Russian and foreign literature. Moscow: "Kalina" 2010; 112 p (in Russian).

5

Stem Cells and Mesothelioma

Bonnie W. Lau
Brown University
USA

1. Introduction

Stem cells are self-renewing cells with the potential to differentiate into other cell types. Physiologically stem cells participate in hematopoiesis, wound healing, neuroregeneration, and many other important biological processes. It has been hypothesized that stem cells play a role in carcinogenesis. Although controversial, stem cell origin of cancers such as breast and prostate carcinomas and glioblastoma have been reported (Al-Hajj, 2003; Collins, 2005; Singh, 2004). In addition, stem cells are reported to be in the tumor microenvironment and potentially contribute to the tumorigenic process (Bergfeld & DeClerck, 2010). Such findings offer potentially new targets for tumor therapy.

Mesothelioma is an aggressive neoplasm of the mesothelial cell layer of pleura, peritoneum, pericardium and tunica vaginalis. Characterized by an aggressive disease course and resistance to current multimodality therapies, mesothelioma needs to be better characterized, including with an understanding of how stem cell biology and mesothelioma pathogenesis intersect. There is evidence for both a stem cell origin of mesothelioma, and a stem cell population in the mesothelioma tumor microenvironment. This review chapter aims to outline the evidence that stem cell biology does indeed intersect with mesothelioma pathogenesis, and that such findings offer important therapeutic targets for tumor therapy.

2. Stem cell origin of cancer

The concept of a stem cell origin of cancer was first described over fifty years ago as a small subset of cells capable of re-initiating a clonal tumor, and the first cancer stem cell population was identified in acute myeloid leukemia (Reya et al., 2001; Huntly & Gilliland, 2005). Cancer stem cells comprise only 0.01-1% of all cells in a tumor, but are capable of re-initiating the tumor while the other cell types cannot. Methods used to define the cancer stem cell vary, however at minimum require prospective selection by lineage; ability to re-initiate tumors that resemble the original tumor in serial tumor xenotransplantation; and display stem cell properties such as self-renewal and multipotential differentiation (Tang et al., 2007). Moreover, these assays most likely underestimate the percentage of cells capable of re-initiating tumor, given that xenotransplantation requires tumor re-initiation in a foreign environment lacking the presence of other cell types that play a supportive role in tumorigenesis (Adams & Strasser, 2008). Cancer stem cells are constituents of tumors that are not only capable of re-initiating tumors, but also likely contribute to resistance to therapy and metastasis. Recent evidence for a stem cell origin of solid tumors provides the impetus to explore such mechanisms of tumorigenesis in mesothelioma (Al-Hajj et al., 2003; Collins et al., 2005; Singh et al., 2004).

It can be argued that a stem cell origin of mesothelioma would be consistent with the pathogenic course of this tumor. Asbestos exposure is reported in over 80% of cases of mesothelioma, and there is a latency period of several decades between exposure and diagnosis. Asbestos does not appear to be a direct mutagen, rather, alveolar macrophages undergo incomplete phagocytosis of the asbestos fibers and induce a chronic release of pro-inflammatory mediators that create a potentially mutagenic environment. Is the pathogenic time course and pro-inflammatory tumor microenvironment consistent with a stem cell origin of mesothelioma?

In 1975 Cairns hypothesized that adult stem cells minimize genetic mutations with asymmetric division that maintains an "immortal DNA strand" in the stem cell population, and passes along any mutations to the daughter cell that will terminally differentiate (Cairns, 1975). Therefore adult stem cells may have developed a protective mechanism against persistence of mutations in the stem cell population. However a dividing stem cell population under chronic mutagenic conditions such as the pro-inflammatory state in asbestos exposure, may be susceptible to mutagenesis and eventual tumorigenesis. The lengthy time course between asbestos exposure and development of mesothelioma may be a reflection of the longer length of time required to overcome the protective mechanism described by the Cairns hypothesis in stem cells (Browne, 1991). Although there is more supportive than conclusive evidence for the Cairns hypothesis, it offers a compelling explanation for a stem cell origin of mesothelioma.

3. Mesothelial progenitor and side population cells

Proliferative tissues such as skin and bone marrow are maintained by a stable population of progenitor cells with self-renewing properties. Tumors are also proliferative tissues, possibly maintained by a self-renewing cancer stem cell population. Therefore leukemia can be viewed as a tumor maintained by a subset of bone marrow progenitor cells that have tumor-initiating properties. Analogously, mesothelioma may be a tumor maintained by a mesothelial progenitor cell population. Normal mesothelium consists of a single layer of simple squamous mesothelial cells of mesodermal origin that function to maintain serosal fluid production in order to provide a frictionless and protective surface for organ movement. Mesothelial cells also participate in material transport across the serosal membrane; and mediate regulatory inflammatory, immune and tissue repair responses (Mutsaers, 2007).

There is evidence for a mesothelial progenitor cell population (Herrick, 2004). First, mesothelial cells express characteristics of mesodermal, epithelial and mesenchymal phenotypes- supportive evidence for multipotential differentiation of a progenitor cell population. In addition, mesothelial cells exhibit plasticity by transforming into tissues such as myofibroblasts and vascular grafts under specific growth conditions (Lv, 2011 & Sparks, 2002). After mesothelial tissue injury, new mesothelium regenerates from both cells at the wound edge and from the surrounding serosal fluid, which may be mesothelial progenitor cells capable of tissue regeneration. Mesothelial progenitor cells with such stem cell-like properties are potentially a source of a cancer stem cell population in mesothelioma.

Another potential cancer stem cell population in mesothelioma is side population (SP) cells. Defined as cells that efflux the DNA-binding dye Hoechst 33342, SP cells can be enriched for using flow cytometry. Side population cells express ATP-binding cassette (ABC) membrane transporters that efflux the Hoechst 33342 dye, and these transporters are also involved in efflux of drugs such as chemotherapeutics. Side population cells are found in both normal and malignant tissues. In cancer, SP cells have been considered a potential cancer stem cell population as well as a cell population responsible for resistance to therapy. SP cells have been identified as a potential cancer stem cell population in various tumors, including ovarian carcinoma and osteosarcoma (Fong, 2010 & Murase, 2009). A group that isolated SP cells from human malignant mesothelioma cell lines illustrated that SP cells had enhanced proliferation and higher expression of stem-cell genes (Kiyonori, 2010). However, the SP cells did not have increased tumorigenic potential in immunodeficiant mice. A more recent study reported that SP cells isolated from malignant pleural mesothelioma not only expressed stem cell markers, but also showed self-renewal, chemoresistance, and tumorigenicity (Frei, 2011). Further the subset of SP cells characterized as WT1 negative/D2-40 positive/CD105 (low) were found to be even more tumorigenic. The increased stem cellness of the SP cells isolated from this study by Frei et al. compared to the study by Kiyonori et al. could be due to their isolation from malignant tissue rather than from mesothelioma cell lines. Since cancer stem cells remain to be fully characterized and defined, a diversity of cell types- including progenitor cells and side population cells- may qualify as cancer stem cells in tumors (Bjerkvig, 2005).

How a normal mesothelial progenitor cell or side population cell transforms into a cancer stem cell remains to be elucidated. Traditional thinking of transformation of a normal differentiated cell into a tumor cell requires multiple hits to the genome resulting in genetic instability and a selective survival advantage. Cancer stem cells may be products of a similar transformative process. Human mesothelial cells exposed to asbestos and SV40 virus were reported to transform via an Akt-mediated cell survival mechanism (Cacciotti, 2005). These authors concluded that mesothelioma originates from a subpopulation of transformed stem cells. More work illustrating this important concept is necessary and offers potential targets for therapy to abrogate this transformation process. Hypothetically, the advantage for a tumor to arise from a transformed stem cell rather than from a transformed differentiated cell includes the ability for the tumor to have multiple phenotypes for growth in different microenvironments; an additional mechanism for a metastatic phenotype; and resistance to current therapies. Interestingly, mesothelioma exhibits aspects of all three of these tumor characteristics.

Diffuse malignant mesothelioma can be classified histologically into three major classes: epithelioid, sarcomatoid, and mixed-type. Epithelioid is the most common phenotype and the mixed-type can be found in 30% of tumors. Sarcomatoid tumors are rare but carry the worst prognosis. There are also rare variants including desmoplastic, undifferentiated and deciduoid types. This wide variety of phenotypes could be explained by a cancer stem cell origin for mesothelioma, such as a transformed mesothelial progenitor cell population that has been shown to differentiate into multiple cell types. Currently, determining the histological subtype is important for diagnosis, prognosis and treatment (Tischoff, 2011). If, however, all the histological subtypes are derived from a single stem cell population, earlier diagnosis could be determined before histological differentiation occurs; prognosis could be improved overall; and treatment could be focused on targeting these stem cells.

Mesothelioma is an aggressive tumor that often metastasizes. In tumor biology epithelial-mesenchymal transition (EMT) is associated with increased tumor invasiveness and metastasis. This transition is reminiscent of the epithelioid versus sarcomatoid type of mesothelioma, and therefore has important implications in the metastatic feature of this tumor. EMT is a transdifferentiation program used in normal embryonic development. Activation of this program in carcinogenesis would confer a metastatic phenotype to the tumor cells. Not only can EMT increase cell invasiveness and migration, but it also contributes to additional properties that promote tumor cell survival; such as resistance to apoptosis and senescence, and increased immunosuppression (Thiery, 2009). In addition, EMT has been shown to induce stem cell-like properties. Many cancer stem cell traits are consistent with a metastatic phenotype- self-renewal, ability to initiate tumors in a new environment, motility, invasiveness, and resistance to apoptosis (Chaffer, 2011). Evidence of EMT occurring in mesothelioma includes expression of proteins involved in the EMT axis in malignant pleural mesothelioma tissue samples from untreated patients, and expression of the periostin protein in particular by sarcomatoid tumors, which in turn correlated with shorter survival in these patients (Schramm, 2010).

Successful colonization of metastatic cells to the distant tissues requires activation of genetic and epigenetic programming for survival in the new tissue environment. This area of research is relatively new, but it is believed that the self-renewal property of stem cells offers one explanation for homing success. Once in the new microenvironment, metastatic cells need to successfully utilize the local growth factors and cytokines to gain mitogenic potential and the ability to self-renew. Subsequently the metastatic cells would need to recruit the stroma to aid in cell survival, such as inducing a blood supply (Chambers, 2002). Distant metastatic lesions of mesothelioma, amongst other tumors both epithelial and non-epithelial, have been reported to highly express the self-renewal gene Bmi-1, suggesting that a state of self-renewal is linked to metastatic potential (Glinsky, 2005). Whether the metastatic cells in mesothelioma represent a cancer stem cell population derived from the primary tumor, or mesothelioma cells that acquired stem cell-like properties such as self-renewal en route to and after homing to the distant metastatic site, remains to be studied. However these finding support a role for stem cells in the pathogenesis of mesothelioma.

Epigenetic mechanisms that do not change the DNA sequence but that do alter gene expression at the mRNA and protein levels are exciting new potential targets for therapy. A number of epigenetic mechanisms have been described in tumors, including microRNA (miRNA) regulation of mRNA expression, histone acetylation/deacetylation, and gene promoter methylation/demethylation. By suppressing expression of tumor suppressor genes or increasing expression of oncogenes, these epigenetic proteins regulate tumorigenesis at an additional level of complexity. A study identifying a panel of miRNAs downregulated in malignant pleural mesothelioma tissue samples found redundant miRNA regulators of Wnt signaling, an important pathway in stem cell self renewal (Gee, 2010). Wnt signaling in mesothelioma suggests a cell population with stemness properties, and whose expression appears to be regulated at an epigenetic level.

The existence of a cancer stem cell population in mesothelioma is supported by evidence of cells with stem cell-like properties in normal mesothelium, primary mesothelial tumors, and metastatic lesions. A definitive cancer stem cell population capable of re-initiating mesotheliomal tumors remains to be identified. If such a cancer stem cell population is discovered, the prospects of earlier diagnosis and novel therapy for malignant mesothelioma would be of utmost importance for further research.

4. Stem cells in the tumor microenvironment

A cancer cell cannot survive without a hospitable microenvironment. If the microenvironment consists of immune cells that attack the cancer, or if the microenvironment does not support cancer cell growth by providing growth factors, cytokines or blood supply, the cancer cell will not survive in the host. Interestingly, stem cells in the tumor microenvironment have been found to support tumor growth by contributing to a hospitable microenvironment. Here we evaluate the evidence for a host-derived stem cell population in the mesothelioma microenvironment, not a tumor-initiating cancer stem cell population as previously discussed.

Stem cells found in the tumor microenvironment include mesenchymal stem cells (MSCs) with multipotential differentiation and self-renewal properties. Initially MSCs were believed to be derived from the bone marrow, and now there is increasing evidence for MSCs existing in other tissues. The bone marrow houses two types of stem cells- hematopoietic and mesenchymal. Hematopoietic stem cells give rise to all the blood cell lineages. Mesenchymal stem cells can differentiate into a number of cells types, including osteoblasts, chondrocytes, and adipocytes. MSCs have been found to travel from bone marrow into the bloodstream and home to sites of tissue injury for repair (Prockop, 2009). MSCs have also been found to home to tumor microenvironments and play a potential role in tumorigenesis. The anti-tumorigenic and pro-tumorigenic roles MSCs play in tumors will be discussed and evidence for MSCs in malignant mesothelioma will be summarized.

The mechanisms by which MSCs travel to tumors are similar to the MSC homing mechanisms to sites of injury and inflammation. Recruitment of MSCs to tumors involves a number of chemokines and growth factors. Tumor-produced vascular endothelial cell growth factor (VEGF), transforming growth factor (TGF), epidermal growth factor (EGF), hepatocyte growth factor (HGF), basic fibroblast growth factor (bFGF) and platelet derived growth factor (PDGF) have been reported to recruit MSCs to tumors (Bergfeld, 2010). Mesothelioma is known to secrete VEGF, EGF, HGF and PDGF; and these growth factors are used as biomarkers for diagnosis as well as potential targets for therapy (Ray, 2009). Chemokines and their receptors such as CCL2 (MCP-1) and CXCL12 (SDF-1) and the cognate receptor CXCR4, as well as extracellular matrix proteases and related interleukins (IL-6) have been shown to recruit MSCs (Spaeth, 2008). Both CCL2 and CXCL12 and the cognate receptor CXCR4, as well as IL-6, are found to be upregulated in mesothelioma (Miselis, 2009). Mesothelioma appears to have a microenvironment rich in growth factors, chemokines, and interleukins conducive for MSC homing.

Many of the factors secreted by malignant mesothelial cells have multiple roles in tumorigenesis, such as in angiogenesis and immunomodulation. The prospect of an additional role of these factors in recruitment of stem cells to the tumor microenvironment is attractive from the standpoint of tumor growth and metastasis. MSCs have been found to be pro-tumorigenic via a number of reported mechanisms. Once in the tumor microenvironment, MSCs differentiate into pericytes, cancer-associated fibroblasts and myofibroblasts (Bexell, 2009; Quante, 2011). Pericytes were first described in the 1870's as cells adjacent to capillaries supporting microvessel growth in normal tissue. Analogously, tumor pericytes support angiogenesis, one of the hallmarks of cancer (Hanahan, 2011). Hence therapies targeting MSCs in the tumor microenvironment are potentially anti-angiogenic therapies.

Cancer-associated fibroblasts (CAFs) and myofibroblasts in the tumor microenvironment appear to play a prominent role in tumor growth and progression. Unlike resting fibroblasts, CAFs and myofibroblasts are activated cells capable of secreting growth factors and extracellular matrix proteins that support tumor growth (Kalluri, 2006). Identifiable by expression of alpha-smooth muscle actin (α-SMA) and fibroblast activation markers such as fibroblast activating protein (FAP), CAFs and myofibroblasts in tumors can be derived from the bone marrow precursors via the same factors known to recruit MSCs (Quante, 2011). The interplay between MSCs and CAFs remains to be fully elucidated, but it does appear there is overlap in the pro-tumorigenic factors secreted by both.

There is recent evidence of a tumor-associated fibroblast population in human malignant pleural mesothelioma (MPM) cell lines orthotopically implanted into SCID mice, as well as in histological analyses of human biopsies of MPM (Li, 2011). These fibroblasts secreted the growth factors FGF, PDGF, and HGF. While this study did not show a MSC origin for these tumor-associated fibroblasts, these growth factors are known to recruit MSCs as well as be secreted by MSCs.

MSCs, staying undifferentiated or differentiating into pericytes or CAFs, appear to be pro-tumorigenic via three mechanisms. First, MSCs secrete growth factors and cytokines that support tumor growth. Second, MSCs secrete many proangiogenic factors, including VEGF, angiopoietin, IL-6, IL-8, TGF-b, PDGF, bFGF, and FGF-7 (Feng, 2009). And three, MSCs contribute to tumor immunotolerance. As previously described, a tumor requires a hospitable environment to grow, and preventing attack of the tumor cells by the host immune system is crucial to promoting tumor survival. MSCs modulate innate immunity by inhibiting natural killer cell activation and dendritic cell maturation (Sotiropoulou, 2007). Acquired immune modulation by MSCs include inhibition of T cell proliferation, inhibition of B cell activation, and increasing the production of regulatory T cells (Sotiropoulou, 2007).

While a MSC population remains to be described in mesothelioma, there is supportive evidence for such a stem cell population given that the mesothelioma microenvironment has been shown to be pro-tumorigenic in similar fashion to the three mechanisms described above. First, there is upregulated expression of growth factors and extracellular matrix proteins in mesothelioma (Miselis, 2010). It could be hypothesized that a stem cell population in the mesothelioma tumor microenvironment is secreting these factors, since MSCs are known to secrete these same factors in other tumors. However, the specific cell types secreting these factors in mesothelioma remain to be fully elucidated.

Secondly, mesothelioma patients have the highest levels of VEGF compared to other patients with solid tumors (Linder, 1998). This pro-angiogenic factor has been targeted for therapy with some success (Zucali, 2011). It could be hypothesized that MSCs in the tumor microenvironment contribute to the high VEGF levels found in mesothelioma patients. Thirdly, mesothelioma in part is such an aggressive tumor secondary to its successful immunosuppressive strategies. Similar to the mechanisms of immunomodulation demonstrated by MSCs, mesothelioma is characterized by inhibition of NK cells, dendritic cells, cytotoxic T cells; while showing upregulation of regulatory T cells, and secretion of the immunosuppressive cytokine TGFβ (Gregoire, 2010). These findings correlate with clinical presentation, where a high lymphocytic infiltration is associated with a better prognosis in patients. It would be interesting to see if an increased infiltration of MSC in the mesothelioma tumor microenvironment would correlate with an immunosuppressive profile leading to poorer prognosis in mesothelioma.

Finally, MSCs have been shown to be pro-metastatic. Distant metastasis of Stage IV malignant mesothelioma is rare compared to other solid tumors that spread to bone, brain, and other metastatic sites. However there are case reports of mesothelioma metastasizing to brain, oral gingiva, and skin (Ishikawa, 2010; Moser, 2011; Terada, 2011). In breast cancer, MSC secretion of CCL5 induced a prometastatic effect on breast cancer cells; and tumors coinjected with MSCs showed multiple fold increase in the number of breast cancer cells metastasized to the lungs (Karnoub, 2007). The chemokine CCL5 is overexpressed by mesothelioma (Miselis, 2010), and one could hypothesize that MSCs in mesothelioma may secrete CCL5 and promote a pro-metastatic state.

5. Conclusion

While many more studies need to be executed in order to elucidate the role of stem cells in mesothelioma, there is mounting evidence that there is a stem cell/progenitor population in mesothelioma. Whether this cell population is a cancer stem cell one capable of repopulating the tumor or host-derived stem cells in the tumor microenvironment capable of promoting tumor growth and metastasis; it is highly likely that stem cells in mesothelioma are a potential target for therapy. With the potential of stem cells playing a role in mesothelioma growth, angiogenesis, immunomodulation, metastasis, resistance to therapy, and even epigenetic control of tumorigenesis; there is great impetus to explore how stem cell biology and malignant mesothelioma tumorigenesis intersect.

6. Acknowledgment

Special thanks to Dr. Agnes Kane who has been a mentor for many years and provided invaluable review and funding for this chapter.

7. References

Adams, J. & Strasser, A. (2008). Is tumor growth sustained by rare cancer stem cells or dominant clones? *Cancer Res*, Vol.68, No.11, pp.4018-4021.
Al-Hajj, M.; Wicha, M.; Benito-Hernandez, A.; Morrison, S. & Clarke, M. (2003). Prospective identification of tumorigenic breast cancer cells. *Proc Natl Acad Sci*, Vol.100, No.7, pp.3983-3988.
Bergfeld, S. & DeClerck, Y. (2010). Bone marrow-derived mesenchymal stem cells and the tumor microenvironment. *Cancer Metastasis Review*, Vol.29, No.2, pp.249-261.

Bexell, D.; Gunnarsson, S.; Tormin, A.; Darabi, A.' Gisselsson, D.; Roybon, L.; Scheding, S.; & Bengzon, J. (2009). Bone marrow multipotent mesenchymal stroma cells act as pericyte-like migratory vehicles in experimental gliomas. *Molecular Therapeutics*, Vol.17, No.1, pp.183-190.

Bjerkvig, R.; Tysnes, B.; Aboody, K.; Najbauer, J.; & Terzis, A. (2005). Opinion: the origin of the cancer stem cell: current controversies and new insights. *Nat Rev Cancer*, Vol.5, No.11, pp.899-904.

Browne, K. (1991). Asbestos related malignancy and the Cairns hypothesis. *Br J Ind Med*, Vol.48, No.2, pp.73-76.

Cacciotti, P.; Barbone, D.; Porta, C.; Altomare, D.; Testa, J.; Mutti, L.; & Gaudino G. (2005). SV40-dependent AKT activity drives mesothelial cell transformation after asbestos exposure. *Cancer Res*, Vol.65, No.12, pp.5256-5262.

Cairns, J. (1975). Mutation selection and the natural history of cancer. *Nature*, Vol.255, No.5505, pp.197-200.

Chaffer, C. & Weinberg, R. (2011). A perspective on cancer cell metastasis. *Science*, Vol.331, No.6024, pp.1559-1564.

Chambers, A.F.; Groom, A.C.; &MacDonald, I.C. (2002). Dissemination and growth of cancer cells in metastatic sites. *Nat Rev Cancer*, Vol.2, No.8, pp.563-572.

Collins, A.; Berry P.; Hyde C.; Stower M. & Maitland N. (2005). Prospective identification of tumorigenic prostate cancer stem cells. *Cancer Research*, Vol.65, No.23, pp.10946-10951.

Feng, B. & Chen, L. (2009). Review of mesenchymal stem cells and tumors: executioner or coconspirator? *Cancer Biotherapy & Radiopharmaceuticals*, Vol.24, pp.717-721.

Fong, M.Y. & Kakar, S.S. (2010). The role of cancer stem cells and the side population in epithelial ovarian cancer. *Histol Histopathol*, Vol.25, No.1, pp.113-120.

Frei, C.; Opitz, I.; Soltermann, A.; Fischer, B.; Moura, U.; Rehrauer, H.; Weder, W.; Stahel, R.; & Felley-Bosco, E. (2011). Pleural mesothelioma side populations have a precursor phenotype. *Carcinogenesis*, epub ahead of print.

Gee, G.; Koestler, D.; Christensen, B.; Sugarbaker, D.; Ugolini, D.; Ivaldi, G.; Resnick, M.; Houseman E.; Kelsey, K.; & Marsit, C. (2010). Downregulated microRNAs in the differential diagnosis of malignant pleural mesothelioma. *Int J Cancer*, Vol.127, No.12, pp.2859-2869.

Glinsky, G.V.; Berezovska, O.; & Glinskli, A.B. (2005). Microarray analysis identifies a death-from-cancer signature predicting therapy failure in patients with multiple types of cancer. *J Clin Invest*, Vol.115, No.6, pp.1503-1521.

Gregoire, M. (2010) What's the place of immunotherapy in malignant mesothelioma treatments? *Cell Adh Migr*, Vol.4, No.1, pp.153-161.

Hanahan, D.& Weinberg, R. (2011). Hallmarks of cancer: the next generation. *Cell*, Vol.144, No.5, pp.646-674.

Herrick, S. & Mutsaers, S. (2004). Mesothelial progenitor cells and their potential in tissue engineering. *Int J Biochem Cell Biol*, Vol.36, No.4, pp.621-642.

Huntly, B. & Gilliland, D. (2005). Leukemia stem cells and the evolution of cancer-stem-cell research. *Nat Rev Cancer*, Vol.5, No.4, pp.311-321.

Ishikawa, T.; Wanifuchi, H.; Abe, K.; Kato, K.; Watanabe, A.; & Okada, Y. (2010). Brain metastasis in malignant pleural mesothelioma presenting as intratumoral hemorrhage. *Neurol Med Chir*, Vol.50, No.11, pp.1027-1030.

Kalluri, R. & Zeisberg, M. (2006). Fibroblasts in cancer. *Nature Rev Cancer*, Vol.6, No.5, pp.392-401.

Karnoub, A.; Dash, A.; Vo, A.; Sullivan, A.; Brooks, M.; Bell, G.; Richardson, A.; Polyak, K.; Tubo, R.; & Weinberg, R. (2007). Mesenchymal stem cells within tumor stroma promote breast cancer metastasis. *Nature*, Vol.449, No.7162, pp.557-563.

Kiyonori, K.; D'Costa, S.; Yoon, B.; Brody, A.R.; Sills, R.C.; & Kim, Y. (2010). Characterization of side population cells in human malignant mesothelioma cell lines. *Lung Cancer*, Vol.70, pp.146-151.

Li, Q.; Wang, W.; Yamada, T.; Matsumoto, K.; Sakai, K.; Bando, Y.; Uehara, H.; Nishioka, Y.; Sone, S.; Iwakiri, S.; Itoi, K.; Utsugi, T.; Yasumoto, K.; & Yano, S. (2011). Pleural mesothelioma instigates tumor-associated fibroblasts to promote progression via a malignant cytokine network. *Am J Pathol*, epub ahead of print.

Linder, C.; Linder, S.; Munck-Wikland, E.; & Strander, H. (1998). Independent expression of serum vascular endothelioal growth factor (VEGF) and basic fibroblast growth factor (bFGF) in patients with carcinoma and sarcoma. *Anticancer Res*, Vol.18, pp.2063-2068.

Miselis, N.; Lau, B.; Wu, Z.; & Kane A. (2010). Kinetics of host cell recruitment during dissemination of diffuse malignant peritoneal mesothelioma. *Cancer Microenvironment*, Vol.4, No.1, pp.39-50.

Moser, S.; Beer, M.; Damerau, G.; Lubbers, H.; Gratz, K.; & Kruse, A. (2011). A case report of metastasis of malignant mesothelioma to the oral gingival. *Head Neck Oncol*, Vol.3, pp.21.

Murase, M.; Kano, M.; Tsukahara, T.; Takahashi, A.; Torigoe, T.; Kawaguchi, S.; Kimura, S.; Wada, T.; Uchihashi, Y.; Kondo, T.; Yamashita, T. & Sato, N. (2009). Side population cells have the characteristics of cancer stem-like cells/cancer-initiating cells in bone sarcomas. *British Journal of Cancer*, Vol.101, pp.1425-1432.

Mutsaers, S. & Wilkosz, S. (2007). Structure and function of mesothelial cells. *Cancer Treat Res*, Vol.134, pp.1-19.

Prockop, D. (2009). Repair of tissues by adult stem/progenitor cells (MSCs): controversies, myths, and changing paradigms. *Molecular Therapy*, Vol.17, pp.939-946.

Quante, M.; Tu, S.; Tomita, H.; Gonda, T.; Wang, S.; Takashi, S.; Baik, G.; Shibata, W.; Diprete, B.; Betz, K.; Friedman, R.;

Varro, A.; Tycko, B.; & Wang, T. (2010) Bone marrow-derived myofibroblasts contribute to the mesenchymal stem cell niche and promote tumor growth. *Cancer Cell*, Vol.19, No.2, pp.257-272.

Ray, M. & Kindler, H. (2009). Malignant pleural mesothelioma: an update on biomarkers and treatment. *Chest*, Vol.136, No.3, pp.888-896.

Reya, T.; Morrison, S.; Clarke, M. & Weissman, I. (2001). Stem cells, cancer, and cancer stem cells. *Nature*, Vol.414, No.6859, pp.105-111.

Schramm, A.; Opitz, I.; Thies, S.; Seifert, B.; Moch, H.; Weder, W. & Soltermann, A. (2010). Prognostic significance of epithelial-mesenchymal transition in malignant pleural mesothelioma. *Eur J Cardiothorac Surg*, Vol.37, No.3, pp.566-572.

Singh, S.; Hawkins C.; Clarke I.; Squire J.; Bayani J.; Hide T.; Henkelman R.; Cusimano M. & Dirks P. (2004). Identification of human brain tumor initiating cells. *Nature*, Vol.432, No.7015, pp.396-401.

Sotiropoulou, P. & Papamichail, M. (2007). Immune properties of mesenchymal stem cells. *Methods in Molecular Biology*, Vol. 407, pp.225-243.

Spaeth, E.; Klopp, A.; Dembinski, J.; Andreeff, M.; & Marini, F. (2008). Inflammation and tumor microenvironments: defining the migratory itinerary of mesenchymal stem cells. *Gene therapy*, Vol.15, No.10, pp.730-738.

Sparks, S.; Tripathy, U.; Broudy, A.; Bergan, J.; Kumins, N. & Owens, E. (2002). Small-caliber mesothelial cell-layered polytetraflouroethylene vascular grafts in New Zealand white rabbits. *Annals of Vascular Surgery*, Vol.16, No.1, pp.73-76.

Tang, D.; Patrawala, L.; Calhoun, T.; Bhatia, B.; Choy, G.; Schneider-Broussard, R. & Jeter, C. (2007). Prostate cancer stem/progenitor cells: identification, characterization, and implications. *Molecular Carcinogenesis*, Vol.46, No.1, pp.1-14.

Terada, T. (2011). Skin metastasis of pleural epitheliod malignant mesothelioma. *Skin metastasis of pleural epithelioid malignant mesothelioma*, Vol.19, No.1, pp.92-93.

Thiery, J.; Acloque, H.; Huang, R. & Nieto, M. (2009). Epithelial-mesenchymal transitions in development and disease. *Cell*, Vol.139, No.5, pp.871-890.

Tischoff, I.; Neld, M.; Neumann, V. & Tannapfel, A. (2011). Pathohistological diagnosis and differential diagnosis. *Recent Results Cancer Res*, Vol.189, pp.57-78.

Zucali, P.; Ceresoli, G.; DeVincenzo, F.; Simonelli, M.; Lorenzi, E.; Gianoncelli, L.; & Santoro, A. (2011). Advances in the biology of malignant pleural mesothelioma. *Cancer Treat Rev*, epub ahead of print.

6

Radiologic Evaluation of Malignant Pleural and Peritoneal Mesothelioma

Elif Aktas[1], Kemal Arda[1], Bora Aktas[2], Sahin Coban[2],
Nazan Çiledağ[1] and Bilgin Kadri Aribas[1]
[1]Ankara Abdurrahman Yurtaslan Oncology Education And Research Hospital
[2]Ankara Yildirim Beyazit Diskapi Education And Research Hospital
Turkey

1. Introduction

Malignant mesothelioma is an asbestos-associated malignancy arising from the mesothelial cells of the pleural and peritoneal cavities, as well as the pericardium and the tunica vaginalis.

Mesothelioma usually presents in the fifth to seventh decades, and 70-80 % of cases occur in men (Moore et al., 2008). Malignant pleural mesothelioma (MPM) is the most widely form of mesothelioma. Patients frequently present with dyspnea, chest pain, cough, and weight loss (Moore et al., 2008, Wang et al., 2004). Although most of the mesotheliomas cover the pleural surface, approximately 35% arise only from peritoneum. Patients with malignant peritoneal mesothelioma may present with abdominal pain, distention, anorexia, and weight loss (Park et al., 2008).

Radiologic modalities play a crucial role in the evaluation of malignant mesothelioma. Computed tomography is the primary imaging method used for the diagnosis and the staging of malignant mesothelioma, but also for guiding biopsy for tissue diagnosis. Magnetic resonans imaging (MRI) is useful for detection of extension of disease, especially to the chest wall and diaphragm (Moore et al., 2008, Wang et al., 2004). In this article we review radiologic findings of malignant pleural and peritoneal mesothelioma with our patient archives. We also wants to give some information about differential diagnosis malignant pleural and peritoneal mesothelioma.

2. Material and methods

We scanned our patient archive of mesothelioma between 2008-2011 years. We accepted patients who had CT or MRI at their initial diagnosis. We have had 135 patient who suffered from mesothelioma but only 35 patient had CT or MRI at the time of diagnosis. Twenty seven of them were pleural mesothelioma, and 8 of them peritoneal mesothelioma.

3. Results

In pleural mesothelioma group, there were 10 women (37%) and 17 men (63%). The avarage age was 55.14±12.47 (min: 29 - max: 87). We found pleural effusion in 23 patients

(85.12%), pleural thickening in 27 patients (100%) (Fig. 1.,2.), pleural calcification in 11 patients (40.7%) (Fig.1.), lymphadenopathy in 11 patients (40.7%) (Fig. 1., 4., 6.), direct extension to mediastinal organs in 10 patients (37%), pericardial effusion in 6 patients (22.2%) (Fig. 5.), extension of chest wall in 7 patients (25.9%), extension of diaphragm in 5 patients (18.5%), thickening of interlober fissur in 11 patients (47.7%)(Fig. 2.), reduction in thoracic volume in 8 patients (29.6%)(Fig. 1.), brain metastases in only one patient (3.7%), pulmonary metastases in 2 patients (%7.4),(Fig. 3) hepatic metastases in 2 patients (7.4%), (Fig. 9) (Table1).

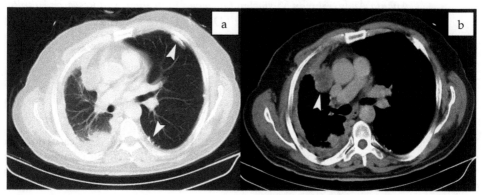

Fig. 1. Axial contrast enhanced CT parenchymal (a.) and mediastinal sections (b.) shows nodular, irregular and circumferantial right sided pleural thickening in 55 year-old man. Note that contracted right hemithorax and anterior mediastinal lymph node (arrow head). We can see pleural calcification on left sided pleural surface (arrow head).

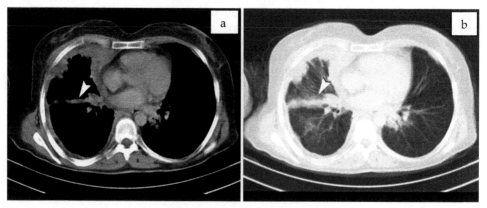

Fig. 2. Axial contrast enhanced CT mediastinal (a.) and parenchymal sections (b.) shows right sided irregular pleural thickening and right major fissur involvement (arrow head).

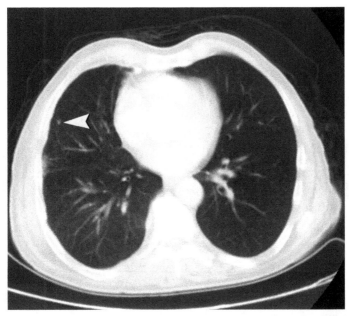

Fig. 3. Axial non- contrast enhanced CT a milimetric parenchymal nodul in right middle lobe (arrow head).

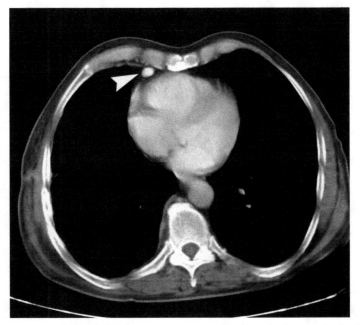

Fig. 4. Axial contrast enhanced CT show 1 cm paracardiac lymphadenopathy in 65 year old man with MPM.

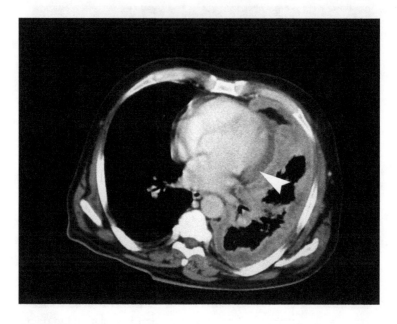

Fig. 5. Axial contrast enhanced CT shows pericardial invasion and pericardial effusion.

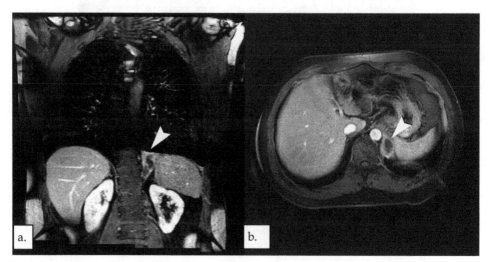

Fig. 6. Coronal (a) and axial (b) postcontrast T1 weighted images show a solitary mass with central necrosis into left retrocrural space at a patient with malignant pleural mesothelioma.

Radiologic Findings	Rates
Pleural Effusion	85.12%
Pleural Thickening	100%
Pleural Calcification	40.7%
Thickening of Interlober Fissur	47.7%
Reduction in Thoracic Volume	29.6%
Mediastinal Lymphadenopathy	40.7%
Direct Extension To Mediastinal Organs	37%
Pericardial Effusion	22.2%
Extension Of Chest Wall	25.9%
Extension Of Diaphragm	18.5%
Metastases	11.1%

Table 1. Pleural mesothelioma radiologic findings

In peritoneal mesothelioma group, the average age 60.75±10.41 (min: 42-max: 73). There were 2 female (25%) and 6 male (75%) patient. We found peritoneal irregularity and nodular thickening in 4 patients (50%)(Fig. 7a.), diffuse peritoneal thickening (omental cake) in 4 patients (50%)(Fig. 7c., 8a., b., c.), ascites in 5 patients (62.5%) (Fig. 7., 8.), extension of adject tissue in only one patient (2.5%) (Table 2).

Radiologic Findings	Rates
Peritoneal irregularity and nodular thickening	50%
Diffuse peritoneal thickening	50%
Ascites	62.5%
Extension of adject tissue	2.5%

Table 2. Malignant peritoneal mesothelioma radiologic findings

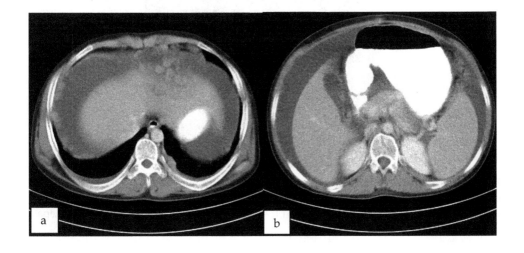

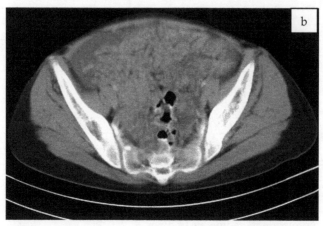

Fig. 7. Malignant peritoneal mesothelioma. a. Contrast enhanced CT scan shows nodular peritoneal thickening. b. Axial contrast enhanced CT shows perisplenic and perihepatic large amount of ascites. c. Axial contrast enhanced CT shows diffuse peritoneal thickening with omental cake.

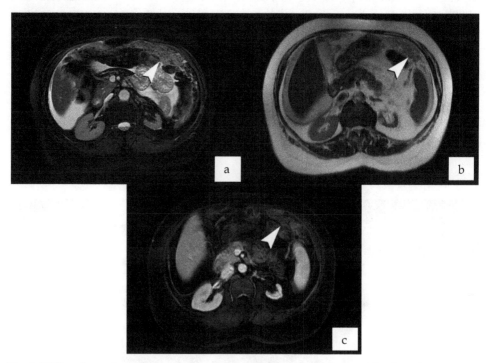

Fig. 8. Diffuse irregular thickening of parietal peritoneum with omental cake is hypointense on axial T2 Weighted images (a), hyperintense on FIESTA sequence (b), shows minimal enhancement on post-gadolinium axial T1 Weighted images (c). We can see perihepatic minimal ascites.

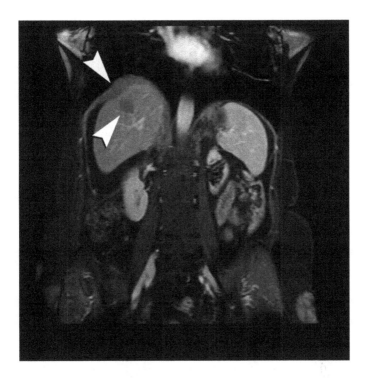

Fig. 9. Coronal post gadolinium T1 weighted image shows perihepatic focal parietal peritoneal thickening and hepatic metastases.

4. Discussion

The association of history, examination, radiology and pathology is essential in the diagnosis of mesothelioma. Radiological imaging is important for the diagnosis, staging and management of mesothelioma.

4.1 Pleural mesothelioma

Intravenous contrast-enhanced CT is the primary imaging modality for suspected malignant mesothelioma. CT can show the whole pleural surface and diaphragm. CT findings that is seen mostly are nodular pleural thickening, unilateral pleural effusion, pleural calcification, thickening of interlobar fissur, reduction of thoracic volume (Wang et al., 2004, Ismail-Khan et al., 2006). Pleural calcification is seen approximately 20% of cases (Moore et al., 2008, Wang et al., 2004). Typically, both the visceral and parietal pleurae are involved. Malignant pleural thickening characteristically is circumferantial, nodular and > 1 cm. Also, mediastinal pleural involvement is often detected (Ismail-Khan et al., 2006). Malignant pleural mesothelioma is locally aggressive with invasion of the chest wall, mediastinum and diaphragm. Obliteration of extrapleural fat planes, invasion of intercostal muscles, displacement of ribs, and bone destruction are findings of chest wall involvement. Heart, esophagus, trachea and major vascular structures of mediastinum may be involved by tumor. Nodular pericardial thickening and pericardial effusion refers to pericardial invasion by malignant pleural mesothelioma. Obliteration of surrounding fat planes of mediastinal organs, covering of vascular structure more than 50% is a strong evidence of invasion (Moore et al., 2008, Wang et al., 2004, Miller et al., 1996, Patz et al., 1992).

Pulmonary metastases of MPM presenting as nodules and masses and, rarely, diffuse miliary nodules may be seen at CT. Chest CT may also rarely demonstrate extrathoracic spread of MPM. Metastasis to the hilar and mediastinal lymph nodes is present at autopsy in approximately 40-45% of patients with MPM (Miller et al., 1996, Patz et al., 1992, Dynes et al., 1992).

MRI screening is not used routinely in the assessment of malignant mesothelioma, however in patients with potentially resectable disease, MRI can help to provide additional staging information over and above CT. Using gadolinium enhancement, MRI can advance the identification of tumor extension into the diaphragm or chest wall. MRI also is preferred in some patients whom intravenous iodinated contrast is contraindicated.

Malignant pleural mesothelioma is typically isointense or slightly hyperintense on T1-weighted images and moderately hyperintense on T2-weighted images relative to adjacent chest wall muscle. After the gadolinium injection, MPM shows enhancement. MR imaging is superior to CT for showing invasion of the diaphragm and invasion of endothoracic fascia or a single chest wall focus (Moore et al., 2008, Miller et al., 1996, Patz et al., 1992).

The radiologic differential diagnosis includes metastatic pleural disease, pleural lymphoma, asbestos releated benign pleural disease, and tuberculous empyema. Pleural rind, nodular pleural thickening, pleural thickening greater than 1 cm, and mediastinal pleural involvement favor malignant pleural disease. Pleural calsification is usually seen in benign process. Mesothelioma can not be distinguished from metastatic pleural disease on CT. Discrimination between epithelial types of mesothelioma and metastatic adenocarcinoma requires histochemical, immunohistochemical, and ultrastructural analysis. The presence of hilar-mediastinal adenopathy may be helpful in differentiating metastases and lymphoma from mesothelioma. The radiologic criteria for unresectability are tumor encasing diaphragm, invasion of extrapleural soft tissue, infiltration, displacement, or seperation of ribs by tumor, or bone destruction (Moore et al., 2008, Dynes et al., 1992, Barreiro et al., 2006, Jeong et al., 2008).

Morphologically malignant pleural mesothelioma can be seen in three forms: epithelial, sarcomatous, and mixed. The mixed form is usually mentioned as biphasic or bimorphic. Mixed tumors are composed of both epithelial and sarcomatous components. Epithelial mesotheliomas have a better diagnosis than sarcomatous and mixed tumors so differential diagnosis is very important for determining the prognosis. Epithelial malignant mesotheliomas consist of cells that are similar to normal mesothelial cells. The cells form a tubulopapillary or trabecular pattern. Epithelial malignant mesothelioma may also show prominent secretory changes, microglandular patterns, signet cell structure, or desmoplastic responses that make these tumors difficult to differentiate from adenocarcinomas based on routine histologic analysis alone. The sarcomatous pattern of malignant mesothelioma is typically consist of closely packed spindle cells. No immunohistochemical markers are spesific for malignant mesotheliomas and so there are some immunohistochemical markers such as calretinin thrombomodulin, and cytokeratin 5/6 to differentiate from metastatic adenocarcinomas and soft tissue sarcomas that have similar to histologic appearances (Levy et al., 2008). (Fig. 10).

4.2 Peritoneal mesothelioma

Approximately 35% of all mesotheliomas arise only from the peritoneum. There are three pathologic subtypes of peritoneal mesothelioma: Malignant mesothelioma, cystic mesothelioma, or well-differentiated papillary mesothelioma. CT findings of these subtypes are different from each other (Park et al., 2008).

Malignant peritoneal mesothelioma is seen at fifth and sixth decades. Asbestos exposure is a predisposing factor. We can see two different apperance at CT. Dry apperence is characterized with peritoneal based masses and wet apperance is characterized ascites, irregular or nodular peritoneal thickening and omental mass may be seen at CT. Peritoneal carcinomatosis, serous papillary carcinoma of peritoneum, tuberculous peritonitis and peritoneal lymphomatosis should be thought in differential diagnosis. It is very difficult to do differential diagnosis by using only CT. Prominent ascites and less severe peritoneal thickening is seen in peritoneal carcinomatosis. The incidence of liver metastasis and lymphadenopathy is also higher in peritoneal carcinomatosis. Serous papillary carcinoma is found predominantly in elderly women and postmenopausal women. We must think tuberculous peritonitis if we see smooth peritoneal thickening, mesenteric lymphadenopathy with central necrosis, ascites with high attenuation, and splenomegaly at CT. Diffuse retroperitoneal and mesenteric lympadenopathy and the lack of omental involvement may misgive about lymphomatosis (Park et al., 2008, Levy et al., 2008).

Cystic mesothelioma is a benign tumor that is occur mainly in young to middle-aged women. It is usually associated with a history of previous abdominal surgery or pelvic inflammatory disease. Relationship between asbestos exposure and cystic mesothelioma has not been reported. Involvement of pelvic region is typical. Hormonal therapy is usually useful for treatment of cystic mesothelioma. Multilocular cystic mass, multiple unilocular cystic thin-walled cysts, or a unilocular cystic mass. Cystic lymphangioma, cystic epithelial neoplasms of the ovaries and endometriosis is thought in the differantial diagnosis. Cystic

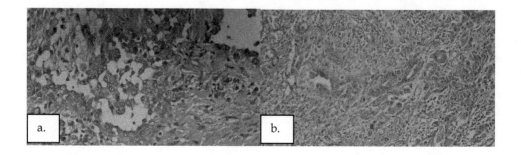

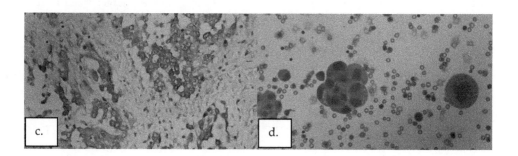

Fig. 10. a. Malignant mesothelioma that shows papillary formation and desmoplastic stromal reaction, b. Biphasic malignant mesothelioma which consists of epitheloid and spindle cells, c. Malignant mesothelioma cells that show immunreactive with calretinen, d. Pleomorphic mesothelial cells (May Gruwald Giemsa)

lymphangioma is seen in younger patients than cystic mesothelioma. It does not show regional predilection. Thick-walled cysts, thick internal septa, and high-attenuation internal debris favor the diagnosis of endometriosis. Well-differentiated papillary mesotheliomas is found reproductive-age women. Peritoneal thickening, multiple peritoneal nodules, omental infiltration and ascites may be seen at CT. It should be thought as the same disease that is thought in malignant peritoneal mesothelioma in differential diagnosis (Park et al., 2008, Levy et al., 2008., Pickhardt et al., 2005).

5. Conclusion

Malignant mesothelioma can be difficult to diagnose. Neither CT scanning nor MRI provides an unequivocal diagnosis of mesothelioma; tissue biopsy is required for the definitive diagnosis (Wang et al., 2004, Miller et al., 1996, Patz et al., 1992, Pickhardt et al., 2005, Zahid I et al. 2011).

6. Acknowledgment

Thanks Nesrin Turhan, M.D., for kind interest and helps

7. References

Barreiro TJ, Katzman PJ.(2006). Malignant mesothelioma: a case presentation and review. *J Am Osteopath Assoc*, Vol.106, No. 12, (December 2006), pp. 699-704.

Dynes MC, White EM, Fry WA. Ghahremani GG. (1992). Imaging manifestations of pleural tumors. *Radiographics,* Vol. 12, No. 6, (November 1992), pp.1191-1201.

Ismail-Khan R, Robinson LA, Williams CC Jr, Garrett CR, Bepler G, Simon GR. (2006). Malignant pleural mesothelioma: a comprehensive review. *Cancer Control*, Vol.13. No 4,(October 2006), pp.255-263.

Jeong YJ, Kim S, Kwak SW, Lee NK, Lee JW, Kim KI, Choi KU, Jeon TY. (2008). Neoplastic and nonneoplastic conditions of serosal membrane origin: CT findings. *Radiographics*, Vol.28, No. 3,(May-June 2008), pp.801-817.

Miller BH, Rosado-de-Christenson ML, Mason AC, Fleming MV, White CC, Krasna MJ. (1996). From the archives of the AFIP. Malignant pleural mesothelioma: radiologic-pathologic correlation. *Radiographics*, Vol.16, No. 3, (May 1996), pp. 613-44

Moore AJ, Parker RJ, Wiggins J. (2008) Malignant mesothelioma. *Orphanet J Rare Dis,* Vol.19, No3, (December 2008), pp. 34.

Park JY, Kim KW, Kwon HJ, Park MS, Kwon GY, Jun SY, Yu ES. (2008) Peritoneal mesotheliomas: clinicopathologic features, CT findings, and differential diagnosis. *AJR Am J Roentgenol,* Vol.191, No.3 (September 2008), pp.814-825.

Patz EF Jr, Shaffer K, Piwnica-Worms DR, Jochelson M, Sarin M, Sugarbaker DJ,Pugatch RD. (1992). Malignant pleural mesothelioma: value of CT and MR imaging in predicting resectability. *AJR Am J Roentgenol,* Vol.159 No. 5, (November 1992), pp. 961-966.

Wang ZJ, Reddy GP, Gotway MB, Higgins CB, Jablons DM, Ramaswamy M, Hawkins RA, Webb WR. (2004). Malignant pleural mesothelioma: evaluation with CT, MR imaging, and PET. *Radiographics*, Vol.24, No.1, (January-February 2004), pp.105-119.

Levy AD, Arnaiz J, Shaw JC, Sobin LH.(2008) From the archives of the AFIP: primary peritoneal tumors: imaging features with pathologic correlation. *Radiographics*, Vol.28, No.2, (March-April 2008), pp.583-607.

Pickhardt PJ, Bhalla S. (2005).Primary neoplasms of peritoneal and sub-peritoneal origin: CT findings. *Radiographic* ,Vol. 25, No. 4, (july-august 2005), pp.983-995.

Zahid I, Sharif S, Routledge T, Scarci M. What is the best way to diagnose and stage malignant pleural mesothelioma? (2011). *Interact Cardiovasc Thorac Surg*, Vol. 12, No. 2 (February 2011), pp.254-259.

7

Mesothelioma in Domestic Animals: Cytological and Anatomopathological Aspects

Winnie A. Merlo and Adriana S. Rosciani
Servicio Diagnóstico Histopatológico y Citológico, Facultad Ciencias Veterinarias
Universidad Nacional del Nordeste
Argentina

1. Introduction

Normal mesothelial cells form a monolayer that covers the serosal surface of pleural, peritoneal and pericardial cavities. When these cells are injured by inflammation or altered in a neoplastic process, they acquire similar cytological characteristics that difficult differentiation between reactive mesothelial cells and neoplastic ones (Ogilvie & Moore, 2008).

Mesotheliomas emerge from the cells that cover serosal cavities (Head et al., 2002). They are really uncommon neoplasms in animals and they are usually malignant (Head et al., 2003). They are more frequent in bovine cattle and dogs, but they represent just 0,2 % of the total of canine neoplasms (Wilson & Dungworth, 2002). There are exceptional reports in horses (Hinrichs et al., 1997), cats, pigs and other species (Brown et al., 2007).

In human beings the relationship between these tumours and asbestos fibre is striking (Butnor et al., 2001; Cantin et al., 1982; Enzinger & Weiss, 1985). In veterinary the presence of asbestos bodies was just established in a few canine reports (Glickman et al., 1983; Harbison & Godlesky, 1983) but controversy exists since many authors consider there is no convincing association between the incidence of mesothelioma and exposure to asbestos (López, 2007). Many other fibres types may cause mesotheliomas probably owing to fibre size and solubility (Brown et al., 2007). It is also related with the exposure to simiam virus 40 (SV40) (Reggetti et al., 2005). Lately, there is emerging evidence of genetic variation in susceptibility to fibre carcinogenesis (Rud, 2010).

Congenital mesotheliomas are described more frecuently in bovine fetuses and young animals (Brown et al., 2007). In canine specie, the average age of onset is 8 years, but there are reports in puppies (Glickman et al., 1983; Kim & Choi, 2002; Leisewitz & Nesbit, 1992). Other authors consider that these tumours are more common in male and spayed bitches, while there does not seem to be any strong breed predilection (Head et al., 2002). Exposure to pesticide is a cofactor that apparently increases the risk of mesothelioma in the animals (Glickman et al., 1983).

The "Histological classification of tumours of the serosal surfaces (pleura, pericardium, peritoneum, and tunica vaginalis) of domestic animals" (Head et al., 2003) considers the existence of benign and malignant mesotheliomas. It describes three varieties for each one: predominantly epithelioid, predominantly fibrous and biphasic or mixed. In human beings, half of malignant mesotheliomas are epithelioid, 20% are fibrous and the remaining 30 % are mixed (De May, 1996). Epitheliod and biphasic mesotheliomas are the most frequent types in dogs (Trigo et al., 1981), horses and cats (Head et al., 2003). Benign tumours are uncommon, many pathologist think that all the mesotheliomas are potentially malignant as virtually all can spread by implantation rather than metastasis (Brown et al., 2007).

2. Anatomopathological aspects

Mesothelial tumours are local, multifocal or diffuse neoplasms arising from the mesothelial lining of coelomic cavities and consisting of a variable mixture of epithelioid and spindle – shaped cells. (Head et al, 2003). They may involve one of the cavities or all of them simultaneously. Bovine lesions are usually epithelioid and primary in the peritoneum, with spread to other coelomic cavities. In dogs, these tumours involve the pleura, peritoneum, pericardium or tunica vaginalis in decreasing order of frequency. Pleural presentation is typical in swine (Brown et. al., 2007). In animals, pleural location usually causes effusion with resulting respiratory distress, cough, and weight loss (López, 2007). The peritoneal form is usually associated with ascitis as a consequence of blockage and effusion of lymphatic's vessels (Enzinger & Weiss, 1985). In these cases peritoneal fluid may appear bloody or milky (Brown et al., 2007).

They usually appear as multiple firm, sessile, or arborescent nodules, from a few milimeters to 6, to 10 cm in diameter: in villus projections on a thickened mesentery or serosal surface (Figure 1); or as fibrous or sclerosing forms, which are more plaque- like (Brown et al., 2007).

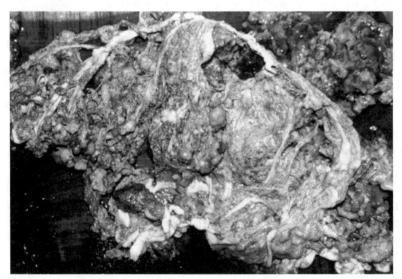

Fig. 1. Macroscopical aspect of a peritoneal predominantly epiteliod malignant mesothelioma in a dog.

3. Histopathological and cytological aspects

Usually mesotheliomas in animals, appear as a solid mass made up of layers of dark, plump cuboidal, columnar or rounded, epithelioid cells with a distintic border and abundant pink cytoplasm, over proliferating fibrocellular stroma. Mitotic figures are typically not numerous. The mesothelial cells form loops and festoons in a papillary pattern, or line cystic spaces and tubular structures (Brown et al., 2007). Asbestos fibres generally form big structures cover by acid mucopolysacharides known as "ferruginous bodies" but they are not always seen in histologic samples (Enzinger & Weiss, 1985). Mesotheliomas can be either benign or malignant. However, usually only the malignant varieties are associated with effusions (De May, 1996). Malignant mesotheliomas frequently start causing effusion, but cytological diagnosis may be difficult because malignant and reactive mesothelial cells are morphologically very similar. During inflammation, mesothelial cells become reactive and not only increase in number, but also become pleomorphic and form multinucleated cells that may be mistaken for a carcinoma (López, 2007).

Three different histological types of these tumors are described (Head et al., 2003). This classification is presented in table 1. The epithelioid malignant and mixed types are most likely to result in an effusion containing diagnostic cells. Predominantly fibrous mesotheliomas seldom cause an effusion and when they do, rarely exfoliate diagnostic cells (Tao, 1989). Therefore, the diagnosis of mesotheliomas is based in two different cytological techniques. The analyses of effusions` sediment is recommended for epithelioid malignant mesothelioma, but for predominantly fibrous and mixed forms, fine needle aspiration is necessary (Koss et al., 1988).

| *Benign mesothelioma* |
| Predominantly epithelioid benign mesothelioma |
| Predominantly fibrous (spindle cell) benign mesothelioma |
| Biphasic (mixed) benign mesothelioma |
| *Malignant mesothelioma* |
| Predominantly epithelioid malignant mesothelioma |
| Predominantly fibrous (spindle cell) malignant mesothelioma |
| Biphasic (mixed) malignant mesothelioma |

Table 1. Histological Classification of Tumours of Serosal Surfaces of Domestic Animals: Tumours of Mesothelium. Head et al., 2003.

3.1 Benign mesothelioma

Benign presentation is rare. Some pathologists think all mesotheliomas are potentially malignant.

3.1.1 Predominantly epithelioid benign mesothelioma

This benign tumor is mainly composed of mesothelial cells resembling epithelium arranged in a papillary, tubular, or solid pattern, either alone or in combination.

When these tumours grow on the surface of serosal membrane, they show papillary branching tree- like outgrowths with a central stromal core. But when the epithelioid cells extend into the underlying stroma in a tubular pattern, microscopically gives a pseudoacinar appearance. Sometimes they grow in solid pattern forming trabeculae or cords (Head et al., 2003).

The fine needle aspiration biopsy specimen is abundantly cellular. Sheets of reactive or atypical mesothelial cells, with windows, are seen in the aspirate specimen (Tao, 1989). Mesothelial cells are cuboidal or polygonal and have distinct outlines, a few may show a hair like brush border. The cytoplasm exhibits vacuoles sometimes of glycogen (Head et al., 2003). The nuclei are central, round to oval and relatively regular and uniform. The chromatin is fine and there may be small, inconspicuous nucleoli (De May, 1996).

They are difficult to differentiate from a reactive mesothelium, and from well differentiated malignant mesotheliomas because cells have similar appearance. So, differential diagnosis may require clinical and other complementary diagnostic techniques correlation (De May, 1996).

3.1.2 Predominantly fibrous (spindle cell) benign mesothelioma

This is the less common variant of mesotheliomas in animals. It is mainly composed of spindle-shaped mesothelial cells with elongated nuclei, sometimes forming a whorled pattern, resembling a fibroma (Head et al., 2003).

Fine needle samples show variable cellularity, usually scarce and may be bloody. The cells are spindle shaped and resemble fibroblasts with a poorly defined cytoplasm. The nuclei are small, oval to elongated, and have fine chromatin and inconspicuous nucleoli (Dusenbery et al., 1992). Naked nuclei may be numerous. Metachromatic stromal fragments are frequently present. No mitoses are seen (De May, 1996).

3.1.3 Biphasic (mixed) bening mesothelioma

This type may show a mixture of variable proportions of epithelial and spindle cells. In such cases, the epithelial component may be reactive while the spindle component is neoplastic (De May, 1996).

3.2 Malignant mesothelioma

Malignant and benign mesotheliomas have a similar basic structure, so that in some cases it can be difficult to establish a diagnosis. The presence of neoplastic cells in lymph vessels at some distance from the deep surface of the tumours and proven lymph node metastases are distinct proof of malignancy. Tumor cells with marked anisocytosis and anisokariosis, arranged in solid masses. Mitosis may be more frequent, but some metastatic mesotheliomas have few mitotic figures. (Head et al., 2003). Usually mesothelial cells show a clear perinuclear region with variable amounts of vacuoles. Sometimes, these vacuoles` fusion leads to formation of mucin lakes producing cellular cohesion loss (Figure 2) (Enzinger & Weiss, 1985). Areas of necrosis may undergo dystrophic mineralization, especially in cattle (Head et al., 2003).

These tumours are frequently associated with a milky or blood- tinged effusion. So, fluid cytology is usually the first diagnostic study performed. Most are exudates (De May, 1996). Effusions are usually present as the result of blocked lymphatics (Brown et al., 2007). The fluid is characteristically viscous to gelatinous, which is primarily due to hyaluronic acid. It could be present in benign diseases but high levels of hyaluronic acid (>8 mg/dl) are more specific for mesothelioma (De May, 1996).

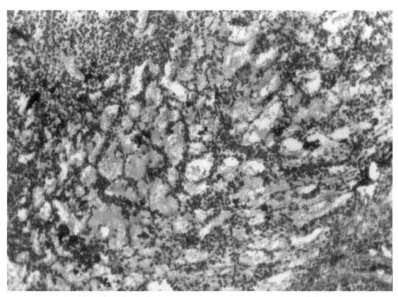

Fig. 2. Predominantly epitheliod mesothelioma. Mesothelial cells forming trabeculae or cords with abundant extracellular mucin lakes. H y E, 100 X.

Fine needle biopsy smears are usually very cellular with abundant papillae, biphasic combination of epithelioid and spindle cells and clinical findings help the diagnosis (Sterret et al., 1987).

3.2.1 Predominantly epithelioid malignant mesothelioma

Is the most common type, not only in humans but also in animals. It is composed of epithelioid mesothelial cells with varying degrees of anaplasia and invasive growth into the underlying tissue (Figure 3), lymphatics and blood vessels (Head et al., 2003).

Cytological samples show neoplastic cells resembling normal mesothelial cells, they may appear in big groups or isolated. There is usually a continuum from bland to malignant-appearing cells, rather than a separate, discrete population of malignant cells, as is seen with metastatic tumor. Occasionally, all the malignant mesothelial cells have only a bland, reactive appearance, that, difficult the diagnosis of malignancy. On the other hand, many cases are composed of anaplastic cells, in which the diagnosis of malignancy is obvious, but the cell of origin is not (De May, 1996).

The cells can form cohesive flat sheets with prominent windows, three-dimensional cell balls or papillae, or tubular/acinar-like structures (Jayaram et al., 1988). Cells in groups are more numerous, bigger and tend to be more irregularly arranged in malignant mesothelioma than in benign proliferations. Cells borders are prominent (Baker & Lumsden,

2000). Thick clusters of cells with highly irregular or knobby outlines are characteristic of mesothelioma (Figure 4). This is important in differential diagnosis from adenocarcinomas since the last one tend to form cell clusters with smooth continuous borders. In some cases, the cells are poorly cohesive, with numerous single cells. Papillary clusters reflect the growth pattern of mesothelioma, so, they are less common in adenocarcinoma and benign effusions. Another common feature in malignant mesotheliomas is long chains of cells known as "cell-embracing", "cell engulfment" and "cannibalism" (De May, 1996).

The cells shape can vary from round to polygonal to angular. A minor component of spindle cells is common (Reuter et al., 1983). The cytoplasm is abundant with relatively well defined cell borders. In Diff Quick, the cells may have raffled cytoplasmic borders corresponding to microvilli, ultrastructurally (Craig et al., 1992). The cytoplasm varies from dense an squamoid (remiscent of immature squamous metaplasia, as seen in the Pap smear) to delicate and vacuolated or foamy. Vacuolated signet ring-like cells may be present. The vacuoles may be degenerative in nature or contain metachromatic, mesenchymal mucin (hyaluronic acid). Some cells contain lipid. The presence of vacuolated, epithelioid cells may suggest adenocarcinoma (Koss et al., 1988).

The nuclei can be centrally or eccentrically located. They are round to oval, and can vary from uniform to pleomorphic (Reuter et al., 1983). Binucleation or multinucleation is common (Cowell et al., 1991). The chromatin ranges from fine to coarse depending on the differentiation. Nucleoli, angular, single or multiple may be prominent (Baker & Lumsden, 2000). Mitotic figures occur, but are not useful in distinguishing benign from malignant mesothelial cells, unless frankly abnormal (De May, 1996). Although psammoma bodies and asbestos bodies can be seen (Tao, 1989), neither is specific for malignant mesothelioma, or even for malignancy.

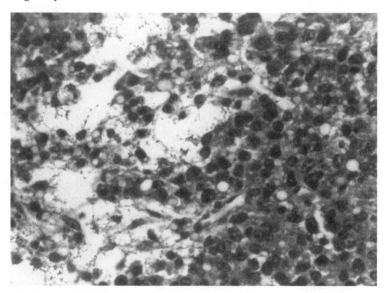

Fig. 3. Neoplastic mesothelial cells proliferation in a solid pattern, with nuclear pleomorphism, coarse chromatin, multiple cytoplasmic vacuoles and extracellular mucus. H y E., 400X

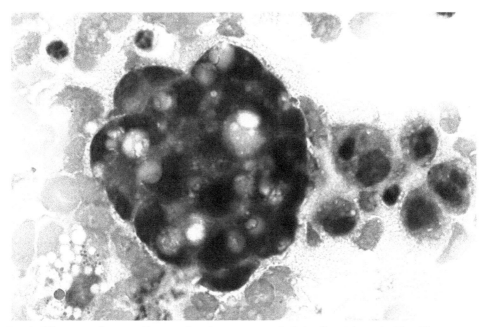

Fig. 4. Effusion sediment. Cluster of malignant mesothelial cells with typical knobby borders. H y E, 1000X.

3.2.2 Predominantly fibrous (spindle cell) malignant mesothelioma

A malignant mesothelial tumor resembling a fibrosarcoma and showing infiltration into the underlying connective tissue (Head et al. 2003). This type is generally localized, rarely cause effusions and its sediment usually shows low cellularity (Enzinger & Weiss, 1985; Tao, 1989). So, fine needle biopsies may be particularly important in the diagnosis of this variety of mesothelioma. These specimens have variable amounts of cells depending on fibrosis degree. The cells may be single or in loose clusters, sometimes forming whorls and storiform patterns. The cells are spindle shaped and may have long cytoplasmic processes. The cells have a moderate amount of cytoplasm that varies from delicate to well defined. The nuclei are relatively large, oval and variably pleomorphic, often with coarse, hyperchromatic chromatin (De May, 1996). Nucleoli are small, but prominent, and frequently multiple. Naked nuclei may be conspicuous (Tao, 1989). Mitoses and necrosis are common (Enzinger & Weiss, 1985). Rarely osseous or cartilaginous metaplasia may occur (De May, 1996).

3.2.3 Biphasic (mixed) malignant mesothelioma

Is rather frequent. Usually the epithelioid pattern predominates in the specimens but that may vary in different areas and cases (De May, 1996).

4. Differential diagnosis

The primary consideration in the differential diagnosis is adenocarcinoma, particularly of the lung, but intestinal and genital metastasis must be also discarded (Head et al., 2003).

Whether, mesothelioma or adenocarcinoma, any malignant tumour with extensive pleural spread is essentially incurable. However, the diagnosis of mesothelioma may be crucial from a medicolegal point of view in humans (De May, 1996).

Special stains, electron microscopy and immuncytochemistry may be helpful in differential diagnosis. Both, mesotheliomas and adenocarcinomas produce mucinous substances that may be differentiated by means of special stains.

Neoplasic mesothelial cells may produce even intra or extracellular acid mucin, hyaluronic acid which have mesenchymal origin (Di Bonito et al., 1993), whereas, adenocarcinomatous cells may secret neutral mucins (epithelial origin). Mesotheliomas very rarely take up neutral mucin stains like mucicarmine and PAS diastase, but they usually have intracellular positive vacuoles to alcian blue (De May, 1996). Acid mucin also stains metachromatically with toluidine blue (Enzinger & Weiss, 1985).

Electron microscopy shows long, slender, abundant, microvilli in mesothelioma, they usually have a length-to-diameter ratio in excess of 12 to 1 (Head et al., 2003) while in adenocarcinoma, microvilli are short and stubby (De May, 1996). The cytoplasm contains numerous bundles of tonofilaments arranged circumferentially around the nucleus (Wilson & Dungworth, 2002).

Immunohistochemistry is also useful in differentiating these tumors since mesothelial cells uniquely express both epithelial cytokeratins and mesenchymal markers such as vimentin (Mc Donough et al., 1992). Mesotheliomas and adenocarcinoma are positive for low molecular weight keratin, while just the former is positive for high-molecular-weight keratin. They are also positive to calretinin, N- cadherin (Abutaily et al., 2002), desmin and P- cadherin (Merlo et al., 2007), but they are negative for carcinoembryonic antigen (CEA) and Leu-M1 (CD 15) (De May, 1996).

There is a report of a peritoneal mesothelioma in a dog of unusual morphologic variant of epithelial mesothelioma, with remarkable cytomorphologic resemblance to decidua. In this case, immunohistochemistry showed strong, diffuse, cytoplasmic staining of neoplastic cells for pancytokeratin and cytokeratin AE1/AE3 and focal, cytoplasmic staining in scattered cells for cytokeratin 5/6. Tumor cells also stained intensely positive for vimentin, whereas anticalretinin, smooth-muscle actin, desmin, S-100 protein and CD117 were negative (Morini et al, 2006).

There is also a description of a lipid rich pleural mesothelioma in a dog, which immunohistochemically, expresses both cytokeratin and vimentin markers as is expected in a mesothelioma. But it also shows S-100 expression, what is consistently found in liposarcoma (Avakian et al., 2008).

5. Conclusion

Mesotheliomas are extremely rare diseases in animals. The relationship between these tumours and exposure to asbestos and other fibres with similar size and solubility is accepted in human beings but in animals there are not many documented proves about this association. Different authors describe congenital mesotheliomas in bovine foetuses and many others consider they are more common in male dogs and spayed bitches.

The histological classification considers benign and malignant mesotheliomas with three different varieties: predominantly epithelioid, predominantly fibrous and biphasic or mixed, but the first one is the commonest. Malignant forms usually cause effusions, so, cytological analysis of the sediment is in general the first approach to diagnosis.

Its differentiation from other entities may be so difficult and may comprise since reactive mesothelial cells responses till adenocarcinomas. So, many complementary diagnostic tools may be required for an accurate diagnosis. Most of histopathological and cytological descriptions are based in human mesotheliomas but its striking features are found in animals neoplasms. Lately, many veterinary cases have been reported, based in different immunohistochemichal analyses aimed at proving mesothelial cells origin.

Even though, "whether, mesothelioma or adenocarcinoma, any malignant tumor with extensive serosal spread is essentially incurable" (De May, 1996) and animal illnesses usually don´t have medicolegal implications, an accurate diagnosis is also expected in veterinary science.

6. References

Abutaily, A.; Addis, B. & Roche, W. (2002). Immunohistochemistry in the distinction between malignant mesothelioma and pulmonary adenocarcinoma: a critical evaluation of new antibodies. *J Clin Pathol,* 55, 662-668.

Avakian, A.; Alroy,J.; Rozanski, E.; Keating, J. & Rosenberg, A. (2008) Lipid-rich pleural mesothelioma in a dog. *J Vet Diagn Invest,* 20, 665–667.

Baker, R. & Lumsden, J. (2000). Pleural and Peritoneal Fluids. In: *Color Atlas of Cytology of the Dog and Cat.* pp. 159-176, Mosby, ISBN 0-8151-0402-2, China.

Brown, C.; Baker, D. & Barker, I. (2007). Alimentary system, In: *Pathology of Domestic Animals. Jubb, Kennedy and Palmer* (Grant Maxie, M Ed), pp. 1-296, Elsevier Saunders, ISBN 13-978 0 7020 2785 7, China.

Butnor, K.; Sporn, T.; Hammar, S. & Roggli, V. (2001). Well differentiated papillary mesothelioma. *Am J Surg Pathol,* 25, 1304-1309.

Cantin, R.; Al-Jabi, M.; Mc Caughey, W. (1982). Desmoplastic diffuse mesothelioma. *Am J Surg Pathol,* 6, 215-222.

Cowell, R.; Tyler, D.& Meinkoth, J. (1993). Abdominal and Thoracic Fluid. In: *Diagnostic Cytology of the dog and cat,* Cowell, RL. & Tyler, DR. pp. 151-166, Edit. American Veterinary Publications, ISBN 0-939674-25-4, California.

Craig, F.; Fishback, NF.; Schwartz, JG. et al. (1992) Occult Metastatic Mesothelioma-Diagnosis by fine- needle aspiration: A Case Report. *Am J Clin Pathol,* 97, 493- 497.

De May, R. (1996). Fluids. In: *The Art and Science of Cytopathology,* pp. 257-290, ASCP Press, ISBN 0-89189-322-9, Chicago, USA.

De May, R. (1996). Pleura. In: *The Art and Science of Cytopathology,* pp. 939-946, ASCP Press, ISBN 0-89189-322-9, Chicago, USA.

DiBonito, L.; Falconieri, G.; Colautti, I.; Bonifacio Gori, D.; Dudine, S. & Giarelli, L. (1993). Cytopathology of malignant mesothelioma: a study of its patterns and histological bases. *Diagn Cytopathol ,* 9, 25-31.

Dusenbery, D.; Grimes, MM.; Frable, WJ. (1992) Fine needle aspiration cytology of localized fibrous tumor of pleura. *Diagn Cytopathol* 8, 444- 450.

Enzinger, F. & Weiss, S. (1985). *Tumores de Tejidos Blandos,* Editorial Médica Panamericana, ISBN 950-06-0615-1, Buenos Aires, Argentina.

Glickman, LT.; Domanski, LM.; Maguire, TG.; Dubielzig, RR.; Churg, A. (1983). Mesothelioma in pet dogs associated with exposure to their owners to asbestos. *Environ Res*, 32, 305–313.

Harbison, M. & Godleski, J. (1983). Malignant mesothelioma in urban dogs. *Vet Pathol* , 20, 531-540.

Head, K.; Else, R. & Dubielzig, R. (2002). Tumors of the alimentary tract, In: *Tumors in Domestic Animals*, Meuten, DJ, pp. 401-481, Blackwell, ISBN-13: 978-0-8138-2652-3, Iowa, USA.

Head, K.; Cullen, J.; Dubielzig, R.; Else, R.; Misdorp, W.; Patnaik, A.; Tateyama, S. & Van der Gaag, I. (2003). *Histological Classification of Tumors of Alimentary System of Domestic Animals*. Armed Forces Institute of Pathology American Registry of Pathology .The World Health Organization, ISBN 1-881041-86-7, Washington, D.C., USA.

Hinrichs, U.; Brugmann, M.; Harps, O. & Wohlstein, P. (1997) Malignant biphasic peritoneal mesothelioma in a horse. *Eur J Vet Pathol*, 3, 95-97.

Jayaram G.; Ashok, S. (1988). Fine needle aspiration cytology of well differentiated papillary peritoneal mesothelioma: Report of a case. *Acta Cytol*, 32, 563- 566.

Kim, J. & Choi, Y. (2002). Juvenile malignant mesothelioma in a dog. *J Vet Med Sci* , 64, 269-271.

Koss, LG.; Woike, S.; Olszewski, W. (1988). Pulmones pleura y mediastino. En: *Biopsia por aspiración*. Koss, LG.; Woike, S.; Olszewski, W. pp.315-383, Lippincott, ISBN 950-06-1233-X, Buenos Aires.

Leisewitz, A. & Nesbit, J. (1992). Malignant mesothelioma in a seven-week-old puppy. *J S Afr Vet Assoc* ,63, 70-73.

López, A. (2007). Respiratory System, In: *Pathology Basis of Veterinary Disease*, McGavin & Zachary, pp. 463-558, Mosby Elsevier, ISBN- 13: 978-0-323-02870-7, China.

Mc Donough, S.; Mac Lachlan, N. & Tobias, A. (1992). Canine pericardial mesothelioma. *Vet Pathol*, 29, 256-260.

Merlo, W.; Rosciani, A.; Koscinczuk, P.; Ortega, H.; Insfrán, R. & Macció, O. (2007). Mesotelioma peritoneal en un canino. *Revista Veterinaria*, 18, 1, 54-57, ISSN 1668-4834.

Morini, M.; Bettini, F.; Morandi, R.; Burdisso, R. &. Marcato, P. (2006). Deciduoid peritoneal mesothelioma in a dog. *Vet Pathol* , 43, 198–201.

Ogilvie, G. & Moore, A. (2008). *Manejo del Paciente Canino Oncológico: Guía práctica para la atención compasiva*, Inter-Médica, ISBN 978-950-555-335-8, Buenos Aires, Argentina.

Reggeti, F.; Brisson, B.; Ruotsalo, K.; Southorn, E.; Bienzle, D. (2005). Invasive epithelial mesothelioma in a dog. *Vet Pathol* , 42, 77-81.

Reuter, K.; Paptopoulos, V.; Reale, F. et al. (1983) Diagnosis of peritoneal mesothelioma: Computed tomography, sonography and fine needle aspiration biopsy. *AJR*, 140: 1189- 1194.

Rudd, R. (2010). Malignant mesothelioma .British Medical Bulletin, 93, 105–123. DOI:10.1093/bmb/ldp047

Sterrett, GF.; Whitaker, D.; Shilkin, KB., et al. (1987) Fine needle aspiration cytoloty of malignant mesothelioma. *Acta Cytol*, 31:185- 193.

Tao, LC. (1989) Aspiration biopsy cytology of mesothelioma. *Diagn Cytopathol*, 5: 14- 21.

Trigo, F.; Morrison, W. & Breeze, R. (1981). An ultraestructural study of canine mesothelioma. *J Com Pathol*, 91, 531-537.

Wilson, D. & Dungworth, D. (2002). Tumors of the respiratory tract. In: *Tumors in Domestic Animals* (Meuten, D.J.), pp. 365-399, Blackwell, ISBN-13:978-0-8138-2652-3, Iowa, USA.

8

Immuno-Oncology and Immunotherapy

R. Cornelissen, J.G.J.V. Aerts and J.P.J.J. Hegmans
Erasmus Medical Centre, Rotterdam
The Netherlands

1. Introduction

The route that mesothelial cells take on their way to becoming malignant is unknown and probably highly variable depending on several environmental and host factors, including polymorphisms and mutations in susceptibility genes, age and immunity. Links between cancer and inflammation were first noted by Rudolf Virchow in 1863, on the basis of observations that tumours often arose at sites of chronic inflammation and that inflammatory cells were present in biopsy samples from tumours (Balkwill & Mantovani 2001). In a SCID mouse xenograft model, it has recently been shown that inflammation precedes the development of human malignant mesothelioma (Hillegass e.a. 2010). Also, epidemiological studies have revealed that chronic inflammation caused by chemical and physical agents, autoimmune and by inflammatory reactions of uncertain aetiology, predisposes for certain forms of cancer (Coussens & Werb 2002). Increasing evidence indicates that the "inflammation-cancer" connection is not only restricted to the initiation of the cancer process, since all types of clinically manifested cancers appear to have an active inflammatory component in their microenvironment. These experimental findings and clinical observations have led to cancer–related inflammation being acknowledged as one of the hallmarks of cancer (Colotta e.a. 2009).

2. Cancer-related immunology

2.1 Tumour-immunosurveillance

By investigating murine tumour transplantation models, Llyod Old, George Klein, and others showed that the immune system of healthy recipient mice was able to differentiate transformed malignant cells from normal cells (Old & Boyse 1964; Klein e.a. 1966). Even preceding these publications, Frank MacFarlane Burnet and Lewis Thomas formulated their cancer immunosurveillance hypothesis: "It is by no means inconceivable that small accumulations of tumour cells may develop and because of their possession of new antigenic potentialities provoke an effective immunological reaction with regression of the tumour and no clinical hint of its existence" (Burnet 1957). At that time this hypothesis was controversial, however, with the current knowledge and ongoing research, it's apparent their premise seems to be correct because there is strong evidence from animal studies that cells of the adaptive immune system carry out surveillance and can eliminate nascent tumours, a process called immuno-editing (Dunn e.a. 2004).

Tumour-associated antigens (TAA) are antigens acquired by tumour cells in the process of neoplastic transformation that can elicit a specific immune response by the host. Expression of these antigens is caused by mutations leading to synthesis and over expression of these abnormal proteins. The immune system can discriminate between malignant cells and their normal counterparts through recognition of these TAA. It is known that several immunological cell types are involved in the recognition and destruction of tumours during early stages of development. These include cells and factors of the innate immune system, including macrophages, neutrophils, complement components, γδ T cells, natural killer (NK) cells, NKT cells and certain cytokines (IL-12, IFN-γ) and cells of the adaptive immune system, including B lymphocytes, helper T cells (Th cells) and cytotoxic T lymphocytes (CTLs).

TAA need to be presented to the cells of the adaptive immune system. Dendritic cells (DCs) are widely acknowledged for their potent antigen presenting capacity and play a key role in the initiation of this adaptive immune response by activation and modulation of lymphocyte subsets (Steinman e.a. 1983). DCs originate from bone marrow precursor cells and are found at low frequencies in peripheral tissues where they maintain an immature phenotype and search their surroundings for foreign substances. Immunogenic TAA are secreted or shed by tumour cells or released when tumour cells die. When TAA are taken up by DCs or other antigen presenting cells (APCs), cells mature and migrate to regional draining lymphoid organs. The captured antigen is processed and presented by major histocompatibility complex (MHC) class I and class II molecules on their cell membrane leading to the activation of antigen-specific lymphocytes. This results in antibody production by B lymphocytes and tumour-specific CTLs to assist the innate immune responses in the killing of tumour cells.

2.2 Tumour immune escape

Increasing evidence reveals that when tumour progress in time, tumour cells undergo changes to escape immune surveillance. The process encompasses three phases: Elimination, Equilibrium, and Escape. During the first phase, immune surveillance takes place. However, tumour cells that are not eliminated by the immune system can enter the equilibrium state, in which there is equilibrium between tumour growth and tumour killing by cells of the immune system. In this stage, tumours can persist for years without progressing to more severe tumour stages. During this period, tumour cells undergo mutations caused by their genetic instability; potentially generating variants that can escape the immune system, by either evading the induction of an immune response or by inhibiting anti-tumour responses via a variety of mechanisms.

2.3 Immune suppressive mechanisms

The induction of an immune suppressive tumour microenvironment is an important escape mechanism how tumours can resist immune destruction. In this microenvironment, inflammatory cells and molecules have a major influence on cancer progress. Effective adaptive immune responses are suppressed through the activation of several pathways. For example, the differentiation and activation of dendritic cells, which are the key initiators of adaptive immune responses, are inhibited by signals (such as IL-10 and VEGF) present in the tumour microenvironment. In addition, tumours but also peripheral blood and lymph nodes contain regulatory T cells (Tregs), which suppress both the adaptive and innate immune responses. Also, a heterogeneous population of myeloid-derived suppressor cells (MDSCs) are induced in tumour-bearing hosts; these cells, as well as conventional tumour-associated macrophages (TAMs), are potent suppressors of antitumour immunity. Not only do MDSCs and TAMs suppress the antitumour response, they also assist the malignant behaviour of tumour cells by secreting cytokines, growth factors, matrix-degrading enzymes and proteases, which promote tumour progression or enhance metastasis.

In conclusion, immune cells can either protect the host against cancer development or promote the emergence of tumours with reduced immunogenicity leading to a complex interplay of tumour growth and tumour regression mechanisms (Mantovani e.a. 2008). In the following sections, the presence and functions of MDSCs, TAMs and Tregs are discussed.

2.3.1 Myeloid-derived suppressor cells

MDSCs are a heterogeneous population of bone marrow-derived myeloid cells, comprising of immature monocytes/macrophages, granulocytes, and DCs at different stages of differentiation (Gabrilovich e.a. 2007). A subset of MDSCs, mononuclear MDSCs (MO-MDSCs) is mainly found at the tumour site while polymorph nuclear MDSCs (PMN-MDSCs) subset is found in blood, lymphoid organs and at the tumour site. They express a number of surface markers, that are on themselves not unique but in combination can define MDSCs. MDSCs are increased in cancer patients and it is anticipated that MDSCs play a suppressive role during the innate and adaptive immune responses to cancer, but have also been described in the course of other pathologic processes such as thermal injury, various infectious diseases, sepsis, trauma, after bone marrow transplantation and in some autoimmune disorders.

Activation of MDSCs not only requires tumour-derived factors (e.g. tumour-derived prostaglandin E2 (PGE2)), but also IFN-γ produced by T cells and factors secreted by tumour stromal cells (like IL-1β, IL-4, IL-6, IL-10, IL- 13). Activation of cytokine receptors on MDSCs leads to activation of STAT-signalling pathways, resulting in the production of immune suppressive substances (like TGF-β, ROS and NOS).

MDSCs inhibit the immune response in several ways;

- MDSCs are capable of producing reactive oxygen species (ROS) and peroxynitrite, which is responsible for most of the adverse effects on T cells, linked to ROS. Changes caused by nitration of the T cell receptor makes T cells incapable of interacting with the MHC complex on antigen presenting cells, which is necessary to obtain T cell specific stimulation (Nagaraj & Gabrilovich 2007; Kusmartsev e.a. 2004).
- MDSCs can inhibit the anti-tumour response in an antigen non-specific manner by the high expression of the enzyme inducible nitric oxid synthetase (iNOS), leading to the generation of NO. NO can suppress T cell function though various mechanisms including the inhibition of the cell signalling pathways and inducing DNA-damage to T cells.
- Arginase-I activity by MDSCs depletes L-arginine from the environment, contributing to the induction of T cell tolerance by the downregulation of the CD3ζ-chain expression of the T cell receptor (Bronte e.a. 2003; Rodríguez & Ochoa 2008).

- MDSCs block T-cell activation by sequestering cystine and thus limiting the availability of the essential amino acid cysteine (Srivastava e.a. 2010).
- MDSCs can inhibit T cell proliferation by producing IL-10 and TGF-β (Hequan Li e.a. 2009).
- Anti-tumour cells, like NK- and NKT-cells, can be inhibited by MDSCs via TGF-β1 depending mechanisms. MDSCs can bind to the TGF-β receptor on target cells via membrane bound TGF-β, leading to activation of intra cellular pathways resulting in downregulation of NK specific receptors (Hequan Li e.a. 2009).
- The plasma membrane expression of enzyme ADAM17 on MDSCs cleaves L-selectin on naïve T cells, decreasing their ability to home to sites where they could be activated (Hanson e.a. 2009).
- MDSCs can indirectly enhance immune suppression via the induction of Tregs (Huang e.a. 2006; Pan e.a. 2010; Kusmartsev & Gabrilovich 2006).
- MDSCs differentiate under certain biological conditions into mature functionally competent macrophages or to DCs influencing tumoural responses (Gabrilovich & Nagaraj 2009).

2.3.2 Tumour-associated macrophages

Macrophages are a major component of the leukocyte infiltrate in the tumour micro-environment (Mantovani e.a. 2002). Classically activated (M1) macrophages, following exposure to IFN-γ, have anti-tumour and tissue destructive activity. In response to IL-4 or IL-13, macrophages undergo alternative (M2) activation. M2 macrophages are oriented to tissue repair, tissue remodelling and immunoregulation. TAMs generally have the phenotype and functions similar to M2 macrophages and display a defective NF-κB activation in response to different pro-inflammatory signals (Sica e.a. 2006).

TAM recruitment in tumours is mediated by several cytokines including colony stimulating factor-1 (CSF-1), vascular endothelial growth factor (VEGF) and chemokines (like CCL2) (Mantovani & Sica 2010). It has been shown that MO-MDSCs are capable of differentiating towards TAMs. Therefore, similar recruitment factors are described that contribute to the infiltration of TAMs and MDSCs into tumour tissue (Mantovani & Sica 2010).

In addition, dynamic changes of the tumour microenvironment occur during the transition from early neoplastic events toward advanced tumour stages resulting in local hypoxia, low glucose level and low pH. These events drive the switch from a M1 macrophage toward the M2 type by profound changes occurring in the tumour microphysiology.

TAMs are able to suppress the adoptive immune response through various mechanisms and contribute to angiogenesis and tumour invasiveness:

- TAMS are able to produce immune suppressive cytokines, like CCL17, CCL18, CCL22, IL-1β, IL-6, IL-10 and TGF-β. IL-10 in combination with IL-6 can lead to upregulation of molecules in TAMs, which are implicated in suppression of tumour-specific T cell immunity (Kryczek e.a. 2006).
- TAMs express the enzyme indoleamine 2,3-dioxygenase (IDO), a well-known suppressor of T cell activation. IDO catalyzes the catabolism of tryptophan, an essential amino acid acquired for T cell activation (Grohmann e.a. 2003).

- TAMs contribute to immune suppression via indirect ways. Secretion of CCL18 leads to recruitment of native T cells. Attraction of naive T cells into the tumour microenvironment is likely to induce T cell anergy (Balkwill 2004). Besides CCL18, CCL17 and CCL22 are abundantly expressed. These cytokines interact with CCR4 receptor, expressed by Tregs and induces T-helper 2 polarization (Bonecchi e.a. 1998). Via expression of VEGF, TAMs can block antigen uptake by APCs and attract MDSCs, which can function as TAM precursors but are also actively suppressing T cell function. MDSCs are depending on prostaglandin E2 (PGE2) for their function. PGE2 is secreted by many types of cancer; however TAMs are also capable of producing PGE2 and therefore assist MDSC function (Nagaraj & Gabrilovich 2008).
- In tumour stroma, TAMs produce matrix metalloproteases (MMPs) and other proteases, leading to degradation of the extracellular matrix. During this process several cytokines, chemokines and growth factors are released from the matrix that promotes and facilitates endothelial cell survival and migration and thereby enhances angiogenesis (Mantovani e.a. 2006).
- Besides indirect mechanisms, angiogenesis is also directly stimulated by TAMs. TAMs can produce proangiogenic factors like VEGF and platelet derived growth factors (PDGF). The release of these factors leads to the formation of (lymph)angiogenic structures and subsequent metastasis (Strieter e.a. 2004).

2.3.3 Regulatory T cells

Tregs are a population of CD4+ T cells with a central role in the prevention of autoimmunity and the promotion of tolerance via their suppressive function on a broad repertoire of cellular targets (Baecher-Allan & Hafler 2005). Characteristic of Tregs is the expression of CD25 (IL-2 receptor-α chain), forkhead/winged-helix transcription factor box P3 (Foxp3), glucocorticoid-induced TNF-receptor-related-protein (GITR), lymphocyte activation gene-3 (LAG-3), and cytotoxic T-lymphocyte-associated antigen 4 (CTLA4), however all these markers are not truly Treg-specific (Larmonier e.a. 2007). Tregs can be divided into natural Tregs and adaptive Tregs. Natural Tregs are important in the suppression of autoreactive T cells that slip through selection processes and therefore natural Tregs maintain peripheral tolerance against self-antigens preventing autoimmunity. In humans, these cells represent 2-5% of total circulating CD4+ T cells in peripheral blood (Ormandy e.a. 2005). Adaptive Tregs arise from naive T cells and are triggered by suboptimal antigen stimulation and stimulation with TGF-β. Adaptive Tregs can be subdivided into IL-10 secreting Tregs type I (Tr1) and TGF-β producing Tregs (Th3 Tregs). These cells are characterized by the secretion of immune suppressive cytokines directly inhibiting T cells and converting DCs into suppressive APCs (Wei e.a. 2006).

Tregs were first recognized to infiltrate human cancers and the prevalence of Tregs in tumour-infiltrating lymphocytes is much higher than their proportion in peripheral blood, constituting 20% or more of tumour-infiltrating lymphocytes (H Jonuleit e.a. 2000). Elevated levels of Tregs have been identified in blood of cancer patients compared with normal individuals and their presence predicts for poor survival (Apostolou e.a. 2008). In mesothelioma patients, elevated levels of Tregs have also been identified in pleural fluid, with a clear patient to patient variability (DeLong e.a. 2005).

Natural Tregs are derived in the thymus and migrate into the periphery. It has been proposed that Tregs need to be activated and/or expended from periphery and bone marrow if needed. Since 25% of CD4+ T cells in the bone marrow function as Tregs, it has been suggested that the bone marrow plays an active role in humoral and cellular immune regulation. However, it is poorly understood which factors are involved in trafficking and regulation of Tregs (94). Induction of suppressive activity of both, natural and adaptive Tregs, require T cell receptor triggering by antigen or stimulation with TGF-β (95-96). Weak stimulation or the absence of co-stimulatory molecules leads to the induction of long-lasting suppressive activity. Via this mechanism, Tregs can also be directed against TAA and contribute to T cell anergy against tumours. TAA-specific Tregs accumulate in the peripheral lymphoid organs and at the tumour side. However TAA-specific Tregs are also found in the bone marrow, suggesting that after activation Tregs can migrate back to the bone marrow and inducing T cell tolerance before these cells enter the circulation (Strauss e.a. 2007). Although exact mechanisms are not fully explored, it has been shown that CCR4+ (receptor for CCL22) Tregs migrate toward tumour microenvironments expressing CCL22 (Sakaguchi e.a. 2009). Also CD62L and CCR7 have been described as important homing markers on Tregs (Gondek e.a. 2005). CD62L is critical for the migration of Tregs to draining lymph nodes. CCR7 is expressed by a majority of Tregs and is essential in homing to lymphoid organs and microenvironments expressing CCL19 (the ligand for CCR7) (Nakamura e.a. 2001).

As MDCSs and TAMs, Tregs have several pathways that diminish immune responses to tumour tissue:

- Direct cell-cell interaction between Tregs and target cells is important for tolerance induction by Tregs (Thornton & Shevach 1998). These target cells include CD4+ and CD8+ effector cells, B cells, NK T cells, DCs and monocytes/macrophages. The cell-cell binding leads to apoptosis by activation of programmed cell death-ligands (PDL), the release of perforin (Boissonnas e.a. 2010) and granzyme-B (Nagaraj & Gabrilovich 2007) and by reducing the proliferation through upregulation of intracellular cyclic AMP (Fassbender e.a. 2010; Bopp e.a. 2007).
- Tregs produce themselves or induce other cells to secrete immunosuppressive cytokines such as IL-10 and transforming growth factor (TGF)-β to blunt immune responses (Hawrylowicz & O'Garra 2005), but also other molecules produced by Tregs like carbon monoxide (Lee e.a. 2007) and galectins (Garín e.a. 2007) are reported to play roles in suppression.
- Tregs can inhibit antitumour effector NK and NK T cells via membrane bound TGF-β (Ghiringhelli e.a. 2005). The binding of membrane-bound TGF-β on Tregs to the TGF-β-receptor on target cells leads to the activation of intracellular pathways, which eventually leads to the down regulation of the NKG2D- receptor on NK and NK T cells.
- Tregs are forming aggregates around DCs to prevent contact between DCs and T cells and in this way disturb the induction of the adaptive immune response by preventing proper antigen presentation (Onishi e.a. 2008; Tadokoro e.a. 2006).
- CTLA4+ Tregs induce the expression of indoleamine 2,3-dioxygenase (IDO) in APCs reducing the essential amino acid tryptophan to kynurenine, which is toxic to neighbouring T cells (Fallarino e.a. 2003).
- Treg aggregation leads to decreased upregulation of CD80 and CD86 on immature DCs and down regulate the expression of CD80 and CD86 on mature DCs (Oderup

e.a. 2006). These phenomena are antigen specific and dependent on lymphocyte function-associated antigen 1 (LFA-1) and CTL-associated protein 4 (CTLA-4) (Rooney e.a. 1998).

- Tregs induce B7-H4 expression by APCs, a member of the B7 family that negatively regulates T-cell responses (Kryczek e.a. 2006).
- Activated Tregs, which express higher affinity IL-2R than conventional T cells, may absorb IL-2 from the microenvironment (de la Rosa e.a. 2004).

However, none of these mechanisms can explain all aspects of suppression. It is probable that various combinations of several mechanisms are operating, depending on the milieu and the type of immune responses.

2.4 Conclusion

In short, MDSCs, TAMs and Tregs are capable of suppressing the anti-tumour response with a variety of mechanisms and contribute to a complex interplay between cells that act on behalf or against the tumour. These cells have an essential role in tumor growth or destruction of tumour cells, as pictures in figure 1.

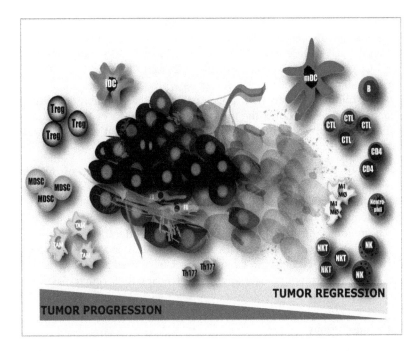

Fig. 1. Interplay between immunological cells that inhibit tumour growth on the right of the tumour and cells that aid in tumour progression on the left. (Tumour is depicted as black cells with a red nucleus in the middle). iDC = immature dendritic cell, mDC = mature dendritic cell, Th17 = helper T lymphocyte 17, M1 MØ= M1 macrophage, FB = fibroblast, B = B cell lymphocyte.

3. Immunotherapy

Cancer immunotherapy attempts to mimic the anti-tumour effects of the immune system of the patient, or it may assist in the capabilities of the immune system to fight cancer. Multiple approaches for immunotherapy have been developed over the years and many are in various stages of (pre-)clinical research. Immunotherapy can be divided into two main categories: passive and active immunotherapy.

3.1 Passive immunotherapy

Passive immunotherapy makes use of *in vitro* produced immunologic effectors that are capable of influencing tumour cell growth. The most common form of passive immunotherapy is called monoclonal antibody therapy. It consists of humanized monoclonal antibodies that are investigated in several human malignancies. Monoclonal antibodies can target cells directly or indirectly. Monoclonal antibodies are also used as immunomodulators to inhibit immune suppressive molecules/cells or activate immune stimulatory molecules. Efficacy of this approach can sometimes be enhanced by linking a toxin to these antibodies (e.g. radionucleotides and anticancer drugs).

In this field, ipilimumab is an interesting newcomer, currently tested mainly in metastatic melanoma. Ipilimumab is a monoclonal antibody against cytotoxic T-lymphocyte antigen (CTLA)-4. It is normally expressed at low levels on the surface of naïve effector T cells, but is upregulated on the cell surface when there is a long-lasting and strong stimulus via the T cell receptor (TCR). CTLA-4 then competes with CD28 for CD80/CD86 on APCs, effectively shutting off TCR signalling and thereby serves as a physiologic "brake" on the activated immune system. Ipilimumab can thus prevent this feedback inhibition, resulting in an unabated immune response against the tumour. The side effects of this therapy, however, can be significant due to the downregulation of tolerance to patient's own normal tissue and colitis is often seen in patients.

Another method of passive immunotherapy uses adaptive transfer of antigen specific effector cells (like T cells and NK cells) that can be expanded and/or activated *ex-vivo* and subsequently administered back into the patient to attack the tumour. This approach showed the potential to reconstitute host immunity against pathogens, like Epstein-Barr virus (EBV) in immune suppressed patients, but more importantly also provides evidence that adaptive T cell transfers can prevent the induction of EBV-associated lymphomas. This led to the concept that antigen specific T cell transfer can be used as an anti-tumour therapy to eradicate established tumours. The approach of adaptive T cell transfer to eradicate malignancies is challenging.

3.2 Active immunotherapy

Active immunotherapeutic approaches aim at inducing or boosting immune effector cells *in vivo* against tumour cells, through the administration of immune mediators capable of activating the immune system.

Several cytokines are capable of activating and recruiting specific immune cells that can enhance anti-tumour immunity (e.g. IL-2, IL-12, IL-15, TNF-α, GM-CSF). These cytokines can be used as an approach as single treatment or in combination with other immunotherapy strategies.

Defined TAA epitopes have been used to vaccinate cancer patients; however this approach is limited by the relatively low number of identified specific epitopes and by the requirement of MHC typing. Nevertheless, some authors have reported the applicability of this approach. By using the whole TAA protein for immunization, the need of peptide identification can be circumvented. These proteins can be taken up by APCs and endogenously processed into epitopes for presentation to T cells. Adjuvants need to be added to induce APCs activation and avoid tolerance induction (Berger e.a. 2005).

DNA sequences coding for specific TAAs can be directly injected into the skin. DNA then needs to be taken up, transcribed into mRNA, translated into a protein and processed into peptides by APCs. An important restriction is the relatively inefficient delivery into APCs. Viruses engineered to express TAAs can be injected directly into the patient. The virus then transduces the host cell, leading to cell death and presentation of antigenic isotopes to the immune system. A wide variety of viral vectors are available. However there are concerns regarding the immuno-dominance of viral antigens over TAAs, resulting in a strong antivirus response leading to virus eradication and attenuation of the anti-tumour immune response.

The ideal source of TAAs is the tumour itself, since it expresses all the TAAs that need to be targeted. Tumour cell-lines are often used as source for this approach. Tumour cell-lines can be genetically modified to co-express cytokines or co-stimulatory molecules to enhance their immunologic capacity. However, in general, tumour cells display a rather weak antigen presentation capacity and because of the need for *ex vivo* tumour cell culture, this approach is rather expensive, time consuming and labour intensive.

Sipuleucel-T is an active cellular immunotherapy consisting of autologous peripheral-blood mononuclear cells (PBMCs), including APCs. Recently, Kantoff *et al.* published a phase III trail where they used *ex vivo* activated Sipuleucel-T with a recombinant fusion protein (PA2024). PA2024 consists of a prostate antigen, prostatic acid phosphatase, that is fused to granulocyte–macrophage colony-stimulating factor (GM-CSF), an immune-cell activator. Sipuleucel-T prolonged survival among men with asymptomatic or minimally symptomatic metastatic castration-resistant prostate cancer (Kantoff e.a. 2010).

DCs have emerged as the most powerful initiators of immune responses. In the natural activation of the adaptive immune system against tumour cells, DCs play a crucial role since they are capable to engulf tumour antigens and activate lymphocytes in an antigen specific manner. Therefore, the application of DCs to therapeutic cancer vaccines has been prompted (Banchereau & Palucka 2005). DCs can be generated in large amounts *ex vivo*, and pulsed with tumour antigens under optimal conditions. Subsequently, the injection of matured tumour antigen-pulsed DCs led to the induction of an anti-tumour response in murine models as well as in patients (Hegmans e.a. 2005). Moreover, DC activation also induces the formation of antibodies against tumour components. Therefore, DC-immunotherapy can potentially induce long lasting immune protection. Over the last decades numerous groups have investigated the safety and applicability of DC-based vaccines in the treatment of cancer in preclinal and clinical studies.

4. DC-based immunotherapy in mesothelioma

We previously investigated the effect of DC-based immunotherapy on the outgrowth of mesothelioma in a murine model (Hegmans e.a. 2005). Because the TAAs are not known for mesothelioma, we used tumour cell lysates as antigen source to pulse DCs. We established that DC-based immunotherapy induced strong tumour-specific CTLs responses leading to prolonged survival in mice. The efficacy of immunotherapy was dependent on the tumour load; most beneficial effects were established at early stages of tumour development.

On the basis of these preclinical animal studies, we have performed the first clinical trial in which autologous tumour lysate–pulsed DCs were administrated in mesothelioma patients (Hegmans e.a. 2010). Patients were eligible for the study when sufficient tumour cells could be obtained from pleural effusion or tumour biopsy material at the time of diagnosis. DC-immunotherapy was planned after completion of the cytoreductive therapy provided that during chemotherapy no major side effects occurred and there was no progressive disease. Concentrated leukocyte fractions were generated through peripheral blood leukapheresis. Peripheral blood mononuclear cells were then enriched, cultured and matured to DCs. Patients received three immunizations with mature DCs, loaded with autologous tumour lysate and keyhole limpet hemocyanin (KLH) as positive control, in 2-week intervals. Each immunization, consisting of 50 x 106 cells, was administered intradermally and intravenously (figure 2).

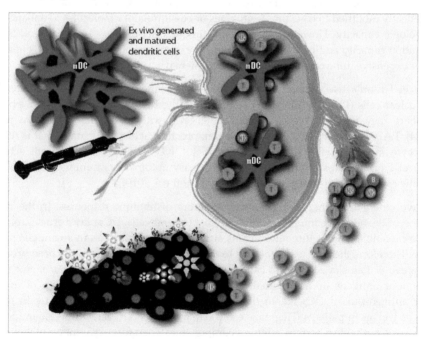

Fig. 2. Schematic representation showing the administration of *ex vivo* maturated autologous dendritic cells into a patient, resulting in antigen presentation in the lymph node and a specific anti-tumour cytotoxic anti-tumour response.

Overall, the vaccination regimen with loaded DCs was well-tolerated in all patients and no CTC grade 3 or 4 toxicities were reported. A local skin rash occurred at the site of the intradermal injection after the first vaccination in 8 of the 10 patients. Subsequent vaccinations (second and third) gave a quicker and increased induration and erythema in all patients suggesting that some form of immunity was induced. Most patients developed mild to severe flu-like symptoms after the vaccination, particularly fever, muscle aches, chills, and tiredness, these symptoms normalized after one day. Since it was a phase I study, no conclusions can be drawn regarding improvement of the progression-free survival or overall survival. However, serum samples from all patients showed a significant increase of pre-vaccine versus post-vaccine antibodies reactive to KLH, both of the immunoglobulin (Ig)G and IgM isotype. No or very low amounts of antibodies against KLH were detected in undiluted serum of all patients before vaccination, illustrating the suitability of this antigen to determine the immunocompetence of the vaccine. Responses against KLH gradually increased with the number of vaccinations suggesting that several vaccinations were necessary to induce a more potent humoral response. Antibodies against KLH in serum could easily be detectable by ELISA in all patients after three vaccinations. The response remained at the same level for several months after the last DC injection and gradually decreased after 6 to 12 months. This proves that a successful immunoreaction was induced by the DC vaccinations. Furthermore chromium release assays were performed in 6 of 10 patients from whom pleural fluid was obtained. In 4 patients a clear inductions of cytotoxicity against autologous tumour cells were measured. The cytotoxicity levels of one patient increased after every vaccination; for the other three patients three vaccinations were necessary to induce cytotoxicity (figure 3).

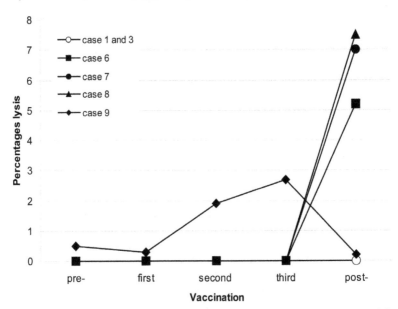

Fig. 3. Percentage of tumour lysis of 6 patients treated with autologous-loaded dendritic cell immunotherapy, showing a clear increase in tumour lysis in half of the patients after the third vaccination.

5. Improving DC-based immunotherapy

While DC-based immunotherapy was proven safe and feasible, it is not "prime time" yet for commencing a larger randomised trial. Because the applied therapy was technically challenging and the efficacy of this therapy was hampered by the presence of immunosuppressive cells in peripheral blood and within the tumour environment, DC-based immunotherapy can be further refined. Several strategies have been tested or are currently tested that target the immunosuppressive cells that diminish the immunoresponse aiming to improve the efficacy of the immunotherapy. In the following sections, we will focus on three populations of suppressive cells, the MDSCs, Tregs and TAMs, that are increased in most cancer patients. It is becoming increasingly clear that these populations contribute to the impaired anti-tumour responses frequently observed in cancer patients. Therefore, combating immunosuppression through modulation of these cell types will be an important key to increase the efficacy of DC-based immunotherapy, and should lead to better prognosis for cancer patients.

5.1 Targeting MDSCs

5.1.1 COX-2 inhibition by celecoxib improves DC-based immunotherapy and is associated with decreased numbers and function of myeloid-derived suppressor cells in mesothelioma

The production of reactive oxygen species (ROS), which is responsible for most of the adverse effects on T cells, by MDSCs is highly depending upon cyclooxygenase-2 (COX-2) enzyme activity (Sinha e.a. 2007). The inducible COX-2 enzyme is essential in the biosynthesis of prostaglandins. Over-expression of COX-2 has been described as an important factor in tumour development. Therefore, high expression of COX-2 has been correlated with poor prognosis in cancer (A Baldi e.a. 2004). In addition, several studies showed the relevance of COX-2 inhibition in cancer progression (Edelman e.a. 2008). Although the relation between COX-2 over-expression and prostaglandin E2 (PGE2) synthesis in cancer has been studied extensively, the impact on the tumour microenvironment is still under investigation (Zha e.a. 2004). Selective inhibition of COX-2 could therefore be a possible strategy for improvement of DC-based immunotherapy. Since celecoxib is a selective COX-2 inhibitor, we investigated the effect of celecoxib treatment on the four MDSC subsets that were identified in the spleen of tumour-bearing mice (Veltman e.a. 2010). Splenocytes from mice that were inoculated with AB1 tumour cells and received celecoxib diet or control diet were analyzed for the presence of the MDSC subsets.

Ten days after tumour inoculation, the absolute number of MDSCs was significantly lower in mice receiving celecoxib diet compared with mice receiving control diet. This difference was even more pronounced at day 22 after tumour injection. Also, dietary celecoxib treatment reduced ROS production in all MDSC subtypes but was most effective in the MO-MDSC and Gr-1low MDSC subset 2 both in percentage as well as the median fluorescence intensity (MFI). Anti-tumour responses induced by DC-treatment were affected by suppressive cells in the spleen of tumour-bearing mice. However, the anti-tumour activity as indicated by AB1 lysis and IFN-g/granzyme B production by CD8+ T cells was no longer influenced when co-cultured with splenocytes of mice receiving celecoxib diet, indicating that COX-2 inhibition leads to a reduction in suppressive immune cells.

When combining DC-based immunotherapy and celecoxib treatment, a significant improvement of the immunotherapy was seen in comparison to no or single modality treatment (figure 4). Treatment of tumour-bearing mice with dietary celecoxib prevented the local and systemic expansion of all MDSC subtypes and also their suppressive function was impaired. Combining celecoxib with DC-based immunotherapy demonstrated highly activated CTLs with superior immunostimulatory potency and anti-tumour activity because of the reduced MDSCs expansion.

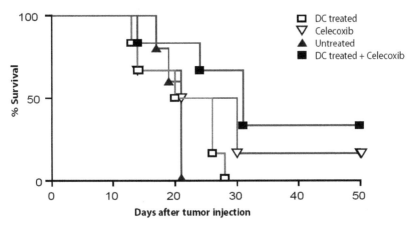

Fig. 4. Improved survival of tumor bearing mice that were treated by dendritic cell-based immunotherapy combined with a diet containing the selective COX-2 inhibitor celecoxib.

5.2 Targeting TAMs

5.2.1 Zoledronic acid impairs myeloid differentiation to tumour-associated macrophages in mesothelioma

We investigated the effect of the depletion of macrophages on tumour progression in a murine model for mesothelioma by treating mice with liposome-encapsulated clodronate (Veltman, e.a. 2010). These liposomes are readily taken up by phagocytic cells, including macrophages, and induce cell-specific apoptosis after clodronate is set free into the cytoplasm of cells (Claassen 1992). Treatment with liposome-encapsulated clodronate significantly reduced the number of macrophages in the peritoneal cavity of tumour inoculated mice. All mice (n=5) treated with control liposome-encapsulated phosphate buffered saline showed profound tumour growth at day 12. Three of the five mice treated with liposome-encapsulated clodronate had no visible tumour. In the case of mice that developed tumours, tumour growth was less profound. Macrophages (M1/M2) were found scattered throughout the tumour of control mice.

These data confirmed that macrophages have a significant role in the onset and progression of tumour in our murine mesothelioma model. We observed an inhibition of myeloid differentiation to macrophages when zoledronic acid (ZA) was added to the culture *in vitro*, conditioned for macrophages. This inhibitory effect on differentiation was dose dependent and led to significant differences in the number of macrophages and immature cells between the different culture conditions on day 6. Furthermore, we showed that tumour-derived factors present in tumour supernatant induced the development of macrophages from bone marrow-derived cells.

No significant differences on tumour progression and survival could be observed between untreated mice and mice treated with ZA, a reduction in the number of macrophages and an increase in the number of immature myeloid cells was detected. We have shown that treatment with ZA reduces the number of macrophages, but at the same time, we observed higher levels of immature myeloid cell types. When we further defined the population of immature myeloid cells, significantly more MO-MDSCs were found. In addition, we found that the expression of CD206 on macrophages was lower in ZA-treated animals. This reduced expression of the M2 macrophage marker was accompanied with a significant reduction in VEGF and CCL-2 (MCP-1) levels and a significant increase in the levels of IL-6 and IL-12.

5.3 Targeting Tregs

5.3.1 Targeting regulatory T cells in clinical studies

Owing to the significant role of Tregs in the failure of immune surveillance and immunotherapy, many attempts to deplete or inhibit Tregs in cancer patients have been made. Many of the strategies to reduce Tregs target CD25, which makes up the alpha-subunit of the IL-2R, that is present on the surface of Tregs and activated cells. An engineered recombinant fusion protein of IL-2 and diphtheria toxin (denileukin diftitox [Ontak]) and other CD25-directed immunotoxins (daclizumab, LMB-2, RFT5-SMPT-dgA) have been investigated for Treg depletion, which seems to kill selectively lymphocytes expressing the IL-2 receptor. However, early human trials have not proven that this approach results in tumor regression and have shown that these strategies may not adequately deplete Foxp3+ Tregs, and may also deplete antitumor effector cells (Attia e.a. 2005; Ruddle e.a. 2006; Attia e.a. 2006; Powell e.a. 2007). Other possible approaches to reduce immunosuppression of Tregs is via CTLA-4 blockade (e.g. ipilimumab)(Fecci e.a. 2007; Phan e.a. 2003), anti GITR agonism (Ko e.a. 2005), and vaccination against Foxp3 (Nair e.a. 2007) and some other suggested approaches, such as the inhibition of IDO, TGF-β, ectonucleotidase (expressed by Tregs and generates immunosuppressive adenosine), or the activation of other agents such as OX40 or Toll-like receptor 8 have not yet proven to be beneficial. IL-7 administration was shown to increase T cell numbers and decrease of the Treg fraction in humans (Rosenberg e.a. 2006), on the contrary, other reports have shown that IL-7 leads to the development of Tregs (Cattaruzza e.a. 2009; Mazzucchelli e.a. 2008). In conclusion, there are many conflicting results in abrogating the action of Tregs, and thus it is unclear which approach holds promise for cancer treatment.

5.3.2 Targeting Tregs with metronomic cyclophosphamide

Low-dose cyclophosphamide (CTX) prevents the development and functionality of the Tregs (Ghiringhelli e.a. 2007), the mechanism behind this effect, however, is not completely understood. We investigated the effect of CTX on immuno-suppression and the combination of CTX and DC-based immunotherapy was studied in a murine MM model (Veltman e.a. 2010). Our data showed that metronomic administration of low-dose CTX has a strong immune-modulating effect *in vivo*, causing a shift in ratio between CD19+/CD3+ cells. Addition of CTX to the drinking water of tumor-bearing mice leads to a significant increase in the proportion of CD3+ T cells in the peripheral blood and the spleen, whereas the proportion of Tregs was reduced. When mice were given drinking water supplemented with 0.13 mg/ml CTX from day 3 till day 10 and day 14 till day 21, an increased survival was measured. However, the combination of DC-based immunotherapy and CTX administration significantly improved survival compared to DC- based immunotherapy or CTX administration alone.

Therefore, we conclude that CTX is a powerful tool to optimize suboptimal DC-based immunotherapy. Although CTX alone also improves survival, the combination of both was significantly better.

Following the murine model trial, we commenced a clinical trial in mesothelioma patients. As in our previous clinical trial, patients received three immunizations with mature DCs, loaded with autologous tumour lysate and KLH (as positive control), in 2-week intervals. Each immunization, consisting of 50×10^6 cells, is administered intradermally and intravenously. Metronomic cyclophosphamide is added in a dosage of 100 mg/day as pictured in figure 5.

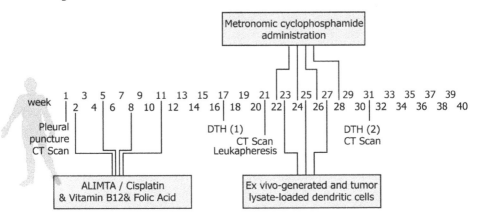

Fig. 5. Treatment plan of the clinical study, starting with diagnosis, followed by chemotherapy treatment. After leukapheresis, dendritic cell therapy with metronomic cyclophosphamide treatment is commenced. DTH = delayed type hypersensitivity, which was performed to test the response against KLH and autologous tumour-lysate.

Primary endpoint of the study is to determine the efficacy of metronomic cyclophosphamide on the modulation of Tregs numbers during DC-based immunotherapy in peripheral blood. Secondary endpoints are the effect on specific anti-tumour activity and clinical and radiological responses. At the moment of publication of this chapter, 8 out of 10 patients have fully completed the immunotherapy treatment. The secondary endpoints are not available yet, but Treg depletion has been confirmed in our first patient (figure 6).

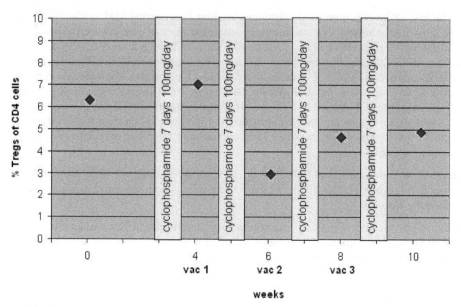

Fig. 6. The first patient in which Tregs were measured during dendritic cell-based therapy treatment combined with metronomic cyclophosphamide, showing a decrease in Treg number in peripheral blood (preliminary data).

6. Future research

6.1 Allogeneic DC-based immunotherapy

In mice, we've observed a distinctive immune response when autologous tumour lysate loaded DC therapy was given after injection of tumour cells. This response was also effective when allogeneic (DCs loaded with mesothelioma cell line lysate derived from other mouse strain) tumour loaded DC therapy was given. This provides opportunities because current clinical trail using autologous lysate loaded DCs are hampered by the amount and quality of tumour lysate available. Most patients already have been diagnosed with mesothelioma before being referred for experimental therapy; often it's not possible to have a patient-friendly way of gathering useful tumour cells. Also, in the future, dendritic cell therapy as a mature anti-tumour therapy would be far more practical if an effective allogeneic tumour cell suspension would be available.

6.2 Response evaluation

Immunotherapy represents a new class of agents in the treatment of mesothelioma. As seen in Sipuleucel-T in prostate cancer and ipilumumab in melanoma improvement in overall survival in patients was seen, however, the agents did not change initial disease progression. Even, a transient worsening of disease manifested either by progression of known lesions or the appearance of new lesions can be seen, before disease stabilizes or tumour regresses.

Commonly accepted treatment paradigm, however, suggests that treatments should initially decrease tumor volume, which can be measured using CT-scan. Also, progression-free survival increasingly is being used as an alternative end-point of studies. This seems to be unfortunate for immunotherapy, which may initiate an immunoresponse that ultimately slows the tumor growth rate, resulting in longer survival, but not a decrease in tumour volume on CT or an increased progression free survival. Future trials are currently planned to investigate these hypotheses, however, clinicians at this moment may need to reconsider how they measure success of their immunotherapy (Madan e.a. 2010).

7. Summary

In conclusion, the role of the immune system in mesothelioma is vast. The tumour uses villainous tricks to evade the immune system and to survive and even abuses immunological cells to harness itself against attack from the immune system. Immunotherapy tries to modulate this immune system to strengthen the anti-tumour effect, this battle however is not yet won and much research lies ahead of us.

8. References

Apostolou, Irina, Panos Verginis, Karsten Kretschmer, Julia Polansky, Jochen Hühn, en Harald von Boehmer. 2008. Peripherally induced Treg: mode, stability, and role in specific tolerance. *Journal of Clinical Immunology* 28, no. 6 (november): 619-624. doi:10.1007/s10875-008-9254-8.

Attia, Peter, Ajay V Maker, Leah R Haworth, Linda Rogers-Freezer, en Steven A Rosenberg. 2005. Inability of a fusion protein of IL-2 and diphtheria toxin (Denileukin Diftitox, DAB389IL-2, ONTAK) to eliminate regulatory T lymphocytes in patients with melanoma. *Journal of Immunotherapy (Hagerstown, Md.: 1997)* 28, no. 6 (december): 582-592.

Attia, Peter, Daniel J Powell Jr, Ajay V Maker, Robert J Kreitman, Ira Pastan, en Steven A Rosenberg. 2006. Selective elimination of human regulatory T lymphocytes in vitro with the recombinant immunotoxin LMB-2. *Journal of Immunotherapy (Hagerstown, Md.: 1997)* 29, no. 2 (april): 208-214. doi:10.1097/01.cji.0000187959.45803.0c.

Baecher-Allan, Clare M, en David A Hafler. 2005. Functional analysis of highly defined, FACS-isolated populations of human regulatory CD4+CD25+ T cells. *Clinical Immunology (Orlando, Fla.)* 117, no. 2 (november): 192; discussion 193. doi:10.1016/j.clim.2005.08.008.

Baldi, A, D Santini, F Vasaturo, M Santini, G Vicidomini, M Pia Di Marino, V Esposito, e.a. 2004. Prognostic significance of cyclooxygenase-2 (COX-2) and expression of cell cycle inhibitors p21 and p27 in human pleural malignant mesothelioma. *Thorax* 59, no. 5 (mei): 428-433.

Balkwill, F, en A Mantovani. 2001. Inflammation and cancer: back to Virchow? *Lancet* 357, no. 9255 (februari 17): 539-545. doi:10.1016/S0140-6736(00)04046-0.

Balkwill, Fran. 2004. Cancer and the chemokine network. *Nature Reviews. Cancer* 4, no. 7 (juli): 540-550. doi:10.1038/nrc1388.

Banchereau, Jacques, en A Karolina Palucka. 2005. Dendritic cells as therapeutic vaccines against cancer. *Nature Reviews. Immunology* 5, no. 4 (april): 296-306. doi:10.1038/nri1592.

Berger, Thomas G, Erwin Strasser, Richard Smith, Curt Carste, Beatrice Schuler-Thurner, Eckhart Kaempgen, en Gerold Schuler. 2005. Efficient elutriation of monocytes within a closed system (Elutra) for clinical-scale generation of dendritic cells. *Journal of Immunological Methods* 298, no. 1-2 (maart): 61-72. doi:10.1016/j.jim.2005.01.005.

Boissonnas, Alexandre, Alix Scholer-Dahirel, Virginie Simon-Blancal, Luigia Pace, Fabien Valet, Adrien Kissenpfennig, Tim Sparwasser, Bernard Malissen, Luc Fetler, en Sebastian Amigorena. 2010. Foxp3+ T cells induce perforin-dependent dendritic cell death in tumor-draining lymph nodes. *Immunity* 32, no. 2 (februari 26): 266-278. doi:10.1016/j.immuni.2009.11.015.

Bonecchi, R, G Bianchi, P P Bordignon, D D'Ambrosio, R Lang, A Borsatti, S Sozzani, e.a. 1998. Differential expression of chemokine receptors and chemotactic responsiveness of type 1 T helper cells (Th1s) and Th2s. *The Journal of Experimental Medicine* 187, no. 1 (januari 5): 129-134.

Bopp, Tobias, Christian Becker, Matthias Klein, Stefan Klein-Hessling, Alois Palmetshofer, Edgar Serfling, Valeska Heib, e.a. 2007. Cyclic adenosine monophosphate is a key component of regulatory T cell-mediated suppression. *The Journal of Experimental Medicine* 204, no. 6 (juni 11): 1303-1310. doi:10.1084/jem.20062129.

Bronte, Vincenzo, Paolo Serafini, Alessandra Mazzoni, David M Segal, en Paola Zanovello. 2003. L-arginine metabolism in myeloid cells controls T-lymphocyte functions. *Trends in Immunology* 24, no. 6 (juni): 302-306.

Burnet, M. 1957. Cancer; a biological approach. I. The processes of control. *British Medical Journal* 1, no. 5022 (april 6): 779-786.

Cattaruzza, Lara, Annunziata Gloghini, Karin Olivo, Raffaele Di Francia, Debora Lorenzon, Rosaria De Filippi, Antonino Carbone, Alfonso Colombatti, Antonio Pinto, en Donatella Aldinucci. 2009. Functional coexpression of Interleukin (IL)-7 and its receptor (IL-7R) on Hodgkin and Reed-Sternberg cells: Involvement of IL-7 in tumor cell growth and microenvironmental interactions of Hodgkin's lymphoma. *International Journal of Cancer. Journal International Du Cancer* 125, no. 5 (september 1): 1092-1101. doi:10.1002/ijc.24389.

Claassen, E. 1992. Post-formation fluorescent labelling of liposomal membranes. In vivo detection, localisation and kinetics. *Journal of Immunological Methods* 147, no. 2 (maart 4): 231-240.

Colotta, Francesco, Paola Allavena, Antonio Sica, Cecilia Garlanda, en Alberto Mantovani. 2009. Cancer-related inflammation, the seventh hallmark of cancer: links to genetic instability. *Carcinogenesis* 30, no. 7 (juli): 1073-1081. doi:10.1093/carcin/bgp127.

Coussens, Lisa M, en Zena Werb. 2002. Inflammation and cancer. *Nature* 420, no. 6917 (december 19): 860-867. doi:10.1038/nature01322.

DeLong, Peter, Richard G Carroll, Adam C Henry, Tomoyuki Tanaka, Sajjad Ahmad, Michael S Leibowitz, Daniel H Sterman, Carl H June, Steven M Albelda, en Robert H Vonderheide. 2005. Regulatory T cells and cytokines in malignant pleural effusions secondary to mesothelioma and carcinoma. *Cancer Biology & Therapy* 4, no. 3 (maart): 342-346.

Dunn, Gavin P, Lloyd J Old, en Robert D Schreiber. 2004. The immunobiology of cancer immunosurveillance and immunoediting. *Immunity* 21, no. 2 (augustus): 137-148. doi:10.1016/j.immuni.2004.07.017.

Edelman, Martin J, Dee Watson, Xiaofei Wang, Carl Morrison, Robert A Kratzke, Scott Jewell, Lydia Hodgson, e.a. 2008. Eicosanoid modulation in advanced lung cancer: cyclooxygenase-2 expression is a positive predictive factor for celecoxib + chemotherapy--Cancer and Leukemia Group B Trial 30203. *Journal of Clinical Oncology: Official Journal of the American Society of Clinical Oncology* 26, no. 6 (februari 20): 848-855. doi:10.1200/JCO.2007.13.8081.

Fallarino, Francesca, Ursula Grohmann, Kwang Woo Hwang, Ciriana Orabona, Carmine Vacca, Roberta Bianchi, Maria Laura Belladonna, Maria Cristina Fioretti, Maria-Luisa Alegre, en Paolo Puccetti. 2003. Modulation of tryptophan catabolism by regulatory T cells. *Nature Immunology* 4, no. 12 (december): 1206-1212. doi:10.1038/ni1003.

Fassbender, Melanie, Bastian Gerlitzki, Nina Ullrich, Corinna Lupp, Matthias Klein, Markus P Radsak, Edgar Schmitt, Tobias Bopp, en Hansjörg Schild. 2010. Cyclic adenosine monophosphate and IL-10 coordinately contribute to nTreg cell-mediated suppression of dendritic cell activation. *Cellular Immunology* 265, no. 2: 91-96. doi:10.1016/j.cellimm.2010.07.007.

Fecci, Peter E, Hidenobu Ochiai, Duane A Mitchell, Peter M Grossi, Alison E Sweeney, Gary E Archer, Thomas Cummings, James P Allison, Darell D Bigner, en John H Sampson. 2007. Systemic CTLA-4 blockade ameliorates glioma-induced changes to the CD4+ T cell compartment without affecting regulatory T-cell function. *Clinical Cancer Research: An Official Journal of the American Association for Cancer Research* 13, no. 7 (april 1): 2158-2167. doi:10.1158/1078-0432.CCR-06-2070.

Gabrilovich, Dmitry I, Vincenzo Bronte, Shu-Hsia Chen, Mario P Colombo, Augusto Ochoa, Suzanne Ostrand-Rosenberg, en Hans Schreiber. 2007. The terminology issue for myeloid-derived suppressor cells. *Cancer Research* 67, no. 1 (januari 1): 425; author reply 426. doi:10.1158/0008-5472.CAN-06-3037.

Gabrilovich, Dmitry I, en Srinivas Nagaraj. 2009. Myeloid-derived suppressor cells as regulators of the immune system. *Nature Reviews. Immunology* 9, no. 3 (maart): 162-174. doi:10.1038/nri2506.

Garín, Marina I, Chung-Ching Chu, Dela Golshayan, Eva Cernuda-Morollón, Robin Wait, en Robert I Lechler. 2007. Galectin-1: a key effector of regulation mediated by CD4+CD25+ T cells. *Blood* 109, no. 5 (maart 1): 2058-2065. doi:10.1182/blood-2006-04-016451.

Ghiringhelli, François, Cedric Menard, Pierre Emmanuel Puig, Sylvain Ladoire, Stephan Roux, François Martin, Eric Solary, Axel Le Cesne, Laurence Zitvogel, en Bruno Chauffert. 2007. Metronomic cyclophosphamide regimen selectively depletes CD4+CD25+ regulatory T cells and restores T and NK effector functions in end stage cancer patients. *Cancer Immunology, Immunotherapy: CII* 56, no. 5 (mei): 641-648. doi:10.1007/s00262-006-0225-8.

Ghiringhelli, François, Cédric Ménard, Magali Terme, Caroline Flament, Julien Taieb, Nathalie Chaput, Pierre E Puig, e.a. 2005. CD4+CD25+ regulatory T cells inhibit natural killer cell functions in a transforming growth factor-beta-dependent manner. *The Journal of Experimental Medicine* 202, no. 8 (oktober 17): 1075-1085. doi:10.1084/jem.20051511.

Gondek, David C, Li-Fan Lu, Sergio A Quezada, Shimon Sakaguchi, en Randolph J Noelle. 2005. Cutting edge: contact-mediated suppression by CD4+CD25+ regulatory cells involves a granzyme B-dependent, perforin-independent mechanism. *Journal of Immunology (Baltimore, Md.: 1950)* 174, no. 4 (februari 15): 1783-1786.

Grohmann, Ursula, Francesca Fallarino, en Paolo Puccetti. 2003. Tolerance, DCs and tryptophan: much ado about IDO. *Trends in Immunology* 24, no. 5 (mei): 242-248.

Hanson, Erica M, Virginia K Clements, Pratima Sinha, Dan Ilkovitch, en Suzanne Ostrand-Rosenberg. 2009. Myeloid-derived suppressor cells down-regulate L-selectin expression on CD4+ and CD8+ T cells. *Journal of Immunology (Baltimore, Md.: 1950)* 183, no. 2 (juli 15): 937-944. doi:10.4049/jimmunol.0804253.

Hawrylowicz, C M, en A O'Garra. 2005. Potential role of interleukin-10-secreting regulatory T cells in allergy and asthma. *Nature Reviews. Immunology* 5, no. 4 (april): 271-283. doi:10.1038/nri1589.

Hegmans, J. P. J. J. 2005. Immunotherapy of Murine Malignant Mesothelioma Using Tumor Lysate-pulsed Dendritic Cells. *American Journal of Respiratory and Critical Care Medicine* 171, no. 10 (februari): 1168-1177. doi:10.1164/rccm.200501-057OC.

Hegmans, Joost P, Joris D Veltman, Margaretha E Lambers, I Jolanda M de Vries, Carl G Figdor, Rudi W Hendriks, Henk C Hoogsteden, Bart N Lambrecht, en Joachim G Aerts. 2010. Consolidative dendritic cell-based immunotherapy elicits cytotoxicity against malignant mesothelioma. *American Journal of Respiratory and Critical Care Medicine* 181, no. 12 (juni 15): 1383-1390. doi:10.1164/rccm.200909-1465OC.

Hillegass, Jedd M, Arti Shukla, Sherrill A Lathrop, Maximilian B MacPherson, Stacie L Beuschel, Kelly J Butnor, Joseph R Testa, e.a. 2010. Inflammation precedes the development of human malignant mesotheliomas in a SCID mouse xenograft model. *Annals of the New York Academy of Sciences* 1203 (augustus): 7-14. doi:10.1111/j.1749-6632.2010.05554.x.

Huang, Bo, Ping-Ying Pan, Qingsheng Li, Alice I Sato, David E Levy, Jonathan Bromberg, Celia M Divino, en Shu-Hsia Chen. 2006. Gr-1+CD115+ immature myeloid suppressor cells mediate the development of tumor-induced T regulatory cells and T-cell anergy in tumor-bearing host. *Cancer Research* 66, no. 2 (januari 15): 1123-1131. doi:10.1158/0008-5472.CAN-05-1299.

Jonuleit, H, E Schmitt, G Schuler, J Knop, en A H Enk. 2000. Induction of interleukin 10-producing, nonproliferating CD4(+) T cells with regulatory properties by repetitive stimulation with allogeneic immature human dendritic cells. *The Journal of Experimental Medicine* 192, no. 9 (november 6): 1213-1222.

Kantoff, Philip W, Celestia S Higano, Neal D Shore, E Roy Berger, Eric J Small, David F Penson, Charles H Redfern, e.a. 2010. Sipuleucel-T immunotherapy for castration-resistant prostate cancer. *The New England Journal of Medicine* 363, no. 5 (juli 29): 411-422. doi:10.1056/NEJMoa1001294.

Klein, J J, A L Goldstein, en A White. 1966. Effects of the thymus lymphocytopoietic factor. *Annals of the New York Academy of Sciences* 135, no. 1 (januari 26): 485-495.

Ko, Kuibeom, Sayuri Yamazaki, Kyoko Nakamura, Tomohisa Nishioka, Keiji Hirota, Tomoyuki Yamaguchi, Jun Shimizu, Takashi Nomura, Tsutomu Chiba, en Shimon Sakaguchi. 2005. Treatment of advanced tumors with agonistic anti-GITR mAb and its effects on tumor-infiltrating Foxp3+CD25+CD4+ regulatory T cells. *The Journal of Experimental Medicine* 202, no. 7 (oktober 3): 885-891. doi:10.1084/jem.20050940.

Kryczek, Ilona, Shuang Wei, Linhua Zou, Gefeng Zhu, Peter Mottram, Huanbin Xu, Lieping Chen, en Weiping Zou. 2006. Cutting edge: induction of B7-H4 on APCs through

IL-10: novel suppressive mode for regulatory T cells. *Journal of Immunology (Baltimore, Md.: 1950)* 177, no. 1 (juli 1): 40-44.

Kryczek, Ilona, Linhua Zou, Paulo Rodriguez, Gefeng Zhu, Shuang Wei, Peter Mottram, Michael Brumlik, e.a. 2006. B7-H4 expression identifies a novel suppressive macrophage population in human ovarian carcinoma. *The Journal of Experimental Medicine* 203, no. 4 (april 17): 871-881. doi:10.1084/jem.20050930.

Kusmartsev, Sergei, en Dmitry I Gabrilovich. 2006. Role of immature myeloid cells in mechanisms of immune evasion in cancer. *Cancer Immunology, Immunotherapy: CII* 55, no. 3 (maart): 237-245. doi:10.1007/s00262-005-0048-z.

Kusmartsev, Sergei, Yulia Nefedova, Daniel Yoder, en Dmitry I Gabrilovich. 2004. Antigen-specific inhibition of CD8+ T cell response by immature myeloid cells in cancer is mediated by reactive oxygen species. *Journal of Immunology (Baltimore, Md.: 1950)* 172, no. 2 (januari 15): 989-999.

Larmonier, Nicolas, Marilyn Marron, Yi Zeng, Jessica Cantrell, Angela Romanoski, Marjan Sepassi, Sylvia Thompson, Xinchun Chen, Samita Andreansky, en Emmanuel Katsanis. 2007. Tumor-derived CD4(+)CD25(+) regulatory T cell suppression of dendritic cell function involves TGF-beta and IL-10. *Cancer Immunology, Immunotherapy: CII* 56, no. 1 (januari): 48-59. doi:10.1007/s00262-006-0160-8.

Lee, Soo Sun, Wenda Gao, Silvia Mazzola, Michael N Thomas, Eva Csizmadia, Leo E Otterbein, Fritz H Bach, en Hongjun Wang. 2007. Heme oxygenase-1, carbon monoxide, and bilirubin induce tolerance in recipients toward islet allografts by modulating T regulatory cells. *The FASEB Journal: Official Publication of the Federation of American Societies for Experimental Biology* 21, no. 13 (november): 3450-3457. doi:10.1096/fj.07-8472com.

Li, Hequan, Yanmei Han, Qiuli Guo, Minggang Zhang, en Xuetao Cao. 2009. Cancer-expanded myeloid-derived suppressor cells induce anergy of NK cells through membrane-bound TGF-beta 1. *Journal of Immunology (Baltimore, Md.: 1950)* 182, no. 1 (januari 1): 240-249.

Madan, Ravi A, James L Gulley, Tito Fojo, en William L Dahut. 2010. Therapeutic cancer vaccines in prostate cancer: the paradox of improved survival without changes in time to progression. *The Oncologist* 15, no. 9: 969-975. doi:10.1634/theoncologist.2010-0129.

Mantovani, Alberto, Paola Allavena, Antonio Sica, en Frances Balkwill. 2008. Cancer-related inflammation. *Nature* 454, no. 7203 (juli): 436-444. doi:10.1038/nature07205.

Mantovani, Alberto, en Antonio Sica. 2010. Macrophages, innate immunity and cancer: balance, tolerance, and diversity. *Current Opinion in Immunology* 22, no. 2 (april): 231-237. doi:10.1016/j.coi.2010.01.009.

Mantovani, Alberto, Tiziana Schioppa, Chiara Porta, Paola Allavena, en Antonio Sica. 2006. Role of tumor-associated macrophages in tumor progression and invasion. *Cancer Metastasis Reviews* 25, no. 3 (september): 315-322. doi:10.1007/s10555-006-9001-7.

Mantovani, Alberto, Silvano Sozzani, Massimo Locati, Paola Allavena, en Antonio Sica. 2002. Macrophage polarization: tumor-associated macrophages as a paradigm for polarized M2 mononuclear phagocytes. *Trends in Immunology* 23, no. 11 (november): 549-555.

Mazzucchelli, Renata, Julie A Hixon, Rosanne Spolski, Xin Chen, Wen Qing Li, Veronica L Hall, Jami Willette-Brown, Arthur A Hurwitz, Warren J Leonard, en Scott K

Durum. 2008. Development of regulatory T cells requires IL-7Ralpha stimulation by IL-7 or TSLP. *Blood* 112, no. 8 (oktober 15): 3283-3292. doi:10.1182/blood-2008-02-137414.

Nagaraj, Srinivas, en Dmitry I Gabrilovich. 2007. Myeloid-derived suppressor cells. *Advances in Experimental Medicine and Biology* 601: 213-223.

Nagaraj, S. & Gabrilovich, D.I., 2008. Tumor escape mechanism governed by myeloid-derived suppressor cells. *Cancer Research*, 68(8), pp.2561-2563.

Nair, Smita, David Boczkowski, Martin Fassnacht, David Pisetsky, en Eli Gilboa. 2007. Vaccination against the forkhead family transcription factor Foxp3 enhances tumor immunity. *Cancer Research* 67, no. 1 (januari 1): 371-380. doi:10.1158/0008-5472.CAN-06-2903.

Nakamura, K, A Kitani, en W Strober. 2001. Cell contact-dependent immunosuppression by CD4(+)CD25(+) regulatory T cells is mediated by cell surface-bound transforming growth factor beta. *The Journal of Experimental Medicine* 194, no. 5 (september 3): 629-644.

Oderup, Cecilia, Lukas Cederbom, Anna Makowska, Corrado M Cilio, en Fredrik Ivars. 2006. Cytotoxic T lymphocyte antigen-4-dependent down-modulation of costimulatory molecules on dendritic cells in CD4+ CD25+ regulatory T-cell-mediated suppression. *Immunology* 118, no. 2 (juni): 240-249. doi:10.1111/j.1365-2567.2006.02362.x.

Old, L J, en E A Boyse. 1964. Immunology of experimenal tumors. *Annual Review of Medicine* 15: 167-186. doi:10.1146/annurev.me.15.020164.001123.

Onishi, Yasushi, Zoltan Fehervari, Tomoyuki Yamaguchi, en Shimon Sakaguchi. 2008. Foxp3+ natural regulatory T cells preferentially form aggregates on dendritic cells in vitro and actively inhibit their maturation. *Proceedings of the National Academy of Sciences of the United States of America* 105, no. 29 (juli 22): 10113-10118. doi:10.1073/pnas.0711106105.

Ormandy, Lars A, Tina Hillemann, Heiner Wedemeyer, Michael P Manns, Tim F Greten, en Firouzeh Korangy. 2005. Increased populations of regulatory T cells in peripheral blood of patients with hepatocellular carcinoma. *Cancer Research* 65, no. 6 (maart 15): 2457-2464. doi:10.1158/0008-5472.CAN-04-3232.

Pan, Ping-Ying, Ge Ma, Kaare J Weber, Junko Ozao-Choy, George Wang, Bingjiao Yin, Celia M Divino, en Shu-Hsia Chen. 2010. Immune stimulatory receptor CD40 is required for T-cell suppression and T regulatory cell activation mediated by myeloid-derived suppressor cells in cancer. *Cancer Research* 70, no. 1 (januari 1): 99-108. doi:10.1158/0008-5472.CAN-09-1882.

Phan, Giao Q, James C Yang, Richard M Sherry, Patrick Hwu, Suzanne L Topalian, Douglas J Schwartzentruber, Nicholas P Restifo, e.a. 2003. Cancer regression and autoimmunity induced by cytotoxic T lymphocyte-associated antigen 4 blockade in patients with metastatic melanoma. *Proceedings of the National Academy of Sciences of the United States of America* 100, no. 14 (juli 8): 8372-8377. doi:10.1073/pnas.1533209100.

Powell, Daniel J, Jr, Aloisio Felipe-Silva, Maria J Merino, Mojgan Ahmadzadeh, Tamika Allen, Catherine Levy, Donald E White, e.a. 2007. Administration of a CD25-directed immunotoxin, LMB-2, to patients with metastatic melanoma induces a selective partial reduction in regulatory T cells in vivo. *Journal of Immunology (Baltimore, Md.: 1950)* 179, no. 7 (oktober 1): 4919-4928.

Rodríguez, Paulo C, en Augusto C Ochoa. 2008. Arginine regulation by myeloid derived suppressor cells and tolerance in cancer: mechanisms and therapeutic perspectives. *Immunological Reviews* 222 (april): 180-191. doi:10.1111/j.1600-065X.2008.00608.x.

Rooney, C M, C A Smith, C Y Ng, S K Loftin, J W Sixbey, Y Gan, D K Srivastava, e.a. 1998. Infusion of cytotoxic T cells for the prevention and treatment of Epstein-Barr virus-induced lymphoma in allogeneic transplant recipients. *Blood* 92, no. 5 (september 1): 1549-1555.

de la Rosa, Maurus, Sascha Rutz, Heike Dorninger, en Alexander Scheffold. 2004. Interleukin-2 is essential for CD4+CD25+ regulatory T cell function. *European Journal of Immunology* 34, no. 9 (september): 2480-2488. doi:10.1002/eji.200425274.

Rosenberg, Steven A, Claude Sportès, Mojgan Ahmadzadeh, Terry J Fry, Lien T Ngo, Susan L Schwarz, Maryalice Stetler-Stevenson, e.a. 2006. IL-7 administration to humans leads to expansion of CD8+ and CD4+ cells but a relative decrease of CD4+ T-regulatory cells. *Journal of Immunotherapy (Hagerstown, Md.: 1997)* 29, no. 3 (juni): 313-319. doi:10.1097/01.cji.0000210386.55951.c2.

Ruddle, J B, C A Harper, D Hönemann, J F Seymour, en H M Prince. 2006. A denileukin diftitox (Ontak) associated retinopathy? *The British Journal of Ophthalmology* 90, no. 8 (augustus): 1070-1071. doi:10.1136/bjo.2006.091165.

Sakaguchi, Shimon, Kajsa Wing, Yasushi Onishi, Paz Prieto-Martin, en Tomoyuki Yamaguchi. 2009. Regulatory T cells: how do they suppress immune responses? *International Immunology* 21, no. 10 (oktober): 1105-1111. doi:10.1093/intimm/dxp095.

Sica, Antonio, Tiziana Schioppa, Alberto Mantovani, en Paola Allavena. 2006. Tumour-associated macrophages are a distinct M2 polarised population promoting tumour progression: potential targets of anti-cancer therapy. *European Journal of Cancer (Oxford, England: 1990)* 42, no. 6 (april): 717-727. doi:10.1016/j.ejca.2006.01.003.

Sinha, Pratima, Virginia K Clements, Amy M Fulton, en Suzanne Ostrand-Rosenberg. 2007. Prostaglandin E2 promotes tumor progression by inducing myeloid-derived suppressor cells. *Cancer Research* 67, no. 9 (mei 1): 4507-4513. doi:10.1158/0008-5472.CAN-06-4174.

Srivastava, Minu K, Pratima Sinha, Virginia K Clements, Paulo Rodriguez, en Suzanne Ostrand-Rosenberg. 2010. Myeloid-derived suppressor cells inhibit T-cell activation by depleting cystine and cysteine. *Cancer Research* 70, no. 1 (januari 1): 68-77. doi:10.1158/0008-5472.CAN-09-2587.

Steinman, R M, B Gutchinov, M D Witmer, en M C Nussenzweig. 1983. Dendritic cells are the principal stimulators of the primary mixed leukocyte reaction in mice. *The Journal of Experimental Medicine* 157, no. 2 (februari 1): 613-627.

Strauss, Laura, Theresa L Whiteside, Ashley Knights, Christoph Bergmann, Alexander Knuth, en Alfred Zippelius. 2007. Selective survival of naturally occurring human CD4+CD25+Foxp3+ regulatory T cells cultured with rapamycin. *Journal of Immunology (Baltimore, Md.: 1950)* 178, no. 1 (januari 1): 320-329.

Strieter, Robert M, John A Belperio, Roderick J Phillips, en Michael P Keane. 2004. CXC chemokines in angiogenesis of cancer. *Seminars in Cancer Biology* 14, no. 3 (juni): 195-200. doi:10.1016/j.semcancer.2003.10.006.

Tadokoro, Carlos E, Guy Shakhar, Shiqian Shen, Yi Ding, Andreia C Lino, Antonio Maraver, Juan J Lafaille, en Michael L Dustin. 2006. Regulatory T cells inhibit stable contacts between CD4+ T cells and dendritic cells in vivo. *The Journal of Experimental Medicine* 203, no. 3 (maart 20): 505-511. doi:10.1084/jem.20050783.

Thornton, A M, en E M Shevach. 1998. CD4+CD25+ immunoregulatory T cells suppress polyclonal T cell activation in vitro by inhibiting interleukin 2 production. *The Journal of Experimental Medicine* 188, no. 2 (juli 20): 287-296.

Veltman, J D, M E H Lambers, M van Nimwegen, R W Hendriks, H C Hoogsteden, J P J J Hegmans, en J G J V Aerts. 2010. Zoledronic acid impairs myeloid differentiation to tumour-associated macrophages in mesothelioma. *British Journal of Cancer* 103, no. 5 (juli): 629-641. doi:10.1038/sj.bjc.6605814.

Veltman, J. D, M. E.H Lambers, M. van Nimwegen, R. W Hendriks, H. C Hoogsteden, J. G.J.V Aerts, en J. P.J.J Hegmans. 2010. COX-2 inhibition improves immunotherapy and is associated with decreased numbers of myeloid-derived suppressor cells in mesothelioma. *BMC cancer* 10, no. 1: 464.

Veltman, Joris D, Margaretha E H Lambers, Menno van Nimwegen, Sanne de Jong, Rudi W Hendriks, Henk C Hoogsteden, Joachim G J V Aerts, en Joost P J J Hegmans. 2010. Low-dose cyclophosphamide synergizes with dendritic cell-based immunotherapy in antitumor activity. *Journal of Biomedicine & Biotechnology* 2010: 798467. doi:10.1155/2010/798467.

Wei, Shuang, Ilona Kryczek, en Weiping Zou. 2006. Regulatory T-cell compartmentalization and trafficking. *Blood* 108, no. 2 (juli 15): 426-431. doi:10.1182/blood-2006-01-0177.

Zha, Shan, Vasan Yegnasubramanian, William G Nelson, William B Isaacs, en Angelo M De Marzo. 2004. Cyclooxygenases in cancer: progress and perspective. *Cancer Letters* 215, no. 1 (november 8): 1-20. doi:10.1016/j.canlet.2004.06.014.

9

Connexin 43 Enhances the Cisplatin-Induced Cytotoxicity in Mesothelioma Cells

Hiromi Sato and Koichi Ueno

Graduate School of Pharmaceutical Sciences, Chiba University
Japan

1. Introduction

The direct cell-to-cell communication is performed by gap junctions (GJ) composed of connexin (Cx), a large protein family with a number of subtypes. GJ channels allow the propagation of electrical impulse and the transfer of small molecules (up to 1,000 to 1,500 Da) between two neighbouring cells (Figure 1). And it has also become clear that different combination of Cxs are expressed in different tissues with temporal specificity during development or tissue differentiation (Paul, 1995). By such a rigid regulation, Cxs contribute to maintain cellular homeostasis in many organs. On the contrary, expression levels of Cx proteins are often decreased in many cancers, and restoring their levels has been shown to have antitumor effects. In this concept, there is a possibility to establish a new cancer therapy based on tumor-suppressive functions of Cxs for refractory cancers, such as mesothelioma.

Malignant mesothelioma is an aggressive and devastating malignancy of the pleura and peritoneum. Although it has been the subject of intense clinical and scientific interest, the case-fatality rate for mesothelioma remains high, and conventional treatments remain inadequate. Systemic chemotherapy is important since it is a whole-body treatment and is useful for patients who cannot be treated with surgery. Cisplatin (CDDP) has been used in clinical mesothelioma therapy, and its chemotherapeutic effect as a single agent (Ryan et al, 1998) as well as in combination with other drugs such as gemcitabine has been examined (Byrne et al, 1999; van Haarst et al, 2002; Vogelzang et al, 2003).

In this chapter, we introduce the tumor-suppressive effect of Cx gene against mesothelioma, especially with regard to chemotherapeutical sensitivity.

2. The possible involvement of Cx43 in mesothelioma

GJ channels are formed by two hemichannels provided by either of neighboring cells. Each hemichannel is a hexameric pore structure made from 6 protein subunits, Cxs. Cx is a protein with four transmembrane spanning domain, two extracellular and one intracellular loop, and N- and C-terminal at the intracellular side (Kumar & Gilula, 1996). The various Cx isoforms differ with regard to their molecular weight due to different length of their C-terminal region. There are 21 Cx morecules which were identified in human so far. With regard to mesothelioma, dysfunction of gap junctional intercellular communication (GJIC) has been observed in several malignant mesotheliomas cells or tissues (Linnainmaa et al, 1993), and among the many Cx proteins, Cx43 is prominently expressed in nontumorigenic mesothelial tissues (Pelin et al, 1994). Besides that, we found that Cx43 expression was very low in human malignant mesothelioma cells (Figure 2A, left). We also examined GJIC ability using fluorescent dye, Lucifer yellow. The molecular size of Lucifer yellow is small enough to pass through GJ, so the spreading distance of this dye tells the GJIC ability (el-Fouly, 1987). By using this method, it became clear that GJIC function was almot dysfunctional in mesothelioma cells (Figure 2B, above). Taken together, it seems that Cx43 has an important role in the parental mesothelial cells and upregulation of Cx43 could reduce malignancy of mesothelioma.

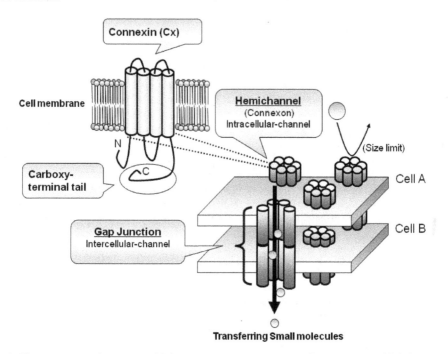

Fig. 1. The structure of connexin (Cx) protein as a component of gap junction (GJ), hemi-channel, and as a membrane protein.

Gap junctions (GJ) provide a pathway for communication between neighboring cells. GJ are organized in plaques at the cell membrane surface and arise from 2 connexons (hemichannels) from neighboring cells. Connexons are composed of 6 connexin (Cx) proteins. GJ channels can be permeable to only small molecules (around 1,000 Da), which contribute to keep cellular homeostasis. It has been suggested that the down-regulation of Cx genes is associated with the development of cancers. Besides GJ, hemichannels provide a pathway for the extracellular release of essential homeostasis regulators, like ATP. Moreover, carboxy-terminal (C-tail) of Cx protein has a possibility to modulate gene expression via binding proteins, which can be also modulated by other proteins. Ex) C-tail of Cx43 includes target sites of Src phosphorylation (Giepmans, 2004)

3. Effect of Cx43 mono-therapy

Recent studies have suggested that not all Cx genes could exert a tumor-suppressive effect on a given tumor but rather than that there seems to be Cx-cell type compatibility for this effect (Yano et al, 2006, as cited in Mesnil et al, 1995). That means Cx can exert growth control only in tissue or cell type in which the particular Cx is naturally expressed. Indeed, overexpression of Cx43 in MDA-MB-231 cells results in downregulation of fibroblast growth factor receptor (FGFR)-3, a member of the FGFR family consisting of potent angiogenic factors, which contribute tumor growth and invasion (Qin et al, 2002). According to this concept, we previously investigated the tumor suppressive role of Cx32 in renal cell carcinoma, in which Cx32 expression is downregulated (Yano et al, 2003), using a forced expression clone of Cx32. As expected, we found that Cx32 acts as a tumor suppressor gene in renal carcinoma cells (Fujimoto et al, 2005).

Here, in order to estimate if Cx43 could suppress malignant phenotype of mesothelioma cells, we arranged a Cx43 transfected clone (Cx43 transfectant) and only mock-tranfected clone (mock), as a control. Naive cell characteristics were compared between Cx43 transfectant and mock. As expected, when attached condition, the growth was significantly inhibited by Cx43 (Figure 2C-i). Next, to examine anchorage-independent growth, the

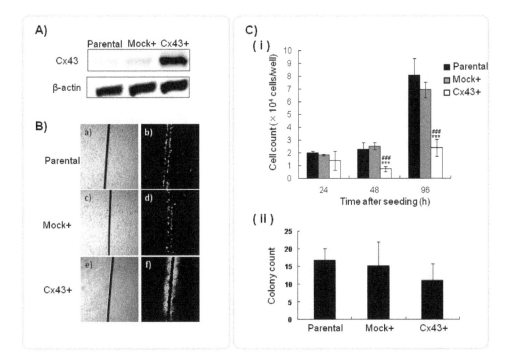

Fig. 2. The naïve role of Cx43 on human mesothelioma cells.
A) and **B)** show characteristics of mesothelioma cells. Cx43 expression **A)** and GJIC activity **B)** in human mesothelioma cells, parental H28 ('Parental'), mock-transfectant ('Mock+'), and

Cx43-transfectant ('Cx43+') are shown. **a)**, **c)**, and **e)**; phase-contrast image, **b)**, **d)**, and **f)**; dye transfer of Lucifer yellow from the scrape lines. **C)** indicates effect of Cx43 on cell growth **i)** when attached condition or **ii)** when non-attached (anchorage independent) condition . Scale shows cell number **(i)** or colony number **(ii)**. Cell growth was significantly inhibited when attached condition in Cx43-transfectant compared to parental (###P <0.001) or mock cells (***P <0.001).

number of cell colonies formed in three-dimentional agarose gels were countted. This time, however, there was almost no difference between cells (Figure 2C-ii). This finding indicates that the proliferation ability of a single cell, which is needed for survival in a nonmatrix environment, is almost the same between different cell types used in this study. There was also no difference in migration ability (data not shown). One possible reason why restoration of Cx43 could not inhibit cell growth enough is disruption of Cx protein traffiking systems. To put it plainly, Cx protein can not be transported from nucleus to cytoplasmic membrane. Under abnormal localization of Cx protein traffiking, Cxs could not exert tumor suppressive effect neither in GJIC dependent or independent manner, although the reason why it happens is unclear (Trosko & Ruch, 2002). Above all, it is suggested that restoring Cx43 expression alone cannot prevent tumor expansion or metastasis competely.

4. Combination effect of Cx43 and CDDP

As mentioned, mesothelioma is very refractory cancer. Radiotherapy and chemotherapeutic agents are ineffective in many cases despite surgery resection is possible only in case the tumor is very early stage or it is very limited focus. Recently, pemetrexed, a novel multitargeted antifolate, has shown modest activity when used as a single agent and in combination with CDDP in mesothelioma patients. However, although pemetrexed is promising, it has yet to be standardized because of the severity of its side effects and the presence of nonresponders. On the other hand, there are several reports of enhancement efficacy of conventional chemotherapy on cancers by Cxs, which are called bystander effect. Actually, we have reported that cytotoxic effects of conventional chemotherapeutic agents on cancer cells are potentiated by Cx32 in lung cancer (Sato et al, 2007a) and renal cell carcinoma (Sato et al, 2007b). Moreover, Cx43-mediated GJIC has been reported as a major mechanism for the transfer of ganciclovir (nucleoside analogue) to neighboring cells (Elshami et al, 1996). Therefore, we examined the combined effect of Cx43 and a chemotherapeutic agent, CDDP.

4.1 Cx43-dependent induction of the CDDP cytotoxicity

As expected, it was confirmed that mesothelioma cells were resistant to CDDP; approximately 80% of cells survived after exposure to high concentrations of CDDP (Fighure 3A). In contrast, Cx43 reduced cell viability and only approximately half of the mesothelioma cells or mock cells survived after being treated with 50 μM of CDDP (Figure 3A). To confirm the contribution of Cx43 to the enhancement of CDDP-induced damage, we knocked down Cx43 expression by using specific siRNA. As a result, sensitivity to CDDP was attenuated by knockdown of Cx43 (Figure 3B); therefore the involvement of Cx43 in CDDP-induced damage was confirmed.

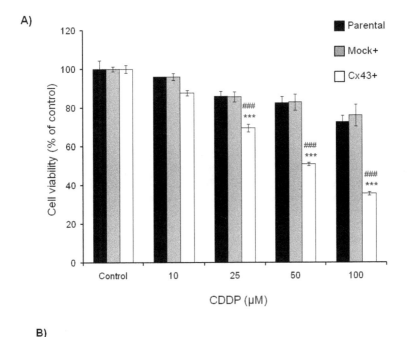

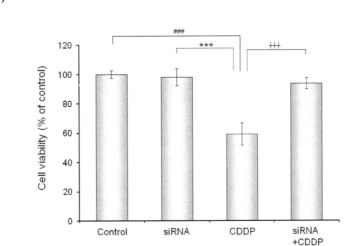

Fig. 3. Effect of Cx43 on CDDP-induced cytotoxicity.
A) shows CDDP cytotoxicic effect on human mesothelioma cells, parental H28 ('Parental'), mock-transfectant ('Mock+'), and Cx43-transfectant ('Cx43+'). The cell viability after CDDP treatment was significantly decreased in Cx43-transfectant compared with parental cells (###P <0.001) or mock cells (***P <0.001). **B)** shows effect of Cx43-knockdown on Cx43-transfectant cell growth after CDDP treatment. The cell viability in cells co-treated with siRNA and CDDP ('siRNA+CDDP') recovered to control level. ###, ***, and +++ P <0.001; Significant differences compared with only treated with CDDP group ('CDDP').

4.2 Molecular mechanism of Cx43 which contributes to the CDDP cytotoxicity

Here, it is confirmed that Cx43 significantly enhances CDDP growth inhibiting effect and apoptosis might be induced, that is, Cx43 upregulates the sensitivity to CDDP in mesothelioma cells. Then considering the involvement of GJIC, molecular mecahnism of this phenomenon was investigated via cell cycle distribution, apoptotic factors, and Src which could interact with Cx43 protein.

4.2.1 Gap junction dependent manner

To determine the influence of GJIC on CDDP-induced cytotoxicity, we usede a GJ blocker, 18β-glycyrrhetinic acid (GA). After 4 h of culturing with GA, CDDP treatment followed, then cell viability was determined using WST-1 Reagent. As a result of Lucifer yellow dye spreading assay, GJIC inhibiting effect by GA was observed in Cx43-transfectant (Figure 4A). However, such inhibition of GJIC had almost no effect on cell viability detected by WST-1 assay (Figure 4B). Thus, inhibition of GJ-dependent function with a specific inhibitor did not abrogate CDDP-induced cytotoxicity. These results suggest that Cx43-mediated enhancement of cytotoxicity might be independent of GJ function.

On the other hand, there are several reports concerning the relation of GJIC and CDDP cytotoxicity. One of the previous reports suggests a posibility that CDDP could affect GJIC, it might be regulated by MAP kinase-dependent phosphorylation of specific sites of Cx43 (Procházka et al, 2007). Because it is known that CDDP toxicity is modulated by a MAP kinase pathway besides the established mechanisms (Park et al, 2002; Woessmann et al, 2002) and that Cxs are regulated by multiple mechanisms, including MAP kinase dependent phosphorylation (Jo et al, 2005; Lampe & Lau, 2004; Wang et al, 2000). Procházka et al showed a new platinum complex, LA-12, had strong GJIC inhibiting effect (Procházka et al, 2007). They also found the inhibitory effect of GJIC was induced by hyperphosphorylation of Cx43 protein which decrease the localization of cell membrane, which correlated with activation of MAP kinase pathway proteins. On the other hand CDDP exerted only a low effect on GJIC though the drug caused activation of MAP kinase protein (Procházka et al, 2007). Another report which supports Procházka et al showed that Cx43 level was elevated in CDDP- resistant cell line (Li et al, 2007). Li et al indicated the conflicting reports in which the role of Cxs in cell survival were different; in case GJ component protein, they have been implicated the bystander effect, but Cx43 protein itself has also been shown to be important in cell survival, although this function is poor characterized. They also suggested that although the selection of CDDP resistance might have favored cells that expressed high level of Cx43, continued expression of this gene might decrease drug resistance by promoting a bystander effect, and finally concluded that Cx43 played a role in drug sensitivity in any case (Li et al, 2007). Meanwhile other reports showed that compounds like CDDP suppressed intercellular communication (Jo et al, 2005; Wang et al, 2000).

Taken together, it is still unclear if GJIC involves to the enhanced effect of CDDP by Cx43. Further investigation of this concern which magnify more elaborate apoptotic pathway field will be needed.

4.2.2 Gap junction independent manner

In this section, several factors which probably concern the mecahnism of Cx43 induced cytotoxicity of CDDP are suggested irrespective of GJIC.

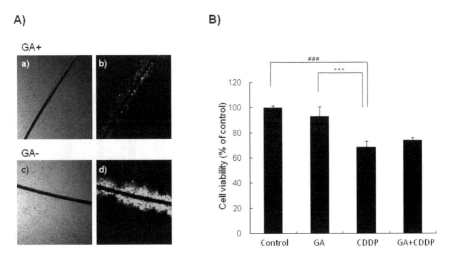

Fig. 4. Effect of GJ blockade on CDDP-induced cytotoxicity.
A); GJ inhibitor (GA) downregulated GJIC in Cx43-transfectant. 'GA+'; cells treated with GA for 4 h, 'GA-'; cells treated with only 0.1%dimethylsulfoxide (DMSO, vehicle for GA). a) and c); phase-contrast image, b) and d); dye transfer of Lucifer yellow from the scraped lines. B); Cell viability after CDDP treatment in Cx43-transfectant was detected by WST-1 assay. Downregulating effect of CDDP did not recover by pre-treamtent of GA 4 h. 'Control'; cells treated with only 0.1% DMSO (vehicle for CDDP), 'GA'; cells pre-treated with GA for 4 h followed 0.1% DMSO treatment for 48 h, 'CDDP'; cells treated with only CDDP for 48 h, and 'GA+CDDP'; cells pre-treated with GA for 4 h followed CDDP treatment for 48 h. ###$P <$ 0.001; Significant difference between 'Control' and 'CDDP', ***$P <$0.001; significant difference between 'GA' and 'CDDP'.

4.2.2.1 Regulation of cell cycle distribution by Cx43

We also checked cell cycle distribution after exposure to CDDP in mesothelioma cells. In both parental mesothelioma cell or Cx43-transfectant, an increase in the G_1-phase population was observed after CDDP treatment for more than 24 h (Figure 5A). On the other hand, the S-phase population increased by Cx43. And we also compared the sub-G_1 peak between cells. A higher sub-G_1 population was induced by Cx43, indicating upregulation of apoptosis. It has been reported that DNA modification by CDDP activates the G_1 checkpoint (Un, 2007). This checkpoint exists to halt cell cycle progression in the event of DNA damage to allow time for repair before initiating DNA replication (Wang et al, 2001). However, even those cells which retain G_1 checkpoint eventually die when they are exposed to persistent treatment. Therefore it is suggested that G_1 arrest represents a critical determinant of CDDP cytotoxicity (Un, 2007). In our study, G_1 arrest was observed in both parental mesothelioma cells and Cx43-transfectant (Sato et al, 2009). Therefore, the G_1 checkpoint does not appear to have broken down in these cells. As expected, an obvious induction of apoptosis was observed by Cx43. This observation might be explained by the additive effect of Cx43 on cell cycle distribution, inducing S-phase arrest. Thus, two surveillance mechanisms possibly work independently in the G_1 and S checkpoints, making it easy to suppress progression of the cell cycle and induce apoptosis in mesothelioma.

A)

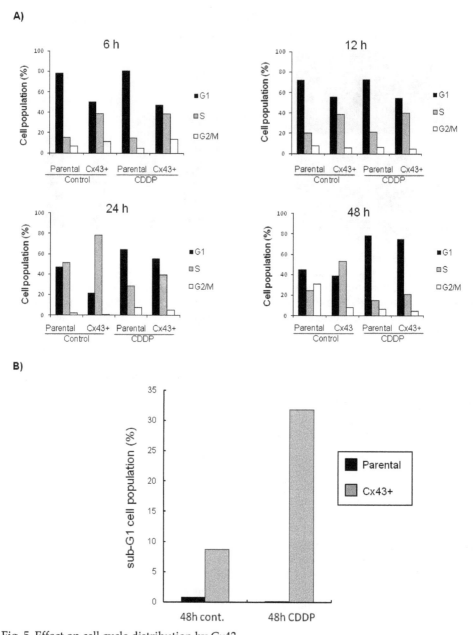

Fig. 5. Effect on cell cycle distribution by Cx43.
A) shows changes in cell cycle distribution in parental mesothelioma cells ('Parental') and in Cx43-transfectant cells ('Cx43+') after 25 μM of CDDP stimulation. Cells were treated with CDDP for the indicated periods, and 20,000 cells of each group were analyzed by flow cytometry. Control cells were treated with only 0.1% dimethylsulfoxide (vehicle for CDDP).

S-phase arrest was observed in Cx43-transfctant. **B)** shows effect on the induction of sub-G_1 population (estimated apoptosis) of mesothelioma cells 48 h CDDP treatment. Strong induction of sub-G_1 population was observed in Cx43 transfectant.

4.2.2.2 Effect of Cx43 on apoptotic factors

Proteins of the Bcl-2 family play an important role in the regulation of programmed cell death. Overexpression of Bcl-2, an anti-apoptotic factor, is associated with resistance to various cytotoxic agents, while the Bax protein is a pro-apoptotic member of the Bcl-2 family. In our study, no differences were noted in the levels of Bcl-2 among parental mesothelioma cells, mock, and Cx43-transfectant (Sato et al, 2009). On the other hand, Bax expression was strongly upregulated in Cx43-transfectant compared to the other two. Thus, the Bcl-2 family balance appeared to lean toward enhancing apoptosis by Cx43.

The Bcl-2 family proteins are invovlved in most of apoptosis pathway, so they are attractive target for cancer therapy (Kim et al, 2004). A previous study reported little or no expression of Bcl-2 but high expression of Bcl-xL and a pro-apoptotic protein, Bax, in mesothelioma histological sections and cells (Soini et al, 1999). Our results showed a different trend: Bcl-2 but not Bcl-xL was detected (data not shown). However, the important finding was the balance between pro- and anti-apoptotic factors. Any approach that changes the balance in favor of apoptosis may have a therapeutic benefit. Our results suggest that Cx43 influences the balance between pro- and anti-apoptotic factors in the direction of apoptosis, possibly contributing to the improved sensitivity of cancer cells to CDDP. However, some studies have reported low Bcl-2 and high Bax expression in mesothelioma samples. A previous study helped the current understanding of apoptosis regulation by raising the following possibilities: one is Bax mutation, which makes it nonfunctional and blocks its pro-apoptotic effect (Narasimhan et al, 1998); and the other is breaking out of antagonists to Bax as previously suggested (Yu et al, 2008). To clarify this issue, a functional assay of Bax in mesothelioma cells that also compares that of Cx43-transfectant is required.

4.2.2.3 Interactive effect of Cx43 with Src

Cx43 is known to interacts with the proto-oncogene product, Src. Src can directly phosphorylate Cx43 (Loo et al, 1995). Including mesothelioma, the Src family of nonreceptor tyrosine kinases are overexpressed in various human tumors, which often involves tumor progression and metastatic potential. In fact, a previous report revealed that total c-Src is highly expressed in some mesothelioma cells (Tsao et al, 2007). On the other hand, it has also shown that Cx43 regulates Src kinase through interaction of the Cx43 C-teminal region, irrespective of GJIC function (Giepmans et al, 2001).

Src activity is regulated by tyrosine phosphorylation. Phosphorylation of Tyr416 in the activation loop of the kinase domain upregulates enzyme activity. We assayed for Src levels and activation in mesothelioma cells using antibodies which recognized total-Src and phospho-Src protein (an activated form, phosphorylated at Tyr416). Tyr416 antibody detects endogenous levels of the Src family proteins, when phosphorylated at Tyr416. As a result, both phospho-Src and total-Src were decreased in Cx43-transfectant, although there were no

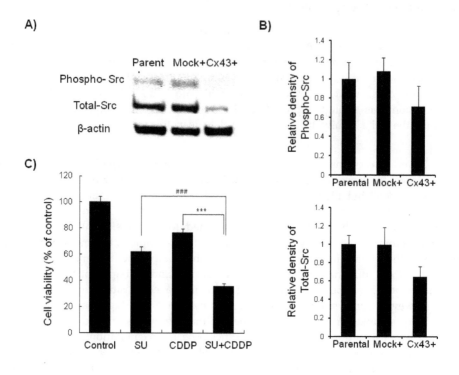

Fig. 6. Downregulation of Src protein level and activity by Cx43.
A) shows expression of total src ('Total Src') and phosphorelated Src (Phospho-Src, active form), in human mesothelioma cells, parental H28 ('Parental') , and only mock-transfected cells ('Mock+'), and Cx43-transfectant ('Cx43+'). β-Actin was used as the internal standard. **B)** shows densitometric data for phosphorelated Src (upper) and total Src (lower). Both Toatl Src and Phosphorelated Src were decreased by Cx43. **C)** shows cell viability after CDDP treatment in parental mesothelioma cells detected by WST-1 assay. CDDP cytotoxic effect was enhanced by Src inhibitor, SU6656. 'Control'; cells treated with only 0.1 % DMSO (vehicle for CDDP), 'SU'; cells treated with only SU6656, 'CDDP'; cells treated with only CDDP, and 'SU + CDDP'; cells co-treated with SU6656 and CDDP. ###$P < 0.001$; Significant difference between 'SU' and 'SU+CDDP', ***$P <0.001$; significant difference between 'CDDP' and 'SU+CDDP'.

significant differences among cells (Figure 6A, 6B). Then, we further investigated whether the inhibition of Src activity affects the cytotoxicity of CDDP in mesothelioma cells by using a specific Src kinase inhibitor, SU6656. It was revealed that when the cells were treated with both CDDP and SU6656, cell viability significantly decreased as compared to that when the cells were treated with CDDP or SU6656 alone (Figure 6C). Our results showed that not only phospho-Src level but also total-Src protein level was decreased in Cx43-transfectant, suggesting that Cx43 somehow suppressed the Src protein expression, which in turn suppressed the total amount of its activation form. One report which supports our results showed that the effect of activated Src on survival after CDDP treatment was reversed by forced overexpression of Cx43 using human Cx43 cDNA transfection model (Peterson-Roth et al). They finally suggested that a novel application for Src kinase inhibitors in combination with CDDP, i.e., one of Src inhibitor, dasatinib has the potential to sensitize tumor cells overexpressing activated Src as well as to sensitize tumor cells without activated Src that are in direct contact with Src-activated cells via GJIC, and also another combination such as proteasome inhibitors with CDDP treatment in order to up-regulate Cx43 expression which sensitize to CDDP.

Interestingly, a previous report showed that some selective inhibitors of Src kinases are specific inhibitors of cell cycle progression into the mid-S phase (Mizenina & Moasser, 2004), which corrrelates with our result of cell cycle distribution. Therefore, Cx43 may inhibit Src activation, which is reflected as S-phase arrest, resulting in the suppression of cell growth which was observed in Cx43-transfectant. Moreover, under the *in vivo* condition, Src upregulates vascular endothelial growth factor (VEGF), the most important factor in angiogenesis. Tumors must undergo angiogenesis for survival and for metastatic spread in a limited physiological environment (Folkman, 1971). Indeed, a previous report showed that a novel Src inhibitor, M475271, significantly inhibited VEGF-induced HUVEC proliferation, migration and angiogenesis (Ali et al, 2005). It is, therefore, possible that Cx43 has a more suppressive role in growth and metastasis *in vivo*, where angiogenesis always contributes to tumor survival.

It has also been indicated that simultaneous inhibition of Src and its downstream factor, signal transducer and activator (Stat) 3, results in synergistic death of mesothelioma cells (Johnson et al, 2007; Tsao et al, 2007). Moreover, CDDP inactivates Stat 3 by modulating Janus kinase (JAK) 2 through dephosphorylation of JAK/Stat in cancer cells (Song et al, 2004). Taken together, inhibition of Src by Cx43 and inactivation of Stat 3 by CDDP could induce synergistic death of mesothelioma cells.

5. Conclusion

From the view of previous studies including our data, we concluded that Cx43 could improve the chemoresistance of mesothelioma cells to CDDP mainly in a GJIC-independent manner (Figure 7). Also there might be another possible factors, such as hemichannel activity. In next step for clinical application, it should be considered that what kind of methodologies can be used which make possible to regulate Cx43 expression and its activities. There are still many concerns, however, this finding will help in overcoming resistance to current chemotherapy for malignant mesothelioma.

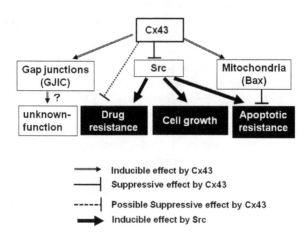

Fig. 7. A scheme of a new potential therapy against mesothelioma using Cx43 functions

6. Acknowledgment

We express our hearty thanks to Dr. Tomohiro Yano, a professor of Toyo University in Japan, and Dr. Christian C. Naus, a professor of the University of British Columbia in Canada, for their valuable advices and technical assistance. This study was supported by Grant-in-Aid for Young Scientists (Start-up) from the Japanese Society for the Promotion of Sciences, and by Special Funds for Education and Research (Development of SPECT Probes for Pharmaceutical Innovation) from the Ministry of Education, Culture, Sports, Sciences, and Technology, Japan.

7. References

Ali, N.; Yoshizumi, M.; Fujita, Y.; Izawa, Y.; Kanematsu, Y.; Ishizawa, K.; Tsuchiya, K.; Yano, S.; Sone, S. & Tamaki, T. (2005). A Novel Src Kinase Inhibitor, M475271, Inhibits VEGF-induced Human Umbilical Vein Endothelial Cell Proliferation and Migration. *Journal of Pharmacological Sciences*, Vol.98, No.2,(June 2005), pp.130–141

Byrne, M. J.; Davidson, J. A.; Musk, A. W; Dewar, J.; van Hazel, G.; Buck, M.; de Klerk, N. H. & Robinson, B. W. (1999). Cisplatin and gemcitabine treatment for malignant mesothelioma: a phase II study. *Journal of Clinical Oncology*, Vol.17, No.1, (January 1999), pp.25–30

El-Fouly, M. H.; Trosko, J. E. & Change, C.C. (1987). Scrape-loading and Dye Transfer. A Rapid and Simple Technique to Study Gap Junctional Intercellular

Communication. *Experimental Cell Research,* Vol.168, No.2, (February 1987), pp.422–430

Elshami, A. A.; Saavedra, A.; Zhang, H.; Kucharczuk, J. C.; Spray, D. C.; Fishman, G. I.; Amin, K. M.; Kaiser, L. R. & Albelda, S. M. (1996) Gap Junctions Play a Role in the 'Bystander Effect' of the Herpes Simplex Virus Thymidine Kinase/Ganciclovir System in vitro. *Gene Therapy,* Vol.3, No.1, (January 1996), pp.85-92

Folkman, J. (1971). Tumor Angiogenesis: Therapeutic Implications. *The New England Journal of Medicine,* Vol.285, No.21, (November 1971), pp.1182–1186

Fujimoto, E.; Sato, H.; Shirai, S.; Nagashima, Y.; Fukumoto, K.; Hagiwara, H.; Negishi, E.; Ueno, K.; Omori, Y.; Yamasaki, H.; Hagiwara, K. & Yano, T. (2005). Connexin32 as a Tumor Suppressor Gene in a Metastatic Renal Cell Carcinoma Cell Line. *Oncogene,* Vol.24, No.22, (May 2005), pp.3684-3690

Giepmans, B. N. G.; Hengeveld, T; Postma, F. R. & Moolenaar, W. H. (2001). Interaction of c-Src with Gap Junction Protein Connexin-43. Role in the Regulation of Cell-Cell Communication. *The Journal of Biological Chemistry,*Vol.276, No.11, (March 2001), pp.8544–8549

Giepmans, B.N. (2004). Gap Junctions and Connexin-Interacting Proteins. *Cardiovascular Research,* Vol.62, No.2, (May 2004), pp.233-245

Johnson, F. M.; Saigal, B.; Tran, H. & Donato, N. J. (2007). Abrogation of Signal Transducer and Activator of Transcription 3 Reactivation After Src Kinase Inhibition Results in Synergistic Antitumor Effects. *Clinical Cancer Research,* Vol.13, No.14, (July 2007), pp.4233–4244

Jo, S. K.; Cho, W. Y.; Sung, S. A.; Kim, H. K, & Won, N. H. (2005). MEK inhibitor, U0126, Attenuates Cisplatin-induced Renal Injury by Decreasing Inflammation and Apoptosis. Kidney International, Vol.67, No.2, (February 2005), pp.458-466

Kim, R.; Emi, M.; Tanabe, K. & Toge, T. (2004). Therapeutic Potential of Antisense Bcl-2 as a Chemosensitizer for Cancer Therapy. *Cancer,* Vol.101, No.11 (December 2004) pp.2491–2502.

Kumar, N. M. & Gilula, N.B. (1996) The Gap Junction Communication Channel. *Cell,* Vol.84, No.3, (February 1996), pp. 381-388

Lampe, P. D. & Lau, A. F. (2004). The Effects of Connexin Phosphorylation on Gap Junctional Communication. *The International Journal of Biochemistry Cell Biology,* Vol.36, No.7, (July 2004), pp.1171-1186

Li, J.; Wood, W. H.; 3rd, Becker, K. G.; Weeraratna, A. T. & Morin, P. J. (2007). Gene Expression Response to Cisplatin Treatment in Drug-Sensitive and Drug-Resistant Ovarian Cancer Cells. *Oncogene,* Vol.26, No.20, (May 2007), pp.2860-2872

Linnainmaa, K.; Pelin, K.; Vanhala, E.; Tuomi, T.; Piccoli, C.; Fitzgerald, D. J. & Yamasaki, H. (1993). Gap Junctional Intercellular Communication of Primary and Asbestos-associated Malignant Human Mesothelial Cells. *Carcinogenesis,* Vol.14, No.8, (August 1993), pp.1597–1602

Loo, L. W; Berestecky, J. M; Kanemitsu, M. Y & Lau, A. F. (1995). pp60src-Mediated Phosphorylation of Connexin 43, a Gap Junction Protein. *The Journal of Biological Chemistry,* Vol.270, No.21 ,(May 1995), pp.12751–12761.

Mizenina, O. A. & Moasser, M. M. (2004). S-phase Inhibition of Cell Cycle Progression by a Novel Class of Pyridopyrimidine Tyrosine Kinase Inhibitors. *Cell Cycle*, Vol.3, No.6, (June 2004), pp.796–803

Narasimhan, S. R.; Yang, L., Gerwin, B. I. & Broaddus, V. C. Resistance of Pleural Mesothelioma Cell Lines to Apoptosis: Relation to Expression of Bcl-2 and Bax. *The American Journal of Physiology*, Vol.275, No.1 Pt 1, (July 1998), pp.L165–L171

Park, M. S.; De Leon, M. & Devarajan, P. (2002). Cisplatin Induces Apoptosis in LLC-PK1 Cells via Activation of Mitochondrial Pathways.*Journal of the American Society of Nephrology*, Vol.13, No.4, (April 2002), pp.858-865

Paul, D. L. (1995) New Functions for Gap Junctions. *The Current Opinion in Cell Biology*, Vol.7, No.5, (Octorber 1995), pp.665-672

Pelin, K.; Hirvonen, A. & Linnainmaa, K. (1994). Expression of Cell Adhesion Molecules and Connexins in Gap Junctional Intercellular Communication Deficient Human Mesothelioma Tumour Cell Lines and Communication Competent Primary Mesothelial Cells. *Carcinogenesis*, Vol.15, No.11, (November 1994), pp.2673-2675

Peterson-Roth, E.; Brdlik, C. M. & Glazer, P. M. (2009). Src-Induced Cisplatin Resistance Mediated by Cell-to-Cell Communication. *Cancer Research*, Vol.69, No.8, (April 2009), pp.3619-3624

Procházka, L.; Turánek, J.; Tesařík, R.; Knotigová, P.; Polásková, P.; Andrysík, Z.; Kozubík, A.; Zák, F.; Sova, P.; Neuzil, J. & Machala, M. (2007). Apoptosis and Inhibition of Gap-junctional Intercellular Communication Induced by LA-12, a Novel Hydrophobic Platinum(IV) Complex. *Archives of Biochemistry and Biophysics*, Vol.462, No.1, (April 2007), pp.54-61

Qin, H.; Shao, Q.; Curtis, H.; Galipeau, J.; Belliveau, D. J.; Wang, T.; Alaoui-Jamali, M. A. & Laird, D. W. (2002). Retroviral Delivery of Connexin Genes to Human Breast Tumor Cells Inhibits in vivo Tumor Growth by a Mechanism That Is Independent of Significant Gap Junctional Intercellular Communication. *The Journal of Biological Chemistry*, Vol.277, No.2, (August 2002), pp.29132-29138

Ryan, C. W.; Herndon, J. & Vogelzang, N. J. (1998). A Review of Chemotherapy Trials for Malignant Mesothelioma. *Chest*, Vol.113, No.1 Supplement, (January 1998), pp.66S–73S

Sato, H.; Senba, H.; Virgona, N.; Fukumoto, K.; Ishida, T.; Hagiwara, H.; Negishi, E.; Ueno, K.; Yamasaki, H. & Yano, T. (2007). Connexin 32 Potentiates Vinblastine-induced Cytotoxicity in Renal Cell Carcinoma Cells. *Molecular Carcinogenesis*, Vol.46, No.3, (March 2007), pp.215–224

Sato, H.; Fukumoto, K.; Hada, S.; Hagiwara, H.; Fujimoto, E.; Negishi, E.; Ueno, K. & Yano, T. (2007). Enhancing Effect of Connexin 32 Gene on Vinorelbine-induced Cytotoxicity in A549 Lung Adenocarcinoma Cells. *Cancer Chemotherapy and Pharmacology*, Vol.60, No.3, (August 2007), pp.449-457

Sato, H.; Iwata, H.; Takano, Y.; Yamada, R.: Okuzawa, H.; Nagashima, Y.;Yamaura, K.; Ueno, K.; Yano, T. (2009) Enhanced Effect of Connexin 43 on Cisplatin-induced

Cytotoxicity in mesothelioma cells. *Journal of Pharmacological Sciences*, Vol.110, (August, 2009), pp.466-475

Soini, Y.; Kinnula, V.; Kaarteenaho-Wiik, R.; Kurttila, E.; Linnainmaa, K. & Pääkkö, P. Apoptosis and Expression of Apoptosis Regulating Proteins bcl-2, mcl-1, bcl-X, and bax in Malignant Mesothelioma. *Clinical Cancer Research*, Vol.5, No.11, (November 1999), pp.3508-3515

Song, H.; Sondak, V. K.; Barber, D. L.; Reid, T. J. & Lin, J. (2004). Modulation of Janus Kinase by Cisplatin in Cancer Cells. *International Journal of Oncology*, Vol.24, No.4, (April 2004), pp.1017-1026

Trosko, J. E. & Ruch, R. J. (2002). Gap Junctions as Targets for Cancer Chemoprevention and Chemotherapy. *Current Drug Targets*, Vol.3, No.6, (December 2002), pp.465-482

Tsao, A. S.; He, D.; Saigal, B.; Liu, S.; Lee, J. J.; Bakkannagari, S.; ez NG, Hong, W. K.; Wistuba, I. & Johnson, F. M. (2007). Inhibition of c-Src Expression and Activation in Malignant Pleural Mesothelioma Tissues Leads to Apoptosis, Cell Cycle Arrest, and Decreased Migration and Invasion. *Molecular Cancer Therapeutics*, Vol.6, No.7, (July 2007), pp.1962-1972

Un F. (2007). G1 Arrest Induction Represents a Critical Determinant for Cisplatin Cytotoxicity in G1 Checkpoint-retaining Human Cancers. *Anti-cancer Drugs*, Vol.18, No.4, (April 2007), pp.411-417

van Haarst, J. M.; Baas, P.; Manegold, Ch.; Schouwink, J. H.; Burgers, J. A.; de Bruin, H. G.; Mooi, W. J.; van Klaveren, R. J.; de Jonge, M. J. & van Meerbeeck, J. P. (2002). Multicentre Phase II Study of Gemcitabine and Cisplatin in Malignant Pleural Mesothelioma. *British Journal of Cancer*, Vol.86, No.3, (February 2002), pp.342-345

Vogelzang, N. J.; Rusthoven, J. J.; Symanowski, J.; Denham, C.; Kaukel, E.; Ruffie, P. Gatzemeier, U.; Boyer, M.; Emri, S.; Manegold, C.; Niyikiza, C. & Paoletti, P. (2003). Phase III Study of Pemetrexed in Combination with Cisplatin versus Cisplatin Alone in Patients with Malignant Pleural Mesothelioma. *Journal of Clinical Oncology*, Vol.15, No.14, (July 2003), pp.2636-2644

Wang, J. Y.; Naderi, S. & Chen, T. T. (2001). Role of Retinoblastoma Tumor Suppressor Protein in DNA Damage Response. *Acta Oncologica*, 2001;Vol.40, No.6, (n.d.), pp.689-695

Wang, X.; Martindale, J. L. & Holbrook, N. J. (2000). Requirement for ERK Activation in Cisplatin-induced Apoptosis. *The Journal of Biological Chemistry*, Vol.275, No.50 (December 2000), pp.39435-39443

Woessmann, W.; Chen, X. & Borkhardt, A. (2002). Ras-mediated Activation of ERK by Cisplatin Induces Cell Death Independently of p53 in Osteosarcoma and Neuroblastoma Cell Lines. *Cancer Chemotherapy and Pharmacology*, Vol.50, No.5, (November 2002), pp.397-404

Yano, T.; Ito, F.; Satoh, H.; Hagiwara, K.; Nakazawa, H.; Toma, H. & Yamasaki, H. (2003). Tumor-suppressive Effect of Connexin 32 in Renal Cell Carcinoma from Maintenance Hemodialysis Patients. *Kidney International*, Vol.63, No.1, (January 2003) pp.683

Yano, T.; Fujimoto, E.; Hagiwara, H.; Sato, H.; Yamasaki, H.; Negishi, E. & Ueno, K. (2006). Connexin 32 as an Anti-invasive and Anti-metastatic Gene in Renal Cell Carcinoma. *Biological & Pharmaceutical Bulletin*, Vol.29, No.10, (Octorber 2006), pp.1991-1994

Yu, J.; Li, X.; Tashiro, S.; Onodera, S. & Ikejima, T. (2008). Bcl-2 Family Proteins were Involved in Pseudolaric Acid B-induced Autophagy in Murine Fibrosarcoma L929 Cells. *Journal of Pharmacological Sciences*, Vol.107, No.3, (July 2008), pp.295–302

10

The Role of Immunotherapy in the Treatment of Mesothelioma

Saly Al-Taei, Jason F. Lester and Zsuzsanna Tabi

Department of Oncology, School of Medicine,
Cardiff University and Velindre NHS Trust, Cardiff,
United Kingdom

1. Introduction

Malignant mesothelioma (MM) is an aggressive and incurable malignancy of the mesothelium which is linked largely to previous asbestos exposure. In 2008, 2,249 people in the UK died from MM and median survival is only 6-18 months. The incidence of MM is still rising and not predicted to peak until 2015 in the UK (Hodgson et al., 2005). However, due to the asbestos content of many homes and public buildings, MM will be present for many more decades.

Pemetrexed-cisplatin chemotherapy is the current standard of care, but treatment results in an improvement in median survival of less than 3 months (Vogelzang et al., 2003). Furthermore, due to the age and co-morbidities of patients, many are not eligible for therapeutic intervention. This dictates an urgent need for improved therapies. Pre-clinical and clinical studies conducted over the years have highlighted the sensitivity of MM to immunotherapy. Immunotherapy offers an alternative to conventional therapies, utilising the patients' own immune system to fight the cancer without severe side effects. It may also confer additional benefits such as long-term immunological memory, which protects against future cancer relapse. Furthermore, in a similar manner to the HPV vaccine which is administered in young women to help prevent cervical cancer, some forms of immunotherapy may be offered in a preventative setting in people with known previous asbestos exposure. Most mesothelioma patients are not systemically immunosuppressed (Jasani et al., 2005) thus expected to respond better to immunotherapy than patients with systemically immunosuppressive cancers, such as ovarian cancer.

This chapter will address the complex relationship between MM and the immune system and review the progress of immunotherapy in the treatment of this disease. Furthermore, we will discuss our clinical trial using the targeted vaccine, Trovax®, for the treatment of pleural MM patients.

2. MM inflammation & tumourigenesis

MM has a strong aetiological link with previous asbestos exposure, although genetic factors may also influence susceptibility of individuals to this disease (Weiner & Neragi-Miandoab, 2009). Asbestos exposure causes DNA damage and death of mesothelial cells. One consequence is the release of the high-mobility group box 1 (HMGB1) protein, a damage-associated molecular pattern molecule which is normally retained in the nucleus by condensed chromatin and is released passively from dead cells. Its release is characteristic of immunogenic cell death (Apetoh et al., 2007) and it actively recruits inflammatory macrophages. HMGB1 and macrophage phagocytosis of asbestos fibres activates the Nalp3 inflammasome and induces secretion of the pro-inflammatory cytokines, interleukin (IL)- 1β and tumour necrosis factor-α (TNF-α) (H. Yang et al., 2010; Dostert et al., 2008). TNF-α is thought to promote malignant transformation of the mesothelium through nuclear factor kappa-light-chain-enhancer of activated B cells (NF-κB; a protein complex which controls DNA transcription)-dependent mechanism, which allows mesothelial cells with asbestos-induced DNA damage to survive rather than die (H. Yang et al., 2006). This localised inflammation alters the permeability of the mesothelial membrane and facilitates the process of pleural effusion whereby proteins and immune cells from the vascular compartment mobilise to the pleural space, establishing a tumour-associated immune environment.

3. MM Immunity

The immunosurveillance theory by Burnet in the 1950s proposed that lymphocytes continuously recognise and eliminate newly transformed malignant cells. With increasing understanding of how the immune system works in cancer, it is now accepted that immunosurveillance is part of a more complex interaction between the immune system and cancer, desribed as immunoediting (Dunn et al., 2002). The concept is supported by observations such as the depletion of T cells or interferon (IFN)-γ resulting in increased tumour incidence in wild type mice (Koebel et al., 2007). Immunoediting is also likely to occur in humans, as tumour infiltration with T cells and natural killer (NK) cells (both effector immune cell types, able to destroy tumour cells by cell-cell killing) is associated with better prognosis in several malignancies, such as colon cancer (Galon et al., 2006) and indeed MM (Anraku et al., 2008). Furthermore, in immunosuppressed transplant recipients, malignancy is the third most common cause of death and not only from cancers of viral origin (Rama & Grinyó, 2010). It is likely that the immune system in MM, similarly to that in other solid tumours, plays an important role during cancer progression and response to traditional treatments.

3.1 MM immune-engagement

The theory of immune-recognition of the tumour is that professional antigen presenting cells (APC), such as dendritic cells (DC) internalise antigen from dying tumour cells and home to the tumour draining lymph nodes (TDLN). In the TDLN, DC cross-present antigen on major histocompatibility complex class I (MHC I) molecules and in the presence of adhesion and co-stimulatory molecules, prime naïve CD8+ T cells resulting in their clonal expansion. Activated antigen-specific CD8+ T cells leave the TDLN, enter the circulation and migrate towards the tumour. At the tumour site these effector or cytotoxic T cells (CTL) recognise tumour antigen expressed on the surface of tumour cells on MHC I molecules and specifically kill those cells.

3.1.1 Tumour-associated antigens in MM

The presence of tumour-associated antigens (TAA), absent or weakly expressed on healthy cells, is crucial for the instigation of a tumour-specific immune response. Many antigens may be expressed by the tumour, however not all will necessarily elicit an immune response (Sommerfeldt et al., 2006). Antigens are largely categorised into 4 groups: i) cancer-testis antigens, e.g. New York-ESO, as the name suggests, are thought to be present selectively on cancer cells or in the testis. ii) Differentiation antigens, e.g. mesothelin, are expressed on both malignant cells and on the normal tissue from which they are derived. iii) Overexpressed antigens, e.g. mucin-1 (Muc-1), Wilms tumor-1 (WT-1), folate receptor-α (FR-α) and survivin, are expressed in a variety of normal tissues, but are overexpressed in tumours. iv) Oncofoetal antigens, e.g. 5T4, are expressed predominantly in the developing foetus and in tumour cells.

Antigen uptake by APC, mainly in the periphery, is crucial for the priming of T cells in the TDLN by these APC. TAA may be taken up when a tumour cell is killed by chemotherapeutic agents or undergoes necrosis in hypoxic regions within the tumour. In MM, antigen uptake may even occur at the time of malignant transformation, when asbestos induces the death of mesothelial cells which share some (e.g. differentiation) antigens with malignant cells. However, as many of these antigens are also 'self antigens' present on normal tissues, they may be subject to self-tolerance, which protects the body from autoimmunity. T cells with high affinity to self antigens are either deleted in the thymus during ontogeny or are regulated by peripheral tolerance mechanisms. However, in tumours a lot of these antigens are overexpressed, which, together with other stimulatory signals, may help to break tolerance, leading to immune recognition.

Several TAA have been identified in MM, all of which are potential immune targets and many have also been exploited for targeted immunotherapies.

Mesothelin is a differentiation antigen that is normally present on mesothelial cells but is highly over-expressed in epithelioid mesothelioma, while absent in sarcomatoid subtypes (Ordóñez, 2003). Its gene encodes a precursor protein which is proteolytically processed into two components; a membrane bound protein, mesothelin, and a secreted protein, megakaryocyte-potentiating factor (Chang & Pastan, 1996). Mesothelin is used as a diagnostic marker in MM, while soluble forms of the protein, the levels of which correlate with clinical stage and tumour burden, can be used as surrogate markers for clinical response to therapy (Creaney et al., 2011). Furthermore, soluble-mesothelin related protein, a member of the mesothelin family of proteins, has been identified as a possible biomarker for MM (Robinson et al., 2005) and has been developed as a commercial assay used in the detection and management of MM (Beyer et al., 2007). The normal biological function of mesothelin is unknown, although it has been implicated in cellular adhesion and mestastatic spread (Hassan et al., 2010). Mesothelin can be targeted on tumour cells by CTL (Yokokawa et al., 2005). Furthermore, mesothelin-specific antibodies were found to be elevated in 39.1% of mesothelioma patients (Ho et al., 2005).

WT-1 is a transcription factor that was originally described as a tumour suppressor gene but is now known to be involved in tumourigenesis. It can positively or negatively regulate the expression of various genes involved in cellular proliferation, differentiation and apoptosis (L. Yang et al., 2007). In normal adult tissue, WT-1 is expressed at low levels on haematopoietic stem cells, myoepithelial progenitor cells, renal podocytes and some cells in the testis and ovary (Mundlos et al., 1993). It is known to be upregulated in epithelioid MM but not in the sarcomatoid subtype and furthermore, its expression does not appear to be of significant prognostic value (Kumar-Singh et al., 1997). However, WT-1 is a relevant immune target in MM (May et al., 2007).

Muc-1, also known as epithelial membrane antigen, is a heavily glycosylated transmembrane protein that is normally found on the apical cell surface of normal glandular epithelium of many tissues, on haematopoietic stem cells and normal mesothelial cells (Baldus et al., 2004). It is overexpressed in the majority of epithelioid MM in an altered glycosylation form (Creaney et al., 2008). While it has been shown that Muc-1+ MM cells are subject to CTL-mediated killing *in vitro* (Roulois et al., 2011), there are currently no Muc-1 targeted therapies under development for MM patients.

Survivin is a member of the inhibitor of apoptosis gene family that is implicated in the control of cell division and apoptotic cell death (Altieri, 2004). It is barely detectable in normal adult tissue but specifically upregulated in tumour cells (Ambrosini et al., 1997). In MM, survivin was observed in 91% of surgical specimens and its knockout with siRNA restored the apoptotic potential of the cells (Zaffaroni et al., 2007). Its expression is a negative prognostic indicator in MM and it may play a role in therapy-refractoriness (GJ Gordon et al., 2007). Survivin is also a target for CTL-mediated killing in patients (Andersen et al., 2001).

FR-α is a glycosyl phosphatidylinositol-anchored glycoprotein that is found on the surface of many epithelial cells (Elnakat & Ratnam, 2004; Weitman et al., 1992). It binds folate at high affinity and mediates its transmembrane transport into the cell cytoplasm for use in purine, pyrimidine and ultimately DNA biosynthesis, a process that is essential for rapidly dividing tumour cells (Antony, 1996; Sierra & Goldman, 1999). FR-α is overexpressed in 72% of MM, regardless of subtypes. Furthermore, the level of expression is 2-4-fold higher in the tumour, compared with normal tissues (Bueno et al., 2001). It has also been shown to be a T cell target (Knutson et al., 2006). While the targeting potential of this antigen has been realised in many studies (Salazar & Ratnam, 2007), it has not been tested in MM.

5T4 is a cell surface oncofoetal glycoprotein (Hole & Stern, 1988). It has restricted expression in normal tissues but is overexpressed in numerous malignancies, such as testicular, breast and colon cancer (Southall et al., 1990). Our studies have identified the presence of this antigen on pleural MM cells and we also demonstrated the presence of 5T4-specific T cells and antibodies in patients (Al-Taei et al., Manuscript). It alters cellular dynamics facilitating metastatic spread (Carsberg et al., 1996; Southgate et al., 2010). Consequently, 5T4-targeted therapies are under development, such as antibody-based therapies, conjugated to cytotoxics such as calicheamicin (Boghaert et al., 2008) or Staphylococcal enterotoxin E (ABR-214936) which proved effective in phase II clinical trials in patients with advanced renal cell carcinoma (Shaw et al., 2007). The cancer vaccine Trovax® (a modified vaccinia Ankara virus encoding 5T4) is also undergoing clinical trials. It has been tested in 500 patients in Phase I, II and III clinical trials in advanced colorectal, renal and prostate cancer. The vaccine was well tolerated and a positive association was observed between the level of vaccine-induced antibody responses and clinical outcome (Harrop et al., 2010; DW Kim et al., 2010).

3.1.2 Antigen presentation by MM cells

Correct functioning of the antigen-processing machinery, transporter for antigen presentation-1 (TAP-1) and MHC I expression by tumour cells is necessary for T cell recognition. One study has shown that in four MM primary cell lines, all cells homogeneously expressed MHC I and II molecules (Mutti et al., 1998). This is in contrast to two further reports, one of which demonstrated the presence of only MHC I molecules on cell lines (Christmas et al., 1991), while the other also found only MHC I and not II expression in 100% of 44 tissue sections from MM patients (Yamada et al., 2010). The widespread detectable expression of MHC I molecules on MM tumour cells is an important feature for immunotherapy as they are downregulated in many cancers to evade immune cell killing (Romero et al., 2005). Furthermore, there are no reports on TAP-1 downregulation in MM.

3.1.3 Clinical relevance of MM immunity

The prognostic value of immune parameters in MM has been reported by independent research groups. Leigh and Webster were the first to report the significance of T cell infiltration on survival in MM patients, demonstrating a positive correlation between T cells and increased survival (9 months vs. 18 months in patients who showed infiltration) (Leigh & Webster, 1982). Later, phenotypic analysis identified that high frequencies of CD8+ tumour infiltrating T cells correlated with significantly increased proportions of apoptotic tumour cells and better progression-free and overall survival than those in patients with low CD8+ T cell frequencies in the tissue (Anraku et al., 2008). In the same study, increased frequencies of CD4+CD25+ T cells and CD45RO+ memory T cells tended to be negative prognostic indicators following induction chemotherapy. Yamada et al. studied T cell infiltration in 44 patients by immunohistochemistry and also reported a correlation between higher levels of CD8+ T cell infiltration and clinical outcome (Yamada et al., 2010). Higher frequencies of infiltrating CD3+ T cells correlated with worse overall survival but only in patients with sarcomatoid or biphasic histology (Burt et al., 2011). However, the authors did not elaborate on the different T cell subsets and potential ratios of regulatory T cells (Treg) to CD8+ T cells in these patients. MM tissues typically contain high numbers of myeloid cells (B Davidson et al., 2007). High myeloid cell counts, such as monocytes and macrophages, are negative prognostic indicators in MM with sarcomatoid and biphasic histology (Burt et al., 2011). Conversely, no correlation was noted between macrophage infiltration and prognosis in epithelioid patients. Tumour infiltration by tryptase expressing proinflammatory mast cells has also been identified as a positive prognostic indicator in patients (Alì et al., 2009). In addition, several reports have documented spontaneous regression in MM patients with a possible immunological basis (Robinson et al., 2001; Pilling et al., 2007; Allen, 2007).

The studies highlighted in this section have demonstrated that MM is a sufficiently immunogenic cancer and it induces immune recognition, immune cell infiltration and immune-mediated killing, the extent of which defines disease prognosis.

3.2 MM immune-escape

In a recent review, the hallmarks of tumour development were described incorporating our most recent knowledge about these events. Integral to all these hallmarks is the genomic instability of tumours, which fosters aberrant tumour phenotypes (Hanahan & Weinberg, 2011). Immune evasion has recently been included in this concept. Immune evasion may arise due to immunological pressure which drives tumour transition from immunosensitive to immunoresistant variants. This was shown in a model where tumours only maintained their immunogenicity in immunodeficient mice (Shankaran et al., 2001).

Localised immune evasion has many different forms. Tumour cells can express immunosuppressive markers and release immunosuppressive soluble factors which may in turn promote the accumulation of regulatory immune cells at the tumour site. Alternatively, the inflammatory tumour environment may non-specifically attract suppressor cells to regulate the level of inflammation (Bunt et al., 2007). The immunosuppressive nature of the tumour environment in MM has been widely reported (DeLong et al., 2005; Hegmans et al., 2006) and will also be addressed in another chapter in this book. Immunosuppressive influences that are relevant to MM immunotherapy are discussed here.

3.2.1 Tumour-mediated immune escape mechanisms

MM tumour cells have been shown to release cytokines and chemokines that cause the preferential accumulation of immunoregulatory cells at the tumour site. Treg are characterised as $CD4^+CD25^+$ T cells that express the transcription factor forkhead box P3 (foxp3). They can inhibit both $CD4^+$ and $CD8^+$ T cells by release of immunosuppressive soluble factors such as IL-10 and transforming growth factor (TGF)-β (Hall et al., 2011). The chemokine CXCL12 was identified in all tissue samples from 6 MM patients and was chemotactic to Treg. MM can therefore actively recruit Treg to the tumour site (Shimizu et al., 2009). Also, cytokines released by tumour cells such as IL-6 and IL-8 have been shown to cause preferential migration of Treg towards the tumour (Eikawa et al., 2010). There are conflicting reports for the role of Treg in the survival of MM patients. One study showed that while patients with a high level of $CD4^+CD25^+$ T cells infiltration demonstrated shorter survival (though not statistically significant), the presence of foxp3, did not affect survival (Anraku et al., 2008). Another study concluded that Treg do not mediate immunosuppression in a MM model (Jackaman et al., 2009), while significant increase in the number of Treg was not seen in MM patients (Meloni et al., 2006). However, in a clinical trial involving 66 patients treated with IL-2, Treg frequency was a significant negative prognostic factor (Alì et al., 2009). The frequencies of infiltrating Treg, rather than those in the periphery, may serve as relevant indicators of disease prognosis.

Normal and malignant mesothelial cells can also release cytokines that are chemotactic for monocytes including macrophage inflammatory protein-1, monocyte chemotactic protein-1, granulocyte-colony stimulating factor and granulocyte-macrophage-colony stimulating factor (GMCSF) (Schmitter et al., 1992). Once monocytes infiltrate the tumour, they can differentiate into tumour-associated macrophages (TAM) that are polarised towards the M2 suppressor phenotype (Sica, 2010).

Myeloid-derived suppressor cells (MDSC) are a phenotypically heterogeneous population of myeloid cells at different stages of maturation. They are well characterised in mouse models but less well studied in humans. MDSC inhibit T cell effector functions through a variety of mechanisms (Ostrand-Rosenberg, 2010). While the significance of these MDSC in MM has not been identified, they have been targeted by immunotherapies with promising results (discussed later).

TGF-β is a homodimeric protein with three isoforms; TGF-β1, TGF-β2 and TGF-β3 (Massagué, 1987). It is secreted by various immune cells such as macrophages, neutrophils, lymphocytes and also by malignant cells, including MM (Kumar-Singh et al., 1999). In cancer, TGF-β is a potent tumour promoter, stimulating angiogenesis and altering the stromal environment and is also a powerful local and systemic immunosuppressor (Mantel & Schmidt-Weber, 2011). TGF-β has been implicated in the cytokine profile shift of T cells which infiltrate the tumour in a mouse model of MM, from pro-inflammatory (interferon; IFN-γ) to anti-inflammatory (IL-4) cytokine-producing cells (Jarnicki et al., 1996).

MM tumours produce vascular endothelial growth factor (VEGF) (Strizzi et al., 2001) that mediates angiogenesis. VEGF production by tumours encourages bulky tumour growth and metastatic spread. High levels of VEGF has also been associated with a resistance to IL-2 immunotherapy (Bonfanti et al., 2000).

3.2.2 Resistance to CTL killing

Tumor cells also develop mechanisms to evade T cell killing, such as suboptimal antigen presentation, resulting in the lack of recognition by CTL (Setiadi et al., 2007). Disregulation of the tumour suppressor, p53, may lead to resistance to apoptotic signals. In MM, merlin is a known regulator of murine double minute 2 degradation (Sekido et al., 1995) with implications on p53 regulation. Cell-cycle checkpoint control defects are frequent in MM (López-Ríos et al., 2006), such as consistent overexpression of checkpoint kinase 1, a DNA damage-induced checkpoint kinase in S and G2/M phases (Romagnoli et al., 2009), serving as another potential CTL resistance mechanism. Upregulation of anti-apoptotic and multi-drug resistance pathways may also impact on CTL sensitivity, such as overexpression of the B-cell CLL/lymphoma 2 family of proteins, especially myeloid cell leukemia sequence 1 (SL O'Kane et al., 2006), and abnormal activation of the Raf/MEK/ERK pathway (de Melo et al., 2006) and the PI3K/AKT pathway (Garland et al., 2007) in MM. CD200 is a potential diagnostic marker of MM (GJ Gordon et al., 2002) with inhibitory effects on mixed lymphocyte reaction and NK-cell cytotoxicity (Wright et al., 2003). B7-H1 (programmed cell death 1 (PD-1) ligand 1) is also expressed on MM (AJ Currie et al., 2009) and negatively regulates the activity of PD-1-expressing T cells (Berthon et al., 2010).

Similar to other solid tumours, MM carries the signs of immunological pressure, as several immune evasion mechanisms can be observed in patients. These not only serve as evidence of engagement between the tumour and the immune system, but also offer potential targets to remove evasion mechanisms and empower the immune system to attack the tumour.

4. Immunological interventions in MM

Immunotherapies can either be non-specific, stimulating the immune system in a general way which may also induce or amplify anti-tumour responses or targeted at a known tumour antigen, generating or boosting specific anti-tumour immune responses. Many immunotherapeutic strategies have been tested in MM.

4.1 Non-specific therapies

The aim of non-specific immunotherapy is to induce general immune stimulation, powerful enough to break immune tolerance induced by the tumour, thereby promoting tumour cell destruction.

4.1.1 Cytokine therapy

Cytokines are best described as messengers of the immune system. They are secreted by both tumour and immune cells and have immunoregulatory roles. IL-2 and IFN-α2b are two cytokines currently approved by the FDA for the treatment of cancer. Both IL-2 and IFN-α2b have demonstrated activity against renal cell carcinoma, melanoma, lymphoma and leukaemia. Cytokines tested in MM are stated in Table 1.

Interferons are a family of cytokines that influence the quality of cellular immune responses and amplify antigen presentation to specific T cells. There are two major classes; IFN-α, IFN-β (the type I interferons secreted by virus infected cells and DC) and IFN-γ (the type II interferon secreted by T cells, NK cells and macrophages). The immunoregulatory effects of IFNs extend to antibody production, NK and T cell activation, macrophage function and MHC antigen expression (Wang et al., 2011). Gene delivery of IFN is the prevalent mode of delivery in patients as it leads to high and prolonged local cytokine concentrations that are sufficient to induce immunogenic tumour cell death, break tolerance and activate anti-tumour immune responses (Vachani et al., 2007).

In preclinical studies IFN-γ has been shown to skew the immunosuppressive M2 phenotype of TAM, converting them into M1-polarised immunostimulatory macrophages (Duluc et al., 2009). IFNs have also been shown to have anti-angiogenic and anti-proliferative effects on the tumour (Rosewicz et al., 2004). The antiproliferative properties of IFN have also been shown in several mesothelioma cell lines (Zeng et al., 1993).

Viral mediated IFN gene-transfer is very popular in IFN immunotherapy. Sterman and colleagues have carried out several clinical trials delivering IFN. Their first trial involved the administration of a single dose of adenovirally encoded IFN-β, where four out of 10 patients showed clinically meaningful responses. Administering two doses rather than one showed no survival benefit due to neutralising antibodies against the viral vector. Subsequently they used a similar adenoviral vector but substituting IFN-β for IFN-α2b and found that to be more potent as six of the nine patients treated displayed clinical responses. Boutin et al. conducted a study involving 89 patients. They showed that there was an overall response rate of 20%. However, this went up to 45% when data from only stage I patients was analysed (Boutin et al., 1991). This trend for better survival in early stage patients was commonly seen with interferon therapy.

Interleukins are another class of cytokines with multiple immunoregulatory properties. **IL-2** is a pro-inflammatory cytokine produced by activated T cells and promotes T cell proliferation, differentiation and survival. It can also enhance NK cells, neutrophil and macrophage function. On the other hand, it can also boost Treg function (Malek, 2008; Foureau et al., 2011).

In MM cell lines, IL-2 was shown to affect the cell cycle, resulting in an accumulation of cells in the G0/G1 phase with subsequent apoptosis (Porta et al., 2000). In the AE17 mouse model, IL-2 markedly enhanced CD8+ CTL activity and decreased tumour vasculature, resulting in tumour regression, with mice remaining tumour free for >2 months (Jackaman et al., 2003). This was mirrored in a clinical trial where IL-2 administered preoperatively induced significantly greater recruitment of CD8+ T cells, tryptase mast cells and also inhibited tumour-associated vasculature (Alì et al., 2009). There have also been reports that

Therapy	Route of Administration	Patients Recruited	Reference
Interferon			
IFN-α2b	Intrapleural via Adenoviral gene transfer	9	(Sterman et al., 2011)
IFN-β Phase I	Intrapleural via Adenoviral gene transfer	10	(Sterman et al., 2010)
IFN-β	Oncolytic vesicular stomatitis virus gene transfer	Murine model	(Willmon et al., 2009)
IFN-β Phase I	Intrapleural via Adenoviral gene transfer	7	(Sterman et al., 2007)
IFN-β	Adenoviral gene transfer	Murine model	(Kruklitis et al., 2004)
IFN-β	Adenoviral gene transfer	Murine model	(Odaka et al., 2002)
IFN-γ	Adenoviral gene transfer	Murine model	(Gattacceca et al., 2002)
IFN-β	Adenoviral gene transfer	Murine model	(Odaka et al., 2001)
IFN-α	Systemic	Murine model	(Bielefeldt-Ohmann et al., 1996)
IFN-α2b Phase II	Systemic	14	(Ardizzoni et al., 1994)
IFN-γ	Intrapleural	89	(Boutin et al., 1994)
IFN-α2a	Systemic	25	(Christmas et al., 1993)
IFN-γ	Intrapleural	22	(Boutin et al., 1991)
IFN-β Phase II	Systemic	14	(Von Hoff et al., 1990)
Interleukin			
IL-2	Pre-operative intrapleural	60	(Alì et al., 2009)
IL-2	Intratumoural	Murine model	(Jackaman et al., 2003)
IL-2	Intrapleural	12	(Porta et al., 2002)
IL-2 Phase II	Combined intravenous and subcutaneous	29	(Mulatero et al., 2001)
IL-2 Phase II	Intrapleural then low dose subcutaneous	31	(Castagneto et al., 2001)
IL-2	Intratumoural via Vaccinia Virus gene transfer	6	(Mukherjee et al., 2000)
IL-2 Phase II	Intrapleural	22	(Astoul et al., 1998)
IL-2	Intrapleural	11	(Astoul et al., 1995)
IL-2 Phase I/II	Intrapleural	23	(Goey et al., 1995)
IL-12	Systemic or intratumoural	Murine model	(Caminschi et al., 1998)
IL-12 Phase I	Intraperitoneal	1	(Lenzi et al., 2002)
GMCSF			
GMCSF	Intratumourally	14	(Davidson et al., 1998)
GMCSF	Intratumourally via Fowlpox gene transfer	Murine model	(Triozzi et al., 2005)

Table 1. Cytokine therapy trials conducted in MM

IL-2 activated non-specific NK-like cells with *in vitro* cytotoxic activity (Astoul et al., 1995). Other effects seen with IL-2 include the resolution of pleural effusion which was observed in 90% of patients receiving intrapleural IL-2 followed by low dose IL-2 maintenance (Castagneto et al., 2001). IL-2 trials in MM have been met with varying successes. Systemic administration was associated with adverse toxicities and suboptimal response rates (Bernsen et al., 1999). More promising results were obtained with localised delivery of IL-2, however it remains more toxic than IFN therapy.

More experimental settings have also been tried, such as the intratumoural administration of IL-2 with a poly-N-acetyl glucosamine-based polymer gel which not only caused slow release of the cytokine, but also triggered inflammation, recruiting inflammatory cells to the tumour site in a mouse model of MM (van Bruggen et al., 2005). A possible reason for the weak responses to IL-2 therapy is that IL-2, like IFN, has a short half-life of around 10 mins and may benefit from viral gene transfer to prolong its effects. Vaccinia virus-mediated gene transfer of IL-2 resulted in direct retardation of tumour growth, as well as the release of IL-2 (Mukherjee et al., 2000; Jackaman & Nelson, 2010). However, as only 6 patients were treated, it is difficult to compare it to recombinant IL-2.

IL-12 is a proinflammatory IL with potent immunoregulatory effects on NK and T cells (Trinchieri, 1995). In a murine model of MM, IL-12 was administered intratumourally, resulting in temporary tumour regression, correlating with the influx of $CD4^+$ and $CD8^+$ T cells. However, tumour regrowth was evident after cessation of treatment indicating that protective memory was not generated (Caminschi et al., 1998). In a mixed patient phase I trial, with one mesothelioma patient included, the MM patient showed a complete response when treated with intraperitoneal IL-12 prior to surgery and remained progression-free at two years after therapy. The response correlated with increased IFN-γ and TNF-α serum levels (Lenzi et al., 2002).

GMCSF enhances the APC activity of DC and macrophages as well as enhancing the tumour cell cytotoxic activity of macrophages (Warren & Weiner, 2000). It also upregulates costimulatory molecules on DC (Larsen et al., 1994). When released by MM cells, in contrast to its immunostimulatory properties, it can increase tumour cell proliferation and recruit suppressor cells (MDSC) to the tumour site (Oshika et al., 1998; Young et al., 1992). In both human and animal studies, GMCSF had very limited anti-tumour efficacy. Intratumoural infusion of GMCSF into 14 patients was associated with systemic toxicity. Tumour necrosis was evident around the catheter in one patient while another showed marked T cell infiltration into the tumour and a partial response. Of the other patients, 10 had progressive disease, and three, including the patient with the necrosis in the tumour, had no response (JA Davidson et al., 1998). The intratumoural administration of GMCSF expressed by fowlpox virus in a mouse model had little effect and GMCSF-treated animals died by day 30 vs. control animals by day 35 (Triozzi et al., 2005). It is not clear whether the tumour-potentiating effects of GMCSF were responsible for this observation. No further GMCSF trials have been pursued in MM patients.

4.1.2 Costimulation strategies

CD40 costimulation is another strategy for immunotherapy. CD40 is a glycoprotein that belongs to the TNF receptor superfamily and is expressed on DC and monocytes

(Banchereau et al., 1994). Its ligand, CD40L, is preferentially expressed on mast cells and CD4+ T cells and has an important role in determining whether the CTL response is initiated or tolerised. Antigen presentation in the absence of CD40 ligation leads to T cell tolerance (Schoenberger et al., 1998). Interaction of CD40 with its ligand during antigen presentation results in production of IL-12 and upregulation of B7-1 and B7-2 costimulatory molecules necessary for generating T cell responses (Schoenberger et al., 1998). Exogenous CD40 ligation has been extensively explored as an immunotherapeutic strategy (Todryk et al., 2001).

In a mouse model of MM, where the CD40L was administered via an adenoviral vector, intratumoural delivery of CD40L resulted in not only the regression of the primary tumour, but also regression at distal sites. This was shown to be mediated by CD8+ T cells (Friedlander et al., 2003). Agonistic CD40 antibody administered intravenously did not generate long-lasting immunological memory and tumour regrowth was evident after cessation of treatment (Stumbles et al., 2004). Agonistic antibody in low doses administered into the tumour-bed resulted in 60% survival rate with most mice cured. In this model, CD8+ T cells were not required for anti-tumour response, but instead B cells were the mediators (Jackaman et al., 2011). No patient trials have been reported for CD40 in MM, however, pre-clinical data sets the precedent for a future trial.

Toll-like receptors (TLR) are mainly expressed on antigen presenting cells and control their activation, maturation and migration. Similarly to CD40, antigen presentation in the absence of TLR ligation may also induce tolerance and so they can alter the context of the immune response. Persistent TLR stimulation has been shown to break tolerance against TAA (Y Yang et al., 2004). In a mouse model of MM, treatment with TLR agonists specific for TLR3, TLR7 and TLR9 resulted in tumour resolution in 40% of mice, with a delay in tumour progression in the other treated mice. The treatment induced type I IFNs and was dependent on the induction of CD8+ T cells at the tumour site (AJ Currie et al., 2008). TLR agonists may represent a promising new agent group to stimulate anti-tumour immune responses, especially in an adjuvant role.

4.1.4 Adoptive cell transfer

Dendritic cell based therapies are an exciting area of research and have shown much promise in MM. These will be discussed in another chapter in this book.

4.1.3 Other strategies

Soluble type II TGF-β receptor, which binds TGF-β1 and TGF-β3, was implemented in three MM mouse models. The AB12 and AC29 models produce large amounts of TGF-β, while the AB1 model does not. Predictably, suppression of tumour growth attributed to the addition of the soluble TGF-β receptor was only evident in the AB12 and AC29 tumours. CD8+ T cells were responsible for tumour cell killing following treatment, but were less efficient in bulky TGF-β secreting tumours. Furthermore, complete regressions were not observed (Suzuki et al., 2004).

SM16 is a small molecule inhibitor of TGF-β type I receptor kinase. When administered locally, it also inhibited tumour growth by a CD8+ T cell-dependent mechanism.

Furthermore, post-surgical administration of SM16 reduced tumour recurrence (Suzuki et al., 2007).

CD26 is a cell surface glycoprotein with dipeptidyl peptidase IV activity in its extracellular domain and is a T cell activation molecule, playing roles in T cell costimulation and signal transduction processes (Ishii et al., 2001; Ohnuma et al., 2004). It is also highly expressed on MM, but not in benign mesothelial tissue, and implicated in tumour growth and metastases (Inamoto et al., 2007). A humanised anti-CD26 antibody was shown to lyse MM cell lines and also prolong survival in a mouse model of MM (Inamoto et al., 2007).

Anti-**CD25** antibody, applied intratumourally to target Treg within the tumour, resulted in 85% depletion of intratumoural Tregs and inhibited tumour growth, which was extended with multiple injections (Needham et al., 2006). These data suggest that removing Treg may contribute to the success of combination therapies.

4.2 Targeted therapy

Tumour-specific markers that have been exploited for targeted therapy either in pre-clinical or clinical settings are described below.

Mesothelin has been shown to be a T cell target as CTL specific for mesothelin peptides can lyse tumour cells (Yokokawa et al., 2005). Furthermore, mesothelin-specific antibodies were elevated in 39.1% of mesothelioma patients (Ho et al., 2005). It is the most widely studied antigen in MM and is at the forefront of many MM-targeted therapies. Antibody-guided targeting of mesothelin accounts for the majority of mesothelin-targeted therapies. In pre-clinical studies, monoclonal antibody induced antibody-dependent cellular cytotoxicity against human MM cell lines in a xenograft model (Inami et al., 2010).

SS1P is a high affinity anti-mesothelin murine antibody which has been genetically combined with a fragment of the potent cytotoxic *Pseudomonas* endotoxin, PE38. A phase I trial established the safe dose of the antibody and showed evidence of modest clinical activity (Kreitman et al., 2009).

MORAb009 (Morphotek Inc.) is a high affinity chimeric (mouse/human) monoclonal antibody. It kills mesothelin positive cell lines via antibody-dependent cellular cytotoxicity (Hassan et al., 2007). A phase I trial administering IV MORAb-009 was carried out in 13 mesothelioma patients and no complete or partial responses were noted (Hassan et al., 2010). Morab009 is currently being evaluated in a phase II trial in patients with unresectable MM, where it is being administered in combination with pemetrexed and cisplatin (ClinicalTrials.gov NCT00738582).

Studies demonstrating mesothelin-specific CD8+ T cell responses in patients (Thomas et al., 2004) have provided a rationale for mesothelin as a tumour vaccine. CRS-207 is a vaccine consisting of a live-attenuated bacterium *Listeria monocytogenes* encoding human mesothelin. A phase I clinical trial of CRS-207 for the treatment of 17 patients with mesothelin-expressing tumours is being conducted.

WT-1 peptide mix, incorporating one CD8 epitope, two CD4 epitopes and one peptide with both CD8 and CD4 epitopes, was developed. The peptides were combined with a Montanide adjuvant before injection and the injection site was primed with GMCSF. Nine MM patients were treated, eight of which developed disease progression and died. One patient however, remained progression-free for 36 months after the start of the study (Krug et al., 2010).

5T4. We are conducting a phase II clinical trial in pleural MM patients due to start later in the year. Patients will be treated with TroVax® (9 injections) in combination with the standard chemotherapy, pemetrexed and cisplatin (4 cycles) according to the scheme shown in Figure 1. Twenty-six chemotherapy-naïve patients with confirmed MM disease and who have normal baseline haematology will be recruited to the trial. The primary endpoint of the trial will be the safety of the regimen and detection of 5T4-specific immune responses either by T cell stimulation assays or the measurement of anti-5T4 antibodies in the patients' plasma. The secondary endpoint will be progression-free survival and overall survival at 6 & 12 months following treatment initiation.

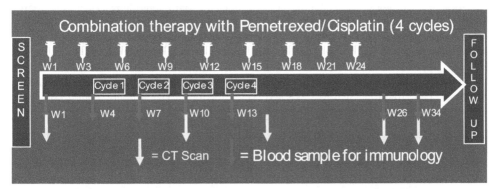

Fig. 1. Schematic diagram of the treatment schedule in the TroVax® trial. Syringes indicate points of vaccine administration. The cycles indicate chemotherapy treatments. W = weeks following trial initiation.

4.3 Combined immunotherapies

As the clinical efficacy of single agent immunotherapies has been limited, combination immunotherapies may induce improved clinical outcomes, particularly if the strategies target both immunosuppressive and immunostimulatory immune mechanisms (Zitvogel et al., 2008). Kim et al. combined SM16, an orally active TGF-β receptor inhibitor, with adenovirally delivered IFN-β in a mouse model of MM and lung cancer. When administered alone, adenoviral IFN-β slowed tumour growth whereas TGF-β inhibition with SM16 alone decreased the size of the tumours and induced one complete regression. However, combination therapy resulted in synergistic effects by shrinking all tumours and inducing complete remissions in four out of five mice. This coincided with significant increases in the frequencies of CD45+ and CD8+ T cells and NK cells (S. Kim et al., 2008).

5. Combination chemo-immunotherapy in MM

Recently, much work has been carried out on the immune-mediated anti-tumour mechanisms of chemotherapy and how chemotherapy could be used to facilitate tumour immunity. Physical destruction of tumour cells by chemotherapy not only makes it a more manageable target for immune attack but also provides tumour antigen for the cross-presentation pathway. The immune-potentiating effects of chemotherapy have become a new focus in the field of tumour targeted immunotherapy (Lake & Robinson, 2005). On the other hand, improving immune parameters prior to chemotherapy can chemosensitise cells and augment the cytotoxic effects of chemotherapy (Radfar et al., 2009).

5.1 Immunogenic effects of chemotherapy

There is a paradoxical relationship between chemotherapy and the immune system whereby lymphodepletion may be reconciled with the induction of effective anti-tumour immunity. Lymphodepletion is a common side effect of chemotherapy at therapeutically relevant concentrations. Lymphodepletion can be beneficial to tumour immunity as it has been shown to enhance T cell homing into tumour-beds and intra-tumoural proliferation of effector cells (Dudley et al., 2002). Some reports claim that chemotherapy actually spares memory T cells (Coleman et al., 2005). Furthermore, following lymphodepletion, there is a repopulation of naïve T cells which are biased towards self-antigen reactivity which could be exploited as there is decreased competition for cytokines and decreased tumour-derived immunosuppressive effects (Dummer et al., 2002). Many studies have also examined the immunological effects of low-dose chemotherapy, demonstrating immune potentiating effects of chemotherapy, such as increased APC function of DC, a phenomenon known as chemomodulation (Zitvogel et al., 2008; Shurin et al., 2009).

Cyclophosphamide was shown to selectively eliminate Tregs in animal models and patients (Ghiringhelli et al., 2004; Ghiringhelli et al., 2007; van der Most et al., 2009). Cyclophosphamide was also found to deplete 75% of total CD8+ T cells while simultaneously conferring a strong CD8+ T cell-dependent anti-tumour response which culminates in 75-100% cure rate in a MM mouse model. Cyclophosphamide sensitised tumour cells to TRAIL (tumour necrosis factor related apoptosis-inducing ligand)-mediated apoptosis induced by CD8+ T cells, in the absence of their expansion (van der Most et al., 2009).

The cyclooxygenase-2 (COX-2) inhibitor, celecoxib, has been shown to inhibit MDSC in a mouse model of MM, preventing the release of reactive oxygen species from MDSC and inhibiting their expansion. This resulted in a reversal of T cell tolerance (Veltman et al., 2010) and will be addressed in more detail in another chapter in this book. Gemcitabine is another chemotherapeutic agent that has been shown to inhibit MDSC and restore CD8+ T cell function (Le et al., 2009).

Melphalan and mitomycin-C upregulate the expression of T cell co-stimulatory molecules, enabling the tumour cells themselves to actively present tumour antigens to T cells (Sojka et al., 2000). 5,6-dimethylxanthenone-4-acetic acid, a vascular disruptive agent, induces activation of TAM, leading to their tumour infiltration and subsequent influx of CD8+ T cell resulting in tumour cell killing in a MM mouse model. This treatment also generated protective immunity against rechallenge (Jassar et al., 2005).

Some chemotherapies can have both immuno-stimulatory and –inhibitory effects which can cancel each other out. In MM mouse model, zoledronic acid was found to impair myeloid cell differentiation, leading to a reduction in the frequency of TAMs. However, this simultaneously led to increased infiltration by immature myeloid cells, resembling MDSC, which might explain the lack of improvement in overall survival (Veltman et al., 2010).

Immunomodulatory roles for the standard first-line chemotherapy with pemetrexed and cisplatin, have also been identified. Patients treated with pemetrexed-cisplatin have more CD8+ tumour infiltrating T cells which correlate with improved survival when compared to that in patients on cisplatin-vinorelbine (Anraku et al., 2008). This demonstrates that pemetrexed and cisplatin may have immune-potentiating effects. Indeed, a study has shown that pemetrexed sensitises cells to immune cell killing by upregulating the death receptor, DR5, on the surface of tumour cells (Su et al., 2011). DR5 is an important mediator of the extrinsic apoptotic signalling pathway and when presented on the cell surface, it binds to TRAIL expressed on T cells (Whiteside, 2007). Cellular FLICE-inhibitory protein (cFLIP), a protein which inhibits caspase mediated apoptosis, was also downregulated by pemetrexed (Su et al., 2011), suggesting that pemetrexed can sensitise tumour cells to TRAIL mediated apoptosis. These effects of pemetrexed may contribute to the dramatic tumour control in a patient on pemetrexed alone (Fasola et al., 2006).

Pemetrexed has also been shown to induce autophagy. Autophagy refers to the sequestration of cytosolic or cellular components in autophagosomes for subsequent degradation. It plays a part in many cellular processes including cell death and antigen processing for MHC II presentation (Deretic, 2006). Pemetrexed promotes autophagy leading to apoptotic cell death, however, whether this leads to antigen presentation remains to be seen (Bareford et al., 2011). Of particular interest is that COX-2 inhibitors, mentioned above, can enhance the cytotoxic effects of pemetrexed (S. L. O'Kane et al., 2010).

Cisplatin has also increased the sensitivity of tumour cells to cell lysis induced by cytotoxic T cells, though the mechanism was not elucidated (Collins & Kao, 1989). More recently, it was reported that cisplatin activates the Fas-ligand (CD95)-related apoptotic pathway in tumour cells. CD95 is widely expressed on MM cell lines but appears to be dysfunctional (Stewart et al., 2002).

5.2 Combination chemoimmunotherapy

As mentioned above, cisplatin sensitises tumour cells to immune cell- mediated killing and has been exploited in several chemo-immunotherapeutic strategies, the majority of which utilise IFN as the immunotherapeutic component. While IFN-α has had limited effectiveness as a single agent, Sklarin et al. showed that IFN-α was able to increase the therapeutic value of cisplatin and mitomycin (Sklarin et al., 1988). This paved the way for several studies that utilised IFN-α in combination with chemotherapeutic agents. A study by Tansan et al. administered cisplatin and mitomycin with IFN-α2b in 19 patients. There was a non-significant difference in the median survival of patients that were treated with this combination (15 months) compared to the control (8 months) (Tansan et al., 1994). In a similar study utilising the same combination but with IFN-α2a in 43 patients, there was no significant survival benefit in the treated group (11.7 months) vs. the untreated group (7 months) (Metintas et al., 1999). Twenty-six patients treated with cisplatin and IFN-α2a showed a similar median survival time of 12 months vs. 8 months (Soulié et al., 1996). While the median survival was not significant between the treatment groups, the survival times of the responders vs. non-responders were significant. A phase II study utilised doxorubicin and IFN-α and showed that while the combination was more effective than either agent alone, survival was not significantly prolonged (Upham et al., 1993). Cisplatin with doxorubicin (shown to elicit immunogenic cell death) (intravenous) and IFN-α2b (subcutaneous) was administered in 37 MM patients in a phase II trial. There were considerable toxicities and an overall response rate of 29%. One and two year survival was 45% and 34%, respectively (Parra et al., 2001). Cisplatin alone with IFN-α 2a in 13 MM patients resulted in clinical responses in 11 patients (one with a complete response), but the regimen was again very toxic.

It would seem that although IFN-therapy is relatively well tolerated, in combination with chemotherapy non-negligible toxicities are evident. Furthermore, mono-IFN-therapies utilised adenoviral IFN, but many of the combination therapies with cisplatin utilised recombinant IFN, which may not be optimal to the regimen.

Cisplatin synergistically inhibited proliferation of mesothelioma cell lines when co-applied with HER-2/neu antibody, Trastuzumab (Toma et al., 2002).

Pemetrexed has been combined with the VEGF antibody, bevacizumab, in a MM immunodeficient mouse model. Bevacizumab alone restricted tumour growth, inhibited the formation of large blood vessels and also prevented the development of pleural effusion. Combination with pemetrexed more effectively suppressed pleural effusion and increased survival in mice (Li et al., 2007).

Combining pemetrexed with Treg blockade in another mouse model of MM was also synergistic in prolonging survival. This combination was associated with decreased numbers of Treg in the tumour, increased IL-2 production, DC maturation and increased numbers of tumour-infiltrating IFN-γ-producing CD8[+] T cells when compared to either agent alone (Anraku et al., 2010).

Although combination of immunotherapy with pemetrexed and/or cisplatin is in an early phase, it is already providing promising results. It remains to be seen however, whether lowering the dose of chemotherapy in order to prevent high grade toxicity diminishes the clinical benefit.

6. Summary and concluding remarks

The importance of applying immunotherapy in combination with other treatments is becoming increasingly obvious from other cancers, mainly melanoma. It has become apparent that generating a transient immune response with a single specificity is not sufficient for clinical benefit; immunosuppressive effects need to be removed and any ensuing broad-specificity immune response needs to be sustained and enhanced.

It has been proposed recently that successful immunotherapy requires multiple elements, such as suppressing or removing tolerance, generating anti-tumour effector immune cells via vaccination, boosting the immune response by inducing immunogenic cancer cell death, checking and compensating for genetic polymorphism which may cause suboptimal immune responses, and finally, adjuvant treatment may be needed to maintain the immune response (Zitvogel et al., 2008).

Immunotherapies administered to MM patients can be analysed from the point of view of these categories. Removing immunosuppression by targeting Treg cells or blocking VEGF in combination with chemotherapy, the latter generating tumour cell death and providing tumour antigens, resulted in impressive results in mouse models. Immunosuppression may vary in patients according to histological subtype. Patients with the sarcomatoid variant of MM have a tendency towards more suppressive haematology (ElGendy et al., 2006). Analysing regulatory cell types in the circulation or in the tissue may provide useful information about the requirement of removing immunosuppression before immunotherapy in some patients.

The largest numbers of clinical trials in MM patients were carried out by applying single cytokines. It does not seem surprising now that addressing only the immune cell stimulation step did not translate to clinical success. It would be interesting to see how combining IL-2 or IFN not only with chemotherapy but also with e.g. a cancer vaccine would improve outcome. On the other hand, some viral vectors delivering tumour antigens, such as vaccinia, trigger considerable IFN-α production by infecting DC in the host (Pascutti et al., 2011).

Combination of chemotherapy and immunotherapy in fact has shown synergy in MM patients, as discussed earlier. However, these combinations are often associated with significant toxicities. These maybe alleviated by using less cytotoxic concentrations of chemotherapeutic agents in combination therapies, as demonstrated in *in vitro* studies (Zitvogel et al., 2008; Shurin et al., 2009)

As MM is a relatively rare disease, multi-arm trials with large patient numbers, comparing several treatment modalities, are challenging to organise. On the other hand, information obtained in mouse models does not always translate well to human studies. The model itself influences the results, as observed e.g. in the AB12 and AC29 models which secrete large amounts of TGF-β, whereas the AB1 mouse model does not. AB12 also produce much more GMCSF than AC29 and AC29 is a much slower growing tumour (Triozzi et al., 2005). The models do not always reflect that many patients have large tumours. In the AE17 mouse model of MM the anti-tumour effect of IL-2/anti-CD40 therapy was only mediated by CD4+ or CD8+ T cells when the mice had large tumours, while with a small tumour burden these cells were not crucial. Thus the results obtained in pre-clinical models may not be reproducible in humans.

Immunotherapy may not lead to tumour shrinkage, however, in an incurable cancer such as MM, stabilisation of the disease and palliation of symptoms are just as important. Bevacizumab in combination with pemetrexed have had profound affects on alleviating pleural effusion, thus improving the quality of life of patients (Li et al., 2007). Thus, clinical trials, although designed for immune-mediated tumour control, should be analysed for improving the quality of life of patients and such treatments maybe provided in palliative situations.

Taken together, it is apparent from the varying success of immunotherapies conducted as monotherapies in MM that the next generation of such treatments need to be designed as combination therapies. The right combination of treatments, timing, dose, patient selection needs to be determined. Disease stage, histological subtype, the patients' general health and relevant genetic polymorphisms also need to be considered. In theory, a well designed therapy addressing all the key immunological steps, as discussed earlier, has the potential to lead to tumour control. It remains to be seen whether immunotherapy can be an effective weapon in controlling mesothelioma.

7. Acknowledgements

SA-T and ZT are supported by the June Hancock Mesothelioma research Fund, Leeds, UK; JFL is supported by the Stepping Stones Appeal, Velindre NHS Trust, Cardiff, UK.

8. References

Alì, G., Boldrini, L., Lucchi, M., Mussi, A., Corsi, V. & Fontanini, G. (2009). Tryptase mast cells in malignant pleural mesothelioma as an independent favorable prognostic factor. *J Thorac Oncol* 4, 3, 348 - 354.

Alì, G., Boldrini, L., Lucchi, M., Picchi, A., Dell'Omodarme, M., Prati, M.C., Mussi, A., Corsi, V. & Fontanini, G. (2009). Treatment with interleukin-2 in malignant pleural mesothelioma: immunological and angiogenetic assessment and prognostic impact. *Br J Cancer* 101, 11, 1869 - 1875.

Allen, R.K. (2007). Apparent spontaneous complete regression of a multifocal malignant mesothelioma of the pleura. *Med J Aust* 187, 7, 413 - 415.

Altieri, D.C. (2004). Molecular circuits of apoptosis regulation and cell division control: the survivin paradigm. *J Cell Biochem* 92, 4, 656 - 663.

Ambrosini, G., Adida, C. & Altieri, D.C. (1997). A novel anti-apoptosis gene, survivin, expressed in cancer and lymphoma. *Nat Med* 3, 8, 917 - 921.

Andersen, M.H., Pedersen, L.O., Becker, J.C. & Straten, P.T. (2001). Identification of a cytotoxic T lymphocyte response to the apoptosis inhibitor protein survivin in cancer patients. *Cancer Res* 61, 3, 869 - 872.

Anraku, M., Cunningham, K.S., Yun, Z., Tsao, M.S., Zhang, L., Keshavjee, S., Johnston, M.R. & de Perrot, M. (2008). Impact of tumor-infiltrating T cells on survival in patients with malignant pleural mesothelioma. *J Thorac Cardiovasc Surg* 135, 4, 823 - 829.

Anraku, M., Tagawa, T., Wu, L., Yun, Z., Keshavjee, S., Zhang, L., Johnston, M.R. & de Perrot, M. (2010). Synergistic antitumor effects of regulatory T cell blockade combined with pemetrexed in murine malignant mesothelioma. *J Immunol* 185, 2, 956 - 966.

Antony, A.C. (1996). Folate receptors. *Annu Rev Nutr* 16, 501 - 521.

Apetoh, L., Ghiringhelli, F., Tesniere, A., Criollo, A., Ortiz, C., Lidereau, R., Mariette, C., Chaput, N., Mira, J.P., Delaloge, S., André, F., Tursz, T., Kroemer, G. & Zitvogel, L. (2007). The interaction between HMGB1 and TLR4 dictates the outcome of anticancer chemotherapy and radiotherapy. *Immunol Rev* 220, 47 - 59.

Ardizzoni, A., Pennucci, M.C., Castagneto, B., Mariani, G.L., Cinquegrana, A., Magri, D., Verna, A., Salvati, F. & Rosso, R. (1994). Recombinant interferon alpha-2b in the treatment of diffuse malignant pleural mesothelioma. *Am J Clin Oncol* 17, 1, 80 - 82.

Astoul, P., Nussbaum, E. & Boutin, C. (1995). Natural-killer cell-mediated cytotoxicity of blood-lymphocytes from patients with malignant mesothelioma treated by intrapleural interleukin-2. *Int J Oncol* 6, 2, 431 - 436.

Astoul, P., Picat-Joossen, D., Viallat, J.R. & Boutin, C. (1998). Intrapleural administration of interleukin-2 for the treatment of patients with malignant pleural mesothelioma: a Phase II study. *Cancer* 83, 10, 2099 - 2104.

Baldus, S.E., Engelmann, K. & Hanisch, F.G. (2004). MUC1 and the MUCs: a family of human mucins with impact in cancer biology. *Crit Rev Clin Lab Sci* 41, 2, 189 - 231.

Banchereau, J., Bazan, F., Blanchard, D., Brière, F., Galizzi, J.P., van Kooten, C., Liu, Y.J., Rousset, F. & Saeland, S. (1994). The CD40 antigen and its ligand. *Annu Rev Immunol* 12, 881 - 922.

Bareford, M.D., Hamed, H.A., Tang, Y., Cruickshanks, N., Burow, M.E., Fisher, P.B., Moran, R.G., Nephew, K.P., Grant, S. & Dent, P. (2011). Sorafenib enhances pemetrexed cytotoxicity through an autophagy-dependent mechanism in cancer cells. *Autophagy* 7, 10.

Bernsen, M.R., Tang, J.W., Everse, L.A., Koten, J.W. & Otter, W.D. (1999). Interleukin 2 (IL-2) therapy: potential advantages of locoregional versus systemic administration. *Cancer Treat Rev* 25, 2, 73 - 82.

Berthon, C., Driss, V., Liu, J., Kuranda, K., Leleu, X., Jouy, N., Hetuin, D. & Quesnel, B. (2010). In acute myeloid leukemia, B7-H1 (PD-L1) protection of blasts from cytotoxic T cells is induced by TLR ligands and interferon-gamma and can be reversed using MEK inhibitors. *Cancer Immunol Immunother* 59, 12, 1839-1849.

Beyer, H.L., Geschwindt, R.D., Glover, C.L., Tran, L., Hellstrom, I., Hellstrom, K.E., Miller, M.C., Verch, T., Allard, W.J., Pass, H.I. & Sardesai, N.Y. (2007). MESOMARK: a potential test for malignant pleural mesothelioma. *Clin Chem* 53, 4, 666 - 672.

Bielefeldt-Ohmann, H., Jarnicki, A.G. & Fitzpatrick, D.R. (1996). Molecular pathobiology and immunology of malignant mesothelioma. *J Pathol* 178, 4, 369 - 378.

Boghaert, E., Sridharan, L., Khandke, K., Armellino, D., Ryan, M., Myers, K., Harrop, R., Kunz, A., Hamann, P., Marquette, K., Dougher, M., DiJoseph, J. & Damle, N. (2008). The oncofetal protein, 5T4, is a suitable target for antibody-guided anti-cancer chemotherapy with calicheamicin. *Int J Oncol* 32, 1, 221-234.

Bonfanti, A., Lissoni, P., Bucovec, R., Rovelli, F., Brivio, F. & Fumagalli, L. (2000). Changes in circulating dendritic cells and IL-12 in relation to the angiogenic factor VEGF during IL-2 immunotherapy of metastatic renal cell cancer. *Int J Biol Markers* 15, 2, 161 - 164.

Boutin, C., Viallat, J.R., Van Zandwijk, N., Douillard, J.T., Paillard, J.C., Guerin, J.C., Mignot, P., Migueres, J., Varlet, F. & Jehan, A. (1991). Activity of intrapleural recombinant gamma-interferon in malignant mesothelioma. *Cancer* 67, 8, 2033 - 2037.

Boutin, C., Nussbaum, E., Monnet, I., Bignon, J., Vanderschueren, R., Guerin, J.C., Menard, O., Mignot, P., Dabouis, G. & Douillard, J.Y. (1994). Intrapleural treatment with recombinant gamma-interferon in early stage malignant pleural mesothelioma. *Cancer* 74, 9, 2460 - 2467.

Bueno, R., Appasani, K., Mercer, H., Lester, S. & Sugarbaker, D. (2001). The alpha folate receptor is highly activated in malignant pleural mesothelioma. *J Thorac Cardiovasc Surg* 121, 2, 225 - 233.

Bunt, S.K., Yang, L., Sinha, P., Clements, V.K., Leips, J. & Ostrand-Rosenberg, S. (2007). Reduced inflammation in the tumor microenvironment delays the accumulation of myeloid-derived suppressor cells and limits tumor progression. *Cancer Res* 67, 20, 10019 - 10026.

Burt, B.M., Rodig, S.J., Tilleman, T.R., Elbardissi, A.W., Bueno, R. & Sugarbaker, D.J. (2011). Circulating and tumor-infiltrating myeloid cells predict survival in human pleural mesothelioma. *Cancer.* Apr 26 (E-pub ahead of print).

Caminschi, I., Venetsanakos, E., Leong, C.C., Garlepp, M.J., Scott, B. & Robinson, B.W. (1998). Interleukin-12 induces an effective antitumor response in malignant mesothelioma. *Am J Respir Cell Mol Biol* 19, 5, 738 - 746.

Carsberg, C., Myers, K. & Stern, P. (1996). Metastasis-associated 5T4 antigen disrupts cell-cell contacts and induces cellular motility in epithelial cells. *Internatl J Cancer* 68, 1, 84-92.

Castagneto, B., Zai, S., Mutti, L., Lazzaro, A., Ridolfi, R., Piccolini, E., Ardizzoni, A., Fumagalli, L., Valsuani, G. & Botta, M. (2001). Palliative and therapeutic activity of IL-2 immunotherapy in unresectable malignant pleural mesothelioma with pleural effusion: Results of a phase II study on 31 consecutive patients. *Lung Cancer* 31, 2-3, 303 - 310.

Chang, K. & Pastan, I. (1996). Molecular cloning of mesothelin, a differentiation antigen present on mesothelium, mesotheliomas, and ovarian cancers. *Proc Natl Acad Sci U S A* 93, 1, 136 - 140.

Christmas, T.I., Manning, L.S., Davis, M.R., Robinson, B.W. & Garlepp, M.J. (1991). HLA antigen expression and malignant mesothelioma. *Am J Respir Cell Mol Biol* 5, 3, 213 - 220.

Christmas, T.I., Manning, L.S., Garlepp, M.J., Musk, A.W. & Robinson, B.W. (1993). Effect of interferon-alpha 2a on malignant mesothelioma. *J Interferon Res* 13, 1, 9 - 12.

Coleman, S., Clayton, A., Mason, M.D., Jasani, B., Adams, M. & Tabi, Z. (2005). Recovery of CD8+ T-cell function during systemic chemotherapy in advanced ovarian cancer. *Cancer Res* 65, 15, 7000 - 7006.

Collins, J.L. & Kao, M.S. (1989). The anticancer drug, cisplatin, increases the naturally occurring cell-mediated lysis of tumor cells. *Cancer Immunol Immunother* 29, 1, 17 - 22.

Creaney, J., Segal, A., Sterrett, G., Platten, M.A., Baker, E., Murch, A.R., Nowak, A.K., Robinson, B.W. & Millward, M.J. (2008). Overexpression and altered glycosylation of MUC1 in malignant mesothelioma. *Br J Cancer* 98, 9, 1562 - 1569.

Creaney, J., Francis, R.J., Dick, I.M., Musk, A.W., Robinson, B.W., Byrne, M.J. & Nowak, A.K. (2011). Serum soluble mesothelin concentrations in malignant pleural mesothelioma: relationship to tumor volume, clinical stage and changes in tumor burden. *Clin Cancer Res* 17, 5, 1181 - 1189.

Currie, A., Prosser, A., McDonnell, A., Cleaver, A., Robinson, B., Freeman, G. & van der Most, R. (2009). Dual control of antitumor CD8 T cells through the programmed death-1/programmed death-ligand 1 pathway and immunosuppressive CD4 T cells: regulation and counterregulation. *J Immunol* 183, 12, 7898-7908.

Currie, A.J., van der Most, R.G., Broomfield, S.A., Prosser, A.C., Tovey, M.G. & Robinson, B.W. (2008). Targeting the effector site with IFN-alphabeta-inducing TLR ligands reactivates tumor-resident CD8 T cell responses to eradicate established solid tumors. *J Immunol* 180, 3, 1535 - 1544.

Davidson, B., Dong, H.P., Holth, A., Berner, A. & Risberg, B. (2007). Chemokine receptors are infrequently expressed in malignant and benign mesothelial cells. *Am J Clin Pathol* 127, 5, 752 - 759.

Davidson, J.A., Musk, A.W., Wood, B.R., Morey, S., Ilton, M., Yu, L.L., Drury, P., Shilkin, K. & Robinson, B.W. (1998). Intralesional cytokine therapy in cancer: a pilot study of GM-CSF infusion in mesothelioma. *J Immunother* 21, 5, 389 - 398.

de Melo, M., Gerbase, M., Curran, J. & Pache, J. (2006). Phosphorylated extracellular signal-regulated kinases are significantly increased in malignant mesothelioma. *J Histochem Cytochem* 54, 8, 855-861.

DeLong, P., Carroll, R.G., Henry, A.C., Tanaka, T., Ahmad, S., Leibowitz, M.S., Sterman, D.H., June, C.H., Albelda, S.M. & Vonderheide, R.H. (2005). Regulatory T cells and cytokines in malignant pleural effusions secondary to mesothelioma and carcinoma. *Cancer Biol Ther* 4, 3, 342 - 346.

Deretic, V. (2006). Autophagy as an immune defense mechanism. *Curr Opin Immunol* 18, 4, 375 - 382.

Dostert, C., Pétrilli, V., Van Bruggen, R., Steele, C., Mossman, B.T. & Tschopp, J. (2008). Innate immune activation through Nalp3 inflammasome sensing of asbestos and silica. *Science* 320, 5876, 674 - 677.

Dudley, M.E., Wunderlich, J.R., Robbins, P.F., Yang, J.C., Hwu, P., Schwartzentruber, D.J., Topalian, S.L., Sherry, R., Restifo, N.P., Hubicki, A.M., Robinson, M.R., Raffeld, M., Duray, P., Seipp, C.A., Rogers-Freezer, L., Morton, K.E., Mavroukakis, S.A., White, D.E. & Rosenberg, S.A. (2002). Cancer regression and autoimmunity in patients after clonal repopulation with antitumor lymphocytes. *Science* 298, 5594, 850 - 854.

Duluc, D., Corvaisier, M., Blanchard, S., Catala, L., Descamps, P., Gamelin, E., Ponsoda, S., Delneste, Y., Hebbar, M. & Jeannin, P. (2009). Interferon-gamma reverses the immunosuppressive and protumoral properties and prevents the generation of human tumor-associated macrophages. *Int J Cancer* 125, 2, 367 - 373.

Dummer, W., Niethammer, A.G., Baccala, R., Lawson, B.R., Wagner, N., Reisfeld, R.A. & Theofilopoulos, A.N. (2002). T cell homeostatic proliferation elicits effective antitumor autoimmunity. *J Clin Invest* 110, 2, 185 - 192.

Dunn, G.P., Bruce, A.T., Ikeda, H., Old, L.J. & Schreiber, R.D. (2002). Cancer immunoediting: from immunosurveillance to tumor escape. *Nat Immunol* 3, 11, 991 - 998.

Eikawa, S., Ohue, Y., Kitaoka, K., Aji, T., Uenaka, A., Oka, M. & Nakayama, E. (2010). Enrichment of Foxp3+ CD4 regulatory T cells in migrated T cells to IL-6- and IL-8-expressing tumors through predominant induction of CXCR1 by IL-6. *J Immunol* 185, 11, 6734 - 6740.

ElGendy, A.M., Abbas Helmy, W.H. & Ezz-ElArab, A. (2006). Flowcytometric immunophenotyping of peripheral-blood leukocytes in relation to immunopathology and cellular proliferation of pleural mesothelioma. *Egypt J Immunol* 13, 1, 87 - 98.

Elnakat, H. & Ratnam, M. (2004). Distribution, functionality and gene regulation of folate receptor isoforms: implications in targeted therapy. *Adv Drug Deliv Rev* 56, 8, 1067 - 1084.

Fasola, G., Puglisi, F., Follador, A., Aita, M., Di Terlizzi, S. & Belvedere, O. (2006). Dramatic tumour response to pemetrexed single-agent in an elderly patient with malignant peritoneal mesothelioma: a case report. *BMC Cancer* 6, 289.

Foureau, D.M., McKillop, I.H., Jones, C.P., Amin, A., White, R.L. & Salo, J.C. (2011). Skin tumor responsiveness to interleukin-2 treatment and CD8 Foxp3+ T cell expansion in an immunocompetent mouse model. *Cancer Immunol Immunother* 60, 9, 1347 - 1356.

Friedlander, P.L., Delaune, C.L., Abadie, J.M., Toups, M., LaCour, J., Marrero, L., Zhong, Q. & Kolls, J.K. (2003). Efficacy of CD40 ligand gene therapy in malignant mesothelioma. *Am J Respir Cell Mol Biol* 29, 3 Pt 1, 321 - 330.

Galon, J., Costes, A., Sanchez-Cabo, F., Kirilovsky, A., Mlecnik, B., Lagorce-Pagès, C., Tosolini, M., Camus, M., Berger, A., Wind, P., Zinzindohoué, F., Bruneval, P., Cugnenc, P.H., Trajanoski, Z., Fridman, W.H. & Pagès, F. (2006). Type, density, and location of immune cells within human colorectal tumors predict clinical outcome. *Science* 313, 5795, 1960 - 1964.

Garland, L., Rankin, C., Gandara, D., Rivkin, S., Scott, K., Nagle, R., Klein-Szanto, A., Testa, J., Altomare, D. & Borden, E. (2007). Phase II study of erlotinib in patients with malignant pleural mesothelioma: a Southwest Oncology Group Study. *J Clin Oncol* 25, 17, 2406-2413.

Gattacceca, F., Pilatte, Y., Billard, C., Monnet, I., Moritz, S., Le Carrou, J., Eloit, M. & Jaurand, M.C. (2002). Ad-IFN gamma induces antiproliferative and antitumoral responses in malignant mesothelioma. *Clin Cancer Res* 8, 10, 3298 - 3304.

Ghiringhelli, F., Larmonier, N., Schmitt, E., Parcellier, A., Cathelin, D., Garrido, C., Chauffert, B., Solary, E., Bonnotte, B. & Martin, F. (2004). CD4+CD25+ regulatory T cells suppress tumor immunity but are sensitive to cyclophosphamide which allows immunotherapy of established tumors to be curative. *Eur J Immunol* 34, 2, 336 - 344.

Ghiringhelli, F., Menard, C., Puig, P.E., Ladoire, S., Roux, S., Martin, F., Solary, E., Le Cesne, A., Zitvogel, L. & Chauffert, B. (2007). Metronomic cyclophosphamide regimen selectively depletes CD4+CD25+ regulatory T cells and restores T and NK effector functions in end stage cancer patients. *Cancer Immunol Immunother* 56, 5, 641 - 648.

Goey, S.H., Eggermont, A.M., Punt, C.J., Slingerland, R., Gratama, J.W., Oosterom, R., Oskam, R., Bolhuis, R.L. & Stoter, G. (1995). Intrapleural administration of interleukin 2 in pleural mesothelioma: a phase I-II study. *Br J Cancer* 72, 5, 1283 - 1288.

Gordon, G., Jensen, R., Hsiao, L., Gullans, S., Blumenstock, J., Ramaswamy, S., Richards, W., Sugarbaker, D. & Bueno, R. (2002). Translation of microarray data into clinically relevant cancer diagnostic tests using gene expression ratios in lung cancer and mesothelioma. *Cancer Res* 62, 17, 4963-4967.

Gordon, G.J., Mani, M., Mukhopadhyay, L., Dong, L., Edenfield, H.R., Glickman, J.N., Yeap, B.Y., Sugarbaker, D.J. & Bueno, R. (2007). Expression patterns of inhibitor of apoptosis proteins in malignant pleural mesothelioma. *J Pathol* 211, 4, 447 - 454.

Hall, B.M., Verma, N.D., Tran, G.T. & Hodgkinson, S.J. (2011). Distinct regulatory CD4(+)T cell subsets; differences between naïve and antigen specific T regulatory cells. *Curr Opin Immunol*.

Hanahan, D. & Weinberg, R.A. (2011). Hallmarks of cancer: the next generation. *Cell* 144, 5, 646 - 674.

Harrop, R., Shingler, W., Kelleher, M., de Belin, J. & Treasure, P. (2010). Cross-trial analysis of immunologic and clinical data resulting from phase I and II trials of MVA-5T4 (TroVax) in colorectal, renal, and prostate cancer patients. *J Immunother* 33, 9, 999-1005.

Hassan, R., Ebel, W., Routhier, E.L., Patel, R., Kline, J.B., Zhang, J., Chao, Q., Jacob, S., Turchin, H., Gibbs, L., Phillips, M.D., Mudali, S., Iacobuzio-Donahue, C., Jaffee,

E.M., Moreno, M., Pastan, I., Sass, P.M., Nicolaides, N.C. & Grasso, L. (2007). Preclinical evaluation of MORAb-009, a chimeric antibody targeting tumor-associated mesothelin. *Cancer Immun* 7, 20.

Hassan, R., Cohen, S.J., Phillips, M., Pastan, I., Sharon, E., Kelly, R.J., Schweizer, C., Weil, S. & Laheru, D. (2010). Phase I clinical trial of the chimeric anti-mesothelin monoclonal antibody MORAb-009 in patients with mesothelin-expressing cancers. *Clin Cancer Res* 16, 24, 6132 - 6138.

Hassan, R., Schweizer, C., Lu, K.F., Schuler, B., Remaley, A.T., Weil, S.C. & Pastan, I. (2010). Inhibition of mesothelin-CA-125 interaction in patients with mesothelioma by the anti-mesothelin monoclonal antibody MORAb-009: Implications for cancer therapy. *Lung Cancer* 68, 3, 455 - 459.

Hegmans, J.P., Hemmes, A., Hammad, H., Boon, L., Hoogsteden, H.C. & Lambrecht, B.N. (2006). Mesothelioma environment comprises cytokines and T-regulatory cells that suppress immune responses. *Eur Respir J* 27, 6, 1086 - 1095.

Ho, M., Hassan, R., Zhang, J., Wang, Q.C., Onda, M., Bera, T. & Pastan, I. (2005). Humoral immune response to mesothelin in mesothelioma and ovarian cancer patients. *Clin Cancer Res* 11, 10, 3814 - 3820.

Hodgson, J.T., McElvenny, D.M., Darnton, A.J., Price, M.J. & Peto, J. (2005). The expected burden of mesothelioma mortality in Great Britain from 2002 to 2050. *Br J Cancer* 92, 3, 587 - 593.

Hole, N. & Stern, P. (1988). A 72 kD trophoblast glycoprotein defined by a monoclonal antibody. *Br J Cancer* 57, 3, 239-246.

Inami, K., Abe, M., Takeda, K., Hagiwara, Y., Maeda, M., Segawa, T., Suyama, M., Watanabe, S. & Hino, O. (2010). Antitumor activity of anti-C-ERC/mesothelin monoclonal antibody in vivo. *Cancer Sci* 101, 4, 969 - 974.

Inamoto, T., Yamada, T., Ohnuma, K., Kina, S., Takahashi, N., Yamochi, T., Inamoto, S., Katsuoka, Y., Hosono, O., Tanaka, H., Dang, N.H. & Morimoto, C. (2007). Humanized anti-CD26 monoclonal antibody as a treatment for malignant mesothelioma tumors. *Clin Cancer Res* 13, 14, 4191 - 4200.

Ishii, T., Ohnuma, K., Murakami, A., Takasawa, N., Kobayashi, S., Dang, N.H., Schlossman, S.F. & Morimoto, C. (2001). CD26-mediated signaling for T cell activation occurs in lipid rafts through its association with CD45RO. *Proc Natl Acad Sci U S A* 98, 21, 12138 - 12143.

Jackaman, C., Bundell, C.S., Kinnear, B.F., Smith, A.M., Filion, P., van Hagen, D., Robinson, B.W. & Nelson, D.J. (2003). IL-2 intratumoral immunotherapy enhances CD8+ T cells that mediate destruction of tumor cells and tumor-associated vasculature: a novel mechanism for IL-2. *J Immunol* 171, 10, 5051 - 5063.

Jackaman, C., Cornwall, S., Lew, A.M., Zhan, Y., Robinson, B.W. & Nelson, D.J. (2009). Local effector failure in mesothelioma is not mediated by CD4+ CD25+ T-regulator cells. *Eur Respir J* 34, 1, 162 - 175.

Jackaman, C. & Nelson, D.J. (2010). Cytokine-armed vaccinia virus infects the mesothelioma tumor microenvironment to overcome immune tolerance and mediate tumor resolution. *Cancer Gene Ther* 17, 6, 429 - 440.

Jackaman, C., Cornwall, S., Graham, P.T. & Nelson, D.J. (2011). CD40-activated B cells contribute to mesothelioma tumor regression. *Immunol Cell Biol* 89, 2, 255 - 267.

Jarnicki, A.G., Fitzpatrick, D.R., Robinson, B.W. & Bielefeldt-Ohmann, H. (1996). Altered CD3 chain and cytokine gene expression in tumor infiltrating T lymphocytes during the development of mesothelioma. *Cancer Lett* 103, 1, 1 - 9.

Jasani, B., Coleman, S., Butchart, E., Evans, E.M., Adams, M., Mason, M., Gibbs, A. & Tabi, Z. (2005). Assessment of immunological competence and SV40 specific recall immunity in malignant pleural mesothelioma. *Vaccine* 23, 17-18, 2399 - 2402.

Jassar, A.S., Suzuki, E., Kapoor, V., Sun, J., Silverberg, M.B., Cheung, L., Burdick, M.D., Strieter, R.M., Ching, L.M., Kaiser, L.R. & Albelda, S.M. (2005). Activation of tumor-associated macrophages by the vascular disrupting agent 5,6-dimethylxanthenone-4-acetic acid induces an effective CD8+ T-cell-mediated antitumor immune response in murine models of lung cancer and mesothelioma. *Cancer Res* 65, 24, 11752 - 11761.

Kim, D., Krishnamurthy, V., Bines, S. & Kaufman, H. (2010). TroVax, a recombinant modified vaccinia Ankara virus encoding 5T4: Lessons learned and future development. *Hum Vacc* 6, 10, 12-19.

Kim, S., Buchlis, G., Fridlender, Z.G., Sun, J., Kapoor, V., Cheng, G., Haas, A., Cheung, H.K., Zhang, X., Corbley, M., Kaiser, L.R., Ling, L. & Albelda, S.M. (2008). Systemic blockade of transforming growth factor-beta signaling augments the efficacy of immunogene therapy. *Cancer Res* 68, 24, 10247 - 10256.

Knutson, K.L., Krco, C.J., Erskine, C.L., Goodman, K., Kelemen, L.E., Wettstein, P.J., Low, P.S., Hartmann, L.C. & Kalli, K.R. (2006). T-cell immunity to the folate receptor alpha is prevalent in women with breast or ovarian cancer. *J Clin Oncol* 24, 26, 4254 - 4261.

Koebel, C.M., Vermi, W., Swann, J.B., Zerafa, N., Rodig, S.J., Old, L.J., Smyth, M.J. & Schreiber, R.D. (2007). Adaptive immunity maintains occult cancer in an equilibrium state. *Nature* 450, 7171, 903 - 907.

Kreitman, R.J., Hassan, R., Fitzgerald, D.J. & Pastan, I. (2009). Phase I trial of continuous infusion anti-mesothelin recombinant immunotoxin SS1P. *Clin Cancer Res* 15, 16, 5274 - 5279.

Krug, L.M., Dao, T., Brown, A.B., Maslak, P., Travis, W., Bekele, S., Korontsvit, T., Zakhaleva, V., Wolchok, J., Yuan, J., Li, H., Tyson, L. & Scheinberg, D.A. (2010). WT1 peptide vaccinations induce CD4 and CD8 T cell immune responses in patients with mesothelioma and non-small cell lung cancer. *Cancer Immunol Immunother* 59, 10, 1467 - 1479.

Kruklitis, R.J., Singhal, S., Delong, P., Kapoor, V., Sterman, D.H., Kaiser, L.R. & Albelda, S.M. (2004). Immuno-gene therapy with interferon-beta before surgical debulking delays recurrence and improves survival in a murine model of malignant mesothelioma. *J Thorac Cardiovasc Surg* 127, 1, 123 - 130.

Kumar-Singh, S., Segers, K., Rodeck, U., Backhovens, H., Bogers, J., Weyler, J., Van Broeckhoven, C. & Van Marck, E. (1997). WT1 mutation in malignant mesothelioma and WT1 immunoreactivity in relation to p53 and growth factor receptor expression, cell-type transition, and prognosis. *J Pathol* 181, 1, 67 - 74.

Kumar-Singh, S., Weyler, J., Martin, M.J., Vermeulen, P.B. & Van Marck, E. (1999). Angiogenic cytokines in mesothelioma: a study of VEGF, FGF-1 and -2, and TGF beta expression. *J Pathol* 189, 1, 72 - 78.

Lake, R.A. & Robinson, B.W. (2005). Immunotherapy and chemotherapy--a practical partnership. *Nat Rev Cancer* 5, 5, 397 - 405.

Larsen, C.P., Ritchie, S.C., Hendrix, R., Linsley, P.S., Hathcock, K.S., Hodes, R.J., Lowry, R.P. & Pearson, T.C. (1994). Regulation of immunostimulatory function and costimulatory molecule (B7-1 and B7-2) expression on murine dendritic cells. *J Immunol* 152, 11, 5208 - 5219.

Le, H.K., Graham, L., Cha, E., Morales, J.K., Manjili, M.H. & Bear, H.D. (2009). Gemcitabine directly inhibits myeloid derived suppressor cells in BALB/c mice bearing 4T1 mammary carcinoma and augments expansion of T cells from tumor-bearing mice. *Int Immunopharmacol* 9, 7-8, 900 - 909.

Leigh, R.A. & Webster, I. (1982). Lymphocytic infiltration of pleural mesothelioma and its significance for survival. *S Afr Med J* 61, 26, 1007 - 1009.

Lenzi, R., Rosenblum, M., Verschraegen, C., Kudelka, A.P., Kavanagh, J.J., Hicks, M.E., Lang, E.A., Nash, M.A., Levy, L.B., Garcia, M.E., Platsoucas, C.D., Abbruzzese, J.L. & Freedman, R.S. (2002). Phase I study of intraperitoneal recombinant human interleukin 12 in patients with Müllerian carcinoma, gastrointestinal primary malignancies, and mesothelioma. *Clin Cancer Res* 8, 12, 3686 - 3695.

Li, Q., Yano, S., Ogino, H., Wang, W., Uehara, H., Nishioka, Y. & Sone, S. (2007). The therapeutic efficacy of anti vascular endothelial growth factor antibody, bevacizumab, and pemetrexed against orthotopically implanted human pleural mesothelioma cells in severe combined immunodeficient mice. *Clin Cancer Res* 13, 19, 5918 - 5925.

López-Ríos, F., Chuai, S., Flores, R., Shimizu, S., Ohno, T., Wakahara, K., Illei, P., Hussain, S., Krug, L., Zakowski, M., Rusch, V., Olshen, A. & Ladanyi, M. (2006). Global gene expression profiling of pleural mesotheliomas: overexpression of aurora kinases and P16/CDKN2A deletion as prognostic factors and critical evaluation of microarray-based prognostic prediction. *Cancer Research* 66, 6, 2970-2979.

Malek, T.R. (2008). The biology of interleukin-2. *Annu Rev Immunol* 26, 453 - 479.

Mantel, P.Y. & Schmidt-Weber, C.B. (2011). Transforming growth factor-beta: recent advances on its role in immune tolerance. *Methods Mol Biol* 677, 303 - 338.

Massagué, J. (1987). The TGF-beta family of growth and differentiation factors. *Cell* 49, 4, 437 - 438.

May, R.J., Dao, T., Pinilla-Ibarz, J., Korontsvit, T., Zakhaleva, V., Zhang, R.H., Maslak, P. & Scheinberg, D.A. (2007). Peptide epitopes from the Wilms' tumor 1 oncoprotein stimulate CD4+ and CD8+ T cells that recognize and kill human malignant mesothelioma tumor cells. *Clin Cancer Res* 13, 15 Pt 1, 4547 - 4555.

Meloni, F., Morosini, M., Solari, N., Passadore, I., Nascimbene, C., Novo, M., Ferrari, M., Cosentino, M., Marino, F., Pozzi, E. & Fietta, A.M. (2006). Foxp3 expressing CD4+ CD25+ and CD8+CD28- T regulatory cells in the peripheral blood of patients with lung cancer and pleural mesothelioma. *Hum Immunol* 67, 1-2, 1 - 12.

Metintas, M., Ozdemir, N., Uçgun, I., Elbek, O., Kolsuz, M., Mutlu, S. & Metintas, S. (1999). Cisplatin, mitomycin, and interferon-alpha2a combination chemoimmunotherapy in the treatment of diffuse malignant pleural mesothelioma. *Chest* 116, 2, 391 - 398.

Mukherjee, S., Haenel, T., Himbeck, R., Scott, B., Ramshaw, I., Lake, R.A., Harnett, G., Phillips, P., Morey, S., Smith, D., Davidson, J.A., Musk, A.W. & Robinson, B. (2000). Replication-restricted vaccinia as a cytokine gene therapy vector in cancer:

persistent transgene expression despite antibody generation. *Cancer Gene Ther* 7, 5, 663 - 670.

Mulatero, C.W., Penson, R.T., Papamichael, D., Gower, N.H., Evans, M. & Rudd, R.M. (2001). A phase II study of combined intravenous and subcutaneous interleukin-2 in malignant pleural mesothelioma. *Lung Cancer* 31, 1, 67 - 72.

Mundlos, S., Pelletier, J., Darveau, A., Bachmann, M., Winterpacht, A. & Zabel, B. (1993). Nuclear localization of the protein encoded by the Wilms' tumor gene WT1 in embryonic and adult tissues. *Development* 119, 4, 1329 - 1341.

Mutti, L., Valle, M.T., Balbi, B., Orengo, A.M., Lazzaro, A., Alciato, P., Gatti, E., Betta, P.G. & Pozzi, E. (1998). Primary human mesothelioma cells express class II MHC, ICAM-1 and B7-2 and can present recall antigens to autologous blood lymphocytes. *Int J Cancer* 78, 6, 740 - 749.

Needham, D.J., Lee, J.X. & Beilharz, M.W. (2006). Intra-tumoural regulatory T cells: a potential new target in cancer immunotherapy. *Biochem Biophys Res Commun* 343, 3, 684 - 691.

Neuzil, J., Dong, L.F., Wang, X.F. & Zingg, J.M. (2006). Tocopherol-associated protein-1 accelerates apoptosis induced by alpha-tocopheryl succinate in mesothelioma cells. *Biochem Biophys Res Commun* 343, 4, 1113 - 1117.

O'Kane, S., Pound, R., Campbell, A., Chaudhuri, N., Lind, M. & Cawkwell, L. (2006). Expression of bcl-2 family members in malignant pleural mesothelioma. *Acta Oncol* 45, 4, 449-453.

O'Kane, S.L., Eagle, G.L., Greenman, J., Lind, M.J. & Cawkwell, L. (2010). COX-2 specific inhibitors enhance the cytotoxic effects of pemetrexed in mesothelioma cell lines. *Lung Cancer* 67, 2, 160 - 165.

Odaka, M., Sterman, D.H., Wiewrodt, R., Zhang, Y., Kiefer, M., Amin, K.M., Gao, G.P., Wilson, J.M., Barsoum, J., Kaiser, L.R. & Albelda, S.M. (2001). Eradication of intraperitoneal and distant tumor by adenovirus-mediated interferon-beta gene therapy is attributable to induction of systemic immunity. *Cancer Res* 61, 16, 6201 - 6212.

Odaka, M., Wiewrodt, R., DeLong, P., Tanaka, T., Zhang, Y., Kaiser, L. & Albelda, S. (2002). Analysis of the immunologic response generated by Ad.IFN-beta during successful intraperitoneal tumor gene therapy. *Mol Ther* 6, 2, 210 - 218.

Ohnuma, K., Yamochi, T., Uchiyama, M., Nishibashi, K., Yoshikawa, N., Shimizu, N., Iwata, S., Tanaka, H., Dang, N.H. & Morimoto, C. (2004). CD26 up-regulates expression of CD86 on antigen-presenting cells by means of caveolin-1. *Proc Natl Acad Sci U S A* 101, 39, 14186 - 14191.

Ordóñez, N.G. (2003). Application of mesothelin immunostaining in tumor diagnosis. *Am J Surg Pathol* 27, 11, 1418 - 1428.

Oshika, Y., Nakamura, M., Abe, Y., Fukuchi, Y., Yoshimura, M., Itoh, M., Ohnishi, Y., Tokunaga, T., Fukushima, Y., Hatanaka, H., Kijima, H., Yamazaki, H., Tamaoki, N. & Ueyama, Y. (1998). Growth stimulation of non-small cell lung cancer xenografts by granulocyte-macrophage colony-stimulating factor (GM-CSF). *Eur J Cancer* 34, 12, 1958 - 1961.

Ostrand-Rosenberg, S. (2010). Myeloid-derived suppressor cells: more mechanisms for inhibiting antitumor immunity. *Cancer Immunol Immunother* 59, 10, 1593 - 1600.

Parra, H.S., Tixi, L., Latteri, F., Bretti, S., Alloisio, M., Gravina, A., Lionetto, R., Bruzzi, P., Dani, C., Rosso, R., Cosso, M., Balzarini, L., Santoro, A. & Ardizzoni, A. (2001). Combined regimen of cisplatin, doxorubicin, and alpha-2b interferon in the treatment of advanced malignant pleural mesothelioma: a Phase II multicenter trial of the Italian Group on Rare Tumors (GITR) and the Italian Lung Cancer Task Force (FONICAP). *Cancer* 92, 3, 650 - 656.

Pascutti, M.F., Rodríguez, A.M., Falivene, J., Giavedoni, L., Drexler, I. & Gherardi, M.M. (2011). Interplay between modified vaccinia virus Ankara and dendritic cells: phenotypic and functional maturation of bystander dendritic cells. *J Virol* 85, 11, 5532 - 5545.

Pilling, J.E., Nicholson, A.G., Harmer, C. & Goldstraw, P. (2007). Prolonged survival due to spontaneous regression and surgical excision of malignant mesothelioma. *Ann Thorac Surg* 83, 1, 314 - 315.

Porta, C., Danova, M., Orengo, A.M., Ferrini, S., Moroni, M., Gaggero, A., Libener, R., Betta, P.G., Ferrari, S., Procopio, A., Strizzi, L. & Mutti, L. (2000). Interleukin-2 induces cell cycle perturbations leading to cell growth inhibition and death in malignant mesothelioma cells in vitro. *J Cell Physiol* 185, 1, 126 - 134.

Porta, C., Rizzo, V., Zimatore, M., Sartore-Bianchi, A., Danova, M. & Mutti, L. (2002). Intrapleural interleukin-2 induces nitric oxide production in pleural effusions from malignant mesothelioma: a possible mechanism of interleukin-2-mediated cytotoxicity? *Lung Cancer* 38, 2, 159 - 162.

Radfar, S., Wang, Y. & Khong, H.T. (2009). Activated CD4+ T cells dramatically enhance chemotherapeutic tumor responses in vitro and in vivo. *J Immunol* 183, 10, 6800 - 6807.

Rama, I. & Grinyó, J.M. (2010). Malignancy after renal transplantation: the role of immunosuppression. *Nat Rev Nephrol* 6, 9, 511 - 519.

Robinson, B.W., Robinson, C. & Lake, R.A. (2001). Localised spontaneous regression in mesothelioma -- possible immunological mechanism. *Lung Cancer* 32, 2, 197 - 201.

Robinson, B.W., Creaney, J., Lake, R., Nowak, A., Musk, A.W., de Klerk, N., Winzell, P., Hellstrom, K.E. & Hellstrom, I. (2005). Soluble mesothelin-related protein--a blood test for mesothelioma. *Lung Cancer* 49 Suppl 1, S109 - 111.

Romagnoli, S., Fasoli, E., Vaira, V., Falleni, M., Pellegrini, C., Catania, A., Roncalli, M., Marchetti, A., Santambrogio, L., Coggi, G. & Bosari, S. (2009). Identification of potential therapeutic targets in malignant mesothelioma using cell-cycle gene expression analysis. *Am J Pathol* 174, 3, 762-770.

Romero, J.M., Jiménez, P., Cabrera, T., Cózar, J.M., Pedrinaci, S., Tallada, M., Garrido, F. & Ruiz-Cabello, F. (2005). Coordinated downregulation of the antigen presentation machinery and HLA class I/beta2-microglobulin complex is responsible for HLA-ABC loss in bladder cancer. *Int J Cancer* 113, 4, 605 - 610.

Rosewicz, S., Detjen, K., Scholz, A. & von Marschall, Z. (2004). Interferon-alpha: regulatory effects on cell cycle and angiogenesis. *Neuroendocrinol* 80 Suppl 1, 85 - 93.

Roulois, D., Vignard, V., Gueugnon, F., Labarrière, N., Grégoire, M. & Fonteneau, J.F. (2011). Recognition of pleural mesothelioma by MUC1(950-958)/HLA-A*0201 specific CD8+ T lymphocyte. *Eur Respir J*.

Salazar, M.D. & Ratnam, M. (2007). The folate receptor: what does it promise in tissue-targeted therapeutics? *Cancer Metastasis Rev* 26, 1, 141 - 152.

Schmitter, D., Lauber, B., Fagg, B. & Stahel, R.A. (1992). Hematopoietic growth factors secreted by seven human pleural mesothelioma cell lines: interleukin-6 production as a common feature. *Int J Cancer* 51, 2, 296 - 301.

Schoenberger, S.P., Toes, R.E., van der Voort, E.I., Offringa, R. & Melief, C.J. (1998). T-cell help for cytotoxic T lymphocytes is mediated by CD40-CD40L interactions. *Nature* 393, 6684, 480 - 483.

Sekido, Y., Pass, H., Bader, S., Mew, D., Christman, M., Gazdar, A. & Minna, J. (1995). Neurofibromatosis type 2 (NF2) gene is somatically mutated in mesothelioma but not in lung cancer. *Cancer Res* 55, 6, 1227-1231.

Setiadi et al, 2007. Epigenetic control of the immune escape mechanisms in malignant carcinomas. *Molecular and cellular biology.* Nov, Vol 27, No.22; p7886-7894.

Shankaran, V., Ikeda, H., Bruce, A.T., White, J.M., Swanson, P.E., Old, L.J. & Schreiber, R.D. (2001). IFNgamma and lymphocytes prevent primary tumour development and shape tumour immunogenicity. *Nature* 410, 6832, 1107 - 1111.

Shaw, D., Connolly, N., Patel, P., Kilany, S., Hedlund, G., Nordle, O., Forsberg, G., Zweit, J., Stern, P. & Hawkins, R. (2007). A phase II study of a 5T4 oncofoetal antigen tumour-targeted superantigen (ABR-214936) therapy in patients with advanced renal cell carcinoma. *Br J Cancer* 96, 4, 567-574.

Shimizu, Y., Dobashi, K., Imai, H., Sunaga, N., Ono, A., Sano, T., Hikino, T., Shimizu, K., Tanaka, S., Ishizuka, T., Utsugi, M. & Mori, M. (2009). CXCR4+FOXP3+CD25+ lymphocytes accumulate in CXCL12-expressing malignant pleural mesothelioma. *Int J Immunopathol Pharmacol* 22, 1, 43 - 51.

Shurin, G.V., Tourkova, I.L., Kaneno, R. & Shurin, M.R. (2009). Chemotherapeutic agents in noncytotoxic concentrations increase antigen presentation by dendritic cells via an IL-12-dependent mechanism. *J Immunol* 183, 1, 137 - 144.

Sica, A. (2010). Role of tumour-associated macrophages in cancer-related inflammation. *Exp Oncol* 32, 3, 153 - 158.

Sierra, E.E. & Goldman, I.D. (1999). Recent advances in the understanding of the mechanism of membrane transport of folates and antifolates. *Semin Oncol* 26, 2 Suppl 6, 11 - 23.

Sklarin, N.T., Chahinian, A.P., Feuer, E.J., Lahman, L.A., Szrajer, L. & Holland, J.F. (1988). Augmentation of activity of cis-diamminedichloroplatinum(II) and mitomycin C by interferon in human malignant mesothelioma xenografts in nude mice. *Cancer Res* 48, 1, 64 - 67.

Sojka, D.K., Donepudi, M., Bluestone, J.A. & Mokyr, M.B. (2000). Melphalan and other anticancer modalities up-regulate B7-1 gene expression in tumor cells. *J Immunol* 164, 12, 6230 - 6236.

Sommerfeldt, N., Schütz, F., Sohn, C., Förster, J., Schirrmacher, V. & Beckhove, P. (2006). The shaping of a polyvalent and highly individual T-cell repertoire in the bone marrow of breast cancer patients. *Cancer Res* 66, 16, 8258 - 8265.

Soulié, P., Ruffié, P., Trandafir, L., Monnet, I., Tardivon, A., Terrier, P., Cvitkovic, E., Le Chevalier, T. & Armand, J.P. (1996). Combined systemic chemoimmunotherapy in advanced diffuse malignant mesothelioma. Report of a phase I-II study of weekly cisplatin/interferon alfa-2a. *J Clin Oncol* 14, 3, 878 - 885.

Southall, P., Boxer, G., Bagshawe, K., Hole, N., Bromley, M. & Stern, P. (1990). Immunohistological distribution of 5T4 antigen in normal and malignant tissues. *Br J Cancer* 61, 1, 89-95.

Southgate, T., McGinn, O., Castro, F., Rutkowski, A., Al-Muftah, M., Marinov, G., Smethurst, G., Shaw, D., Ward, C., Miller, C. & Stern, P. (2010). CXCR4 mediated chemotaxis is regulated by 5T4 oncofetal glycoprotein in mouse embryonic cells. *PLoS ONE* 5, 4, e9982.

Sterman, D.H., Recio, A., Carroll, R.G., Gillespie, C.T., Haas, A., Vachani, A., Kapoor, V., Sun, J., Hodinka, R., Brown, J.L., Corbley, M.J., Parr, M., Ho, M., Pastan, I., Machuzak, M., Benedict, W., Zhang, X.Q., Lord, E.M., Litzky, L.A., Heitjan, D.F., June, C.H., Kaiser, L.R., Vonderheide, R.H., Albelda, S.M. & Kanther, M. (2007). A phase I clinical trial of single-dose intrapleural IFN-beta gene transfer for malignant pleural mesothelioma and metastatic pleural effusions: high rate of antitumor immune responses. *Clin Cancer Res* 13, 15 Pt 1, 4456 - 4466.

Sterman, D.H., Recio, A., Haas, A.R., Vachani, A., Katz, S.I., Gillespie, C.T., Cheng, G., Sun, J., Moon, E., Pereira, L., Wang, X., Heitjan, D.F., Litzky, L., June, C.H., Vonderheide, R.H., Carroll, R.G. & Albelda, S.M. (2010). A phase I trial of repeated intrapleural adenoviral-mediated interferon-beta gene transfer for mesothelioma and metastatic pleural effusions. *Mol Ther* 18, 4, 852 - 860.

Sterman, D.H., Haas, A., Moon, E., Recio, A., Schwed, D., Vachani, A., Katz, S.I., Gillespie, C.T., Cheng, G., Sun, J., Papasavvas, E., Montaner, L.J., Heitjan, D.F., Litzky, L., Friedberg, J., Culligan, M., June, C.H., Carroll, R.G. & Albelda, S.M. (2011). A Trial of Intrapleural Adenoviral-mediated Interferon-{alpha}2b Gene Transfer for Malignant Pleural Mesothelioma. *Am J Respir Crit Care Med*.

Stewart, J.H., Nguyen, D.M., Chen, G.A. & Schrump, D.S. (2002). Induction of apoptosis in malignant pleural mesothelioma cells by activation of the Fas (Apo-1/CD95) death-signal pathway. *J Thorac Cardiovasc Surg* 123, 2, 295 - 302.

Strizzi, L., Catalano, A., Vianale, G., Orecchia, S., Casalini, A., Tassi, G., Puntoni, R., Mutti, L. & Procopio, A. (2001). Vascular endothelial growth factor is an autocrine growth factor in human malignant mesothelioma. *J Pathol* 193, 4, 468 - 475.

Stumbles, P.A., Himbeck, R., Frelinger, J.A., Collins, E.J., Lake, R.A. & Robinson, B.W. (2004). Cutting edge: tumor-specific CTL are constitutively cross-armed in draining lymph nodes and transiently disseminate to mediate tumor regression following systemic CD40 activation. *J Immunol* 173, 10, 5923 - 5928.

Su, L., Liu, G., Hao, X., Zhong, N., Zhong, D., Liu, X. & Singhal, S. (2011). Death Receptor 5 and cellular FLICE-inhibitory protein regulate pemetrexed-induced apoptosis in human lung cancer cells. *Eur J Cancer*.

Suzuki, E., Kapoor, V., Cheung, H.K., Ling, L.E., DeLong, P.A., Kaiser, L.R. & Albelda, S.M. (2004). Soluble type II transforming growth factor-beta receptor inhibits established murine malignant mesothelioma tumor growth by augmenting host antitumor immunity. *Clin Cancer Res* 10, 17, 5907 - 5918.

Suzuki, E., Kim, S., Cheung, H.K., Corbley, M.J., Zhang, X., Sun, L., Shan, F., Singh, J., Lee, W.C., Albelda, S.M. & Ling, L.E. (2007). A novel small-molecule inhibitor of transforming growth factor beta type I receptor kinase (SM16) inhibits murine mesothelioma tumor growth in vivo and prevents tumor recurrence after surgical resection. *Cancer Res* 67, 5, 2351 - 2359.

Tansan, S., Emri, S., Selçuk, T., Koç, Y., Hesketh, P., Heeren, T., McCaffrey, R.P. & Baris, Y.I. (1994). Treatment of malignant pleural mesothelioma with cisplatin, mitomycin C and alpha interferon. *Oncology* 51, 4, 348 - 351.

Thomas, A.M., Santarsiero, L.M., Lutz, E.R., Armstrong, T.D., Chen, Y.C., Huang, L.Q., Laheru, D.A., Goggins, M., Hruban, R.H. & Jaffee, E.M. (2004). Mesothelin-specific CD8(+) T cell responses provide evidence of in vivo cross-priming by antigen-presenting cells in vaccinated pancreatic cancer patients. *J Exp Med* 200, 3, 297 - 306.

Todryk, S.M., Tutt, A.L., Green, M.H., Smallwood, J.A., Halanek, N., Dalgleish, A.G. & Glennie, M.J. (2001). CD40 ligation for immunotherapy of solid tumours. *J Immunol Methods* 248, 1-2, 139 - 147.

Toma, S., Colucci, L., Scarabelli, L., Scaramuccia, A., Emionite, L., Betta, P.G. & Mutti, L. (2002). Synergistic effect of the anti-HER-2/neu antibody and cisplatin in immortalized and primary mesothelioma cell lines. *J Cell Physiol* 193, 1, 37 - 41.

Trinchieri, G. (1995). Interleukin-12: a proinflammatory cytokine with immunoregulatory functions that bridge innate resistance and antigen-specific adaptive immunity. *Annu Rev Immunol* 13, 251 - 276.

Triozzi, P.L., Aldrich, W., Allen, K.O., Lima, J., Shaw, D.R. & Strong, T.V. (2005). Antitumor activity of the intratumoral injection of fowlpox vectors expressing a triad of costimulatory molecules and granulocyte/macrophage colony stimulating factor in mesothelioma. *Int J Cancer* 113, 3, 406 - 414.

Upham, J.W., Musk, A.W., van Hazel, G., Byrne, M. & Robinson, B.W. (1993). Interferon alpha and doxorubicin in malignant mesothelioma: a phase II study. *Aust N Z J Med* 23, 6, 683 - 687.

Vachani, A., Sterman, D.H. & Albelda, S.M. (2007). Cytokine gene therapy for malignant pleural mesothelioma. *J Thorac Oncol* 2, 4, 265 - 267.

van Bruggen, I., Nelson, D.J., Currie, A.J., Jackaman, C. & Robinson, B.W. (2005). Intratumoral poly-N-acetyl glucosamine-based polymer matrix provokes a prolonged local inflammatory response that, when combined with IL-2, induces regression of malignant mesothelioma in a murine model. *J Immunother* 28, 4, 359 - 367.

van der Most, R.G., Currie, A.J., Cleaver, A.L., Salmons, J., Nowak, A.K., Mahendran, S., Larma, I., Prosser, A., Robinson, B.W., Smyth, M.J., Scalzo, A.A., Degli-Esposti, M.A. & Lake, R.A. (2009). Cyclophosphamide chemotherapy sensitizes tumor cells to TRAIL-dependent CD8 T cell-mediated immune attack resulting in suppression of tumor growth. *PLoS One* 4, 9, e6982.

van der Most, R.G., Currie, A.J., Mahendran, S., Prosser, A., Darabi, A., Robinson, B.W., Nowak, A.K. & Lake, R.A. (2009). Tumor eradication after cyclophosphamide depends on concurrent depletion of regulatory T cells: a role for cycling TNFR2-expressing effector-suppressor T cells in limiting effective chemotherapy. *Cancer Immunol Immunother* 58, 8, 1219 - 1228.

Veltman, J.D., Lambers, M.E., van Nimwegen, M., Hendriks, R.W., Hoogsteden, H.C., Aerts, J.G. & Hegmans, J.P. (2010). COX-2 inhibition improves immunotherapy and is associated with decreased numbers of myeloid-derived suppressor cells in mesothelioma. Celecoxib influences MDSC function. *BMC Cancer* 10, 464.

Veltman, J.D., Lambers, M.E., van Nimwegen, M., Hendriks, R.W., Hoogsteden, H.C., Hegmans, J.P. & Aerts, J.G. (2010). Zoledronic acid impairs myeloid differentiation to tumour-associated macrophages in mesothelioma. *Br J Cancer* 103, 5, 629 - 641.

Vogelzang, N.J., Rusthoven, J.J., Symanowski, J., Denham, C., Kaukel, E., Ruffie, P., Gatzemeier, U., Boyer, M., Emri, S., Manegold, C., Niyikiza, C. & Paoletti, P. (2003).

Phase III study of pemetrexed in combination with cisplatin versus cisplatin alone in patients with malignant pleural mesothelioma. *J Clin Oncol* 21, 14, 2636 - 2644.

Von Hoff, D.D., Metch, B., Lucas, J.G., Balcerzak, S.P., Grunberg, S.M. & Rivkin, S.E. (1990). Phase II evaluation of recombinant interferon-beta (IFN-beta ser) in patients with diffuse mesothelioma: a Southwest Oncology Group study. *J Interferon Res* 10, 5, 531 - 534.

Wang, B.X., Rahbar, R. & Fish, E.N. (2011). Interferon: current status and future prospects in cancer therapy. *J Interferon Cytokine Res* 31, 7, 545 - 552.

Warren, T.L. & Weiner, G.J. (2000). Uses of granulocyte-macrophage colony-stimulating factor in vaccine development. *Curr Opin Hematol* 7, 3, 168 - 173.

Weiner, S.J. & Neragi-Miandoab, S. (2009). Pathogenesis of malignant pleural mesothelioma and the role of environmental and genetic factors. *J Cancer Res Clin Oncol* 135, 1, 15 - 27.

Weitman, S.D., Weinberg, A.G., Coney, L.R., Zurawski, V.R., Jennings, D.S. & Kamen, B.A. (1992). Cellular localization of the folate receptor: potential role in drug toxicity and folate homeostasis. *Cancer Res* 52, 23, 6708 - 6711.

Whiteside, T.L. (2007). The role of death receptor ligands in shaping tumor microenvironment. *Immunol Invest* 36, 1, 25 - 46.

Willmon, C.L., Saloura, V., Fridlender, Z.G., Wongthida, P., Diaz, R.M., Thompson, J., Kottke, T., Federspiel, M., Barber, G., Albelda, S.M. & Vile, R.G. (2009). Expression of IFN-beta enhances both efficacy and safety of oncolytic vesicular stomatitis virus for therapy of mesothelioma. *Cancer Res* 69, 19, 7713 - 7720.

Wright, G., Cherwinski, H., Foster-Cuevas, M., Brooke, G., Puklavec, M., Bigler, M., Song, Y., Jenmalm, M., Gorman, D., McClanahan, T., Liu, M., Brown, M., Sedgwick, J., Phillips, J. & Barclay, A. (2003). Characterization of the CD200 receptor family in mice and humans and their interactions with CD200. *J Immunol* 171, 6, 3034-3046.

Yamada, N., Oizumi, S., Kikuchi, E., Shinagawa, N., Konishi-Sakakibara, J., Ishimine, A., Aoe, K., Gemba, K., Kishimoto, T., Torigoe, T. & Nishimura, M. (2010). CD8+ tumor-infiltrating lymphocytes predict favorable prognosis in malignant pleural mesothelioma after resection. *Cancer Immunol Immunother* 59, 10, 1543 - 1549.

Yang, H., Bocchetta, M., Kroczynska, B., Elmishad, A.G., Chen, Y., Liu, Z., Bubici, C., Mossman, B.T., Pass, H.I., Testa, J.R., Franzoso, G. & Carbone, M. (2006). TNF-alpha inhibits asbestos-induced cytotoxicity via a NF-kappaB-dependent pathway, a possible mechanism for asbestos-induced oncogenesis. *Proc Natl Acad Sci U S A* 103, 27, 10397 - 10402.

Yang, H., Rivera, Z., Jube, S., Nasu, M., Bertino, P., Goparaju, C., Franzoso, G., Lotze, M.T., Krausz, T., Pass, H.I., Bianchi, M.E. & Carbone, M. (2010). Programmed necrosis induced by asbestos in human mesothelial cells causes high-mobility group box 1 protein release and resultant inflammation. *Proc Natl Acad Sci U S A* 107, 28, 12611 - 12616.

Yang, L., Han, Y., Suarez Saiz, F., Saurez Saiz, F. & Minden, M.D. (2007). A tumor suppressor and oncogene: the WT1 story. *Leukemia* 21, 5, 868 - 876.

Yang, Y., Huang, C.T., Huang, X. & Pardoll, D.M. (2004). Persistent Toll-like receptor signals are required for reversal of regulatory T cell-mediated CD8 tolerance. *Nat Immunol* 5, 5, 508 - 515.

Yokokawa, J., Palena, C., Arlen, P., Hassan, R., Ho, M., Pastan, I., Schlom, J. & Tsang, K.Y. (2005). Identification of novel human CTL epitopes and their agonist epitopes of mesothelin. *Clin Cancer Res* 11, 17, 6342 - 6351.

Young, M.R., Wright, M.A., Coogan, M., Young, M.E. & Bagash, J. (1992). Tumor-derived cytokines induce bone marrow suppressor cells that mediate immunosuppression through transforming growth factor beta. *Cancer Immunol Immunother* 35, 1, 14 - 18.

Zaffaroni, N., Costa, A., Pennati, M., De Marco, C., Affini, E., Madeo, M., Erdas, R., Cabras, A., Kusamura, S., Baratti, D., Deraco, M. & Daidone, M.G. (2007). Survivin is highly expressed and promotes cell survival in malignant peritoneal mesothelioma. *Cell Oncol* 29, 6, 453 - 466.

Zeng, L., Buard, A., Monnet, I., Boutin, C., Fleury, J., Saint-Etienne, L., Brochard, P., Bignon, J. & Jaurand, M.C. (1993). In vitro effects of recombinant human interferon gamma on human mesothelioma cell lines. *Int J Cancer* 55, 3, 515 - 520.

Zitvogel, L., Apetoh, L., Ghiringhelli, F., André, F., Tesniere, A. & Kroemer, G. (2008). The anticancer immune response: indispensable for therapeutic success? *J Clin Invest* 118, 6, 1991 - 2001.

Zitvogel, L., Apetoh, L., Ghiringhelli, F. & Kroemer, G. (2008). Immunological aspects of cancer chemotherapy. *Nat Rev Immunol* 8, 1, 59 - 73.

11

Cisplatin Resistance in Malignant Pleural Mesothelioma

Parviz Behnam-Motlagh, Andreas Tyler, Thomas Brännström,
Terese Karlsson, Anders Johansson and Kjell Grankvist
Umeå University, Umeå
Sweden

1. Introduction

Malignant pleural mesothelioma (MPM) is an aggressive tumour. Patients have a very short median survival after diagnosis. Inherent but importantly, also induced, tumour survival mechanisms of malignant pleural mesothelioma is a major contributor to the short survival time (Bridda et al., 2007). No curative treatment is available. Mesothelioma has been subject to therapeutic trials, hitherto with little clinical gain. Most targeted therapies have focused on impairing signaling pathways on which cancers depend for survival. However, the efficacy of these approaches is impaired by signaling redundancy, adaptation and activating/silencing mutations.

Apoptosis is a physiological form of cell death that removes mutated and damaged cells. Deregulation of apoptosis in tumour cells allows them to bypass apoptosis during clonal expansion. Cancer-generating mutations disrupt apoptosis, leading to tumor initiation, progression or metastasis. The mutations that suppress apoptosis also reduce the sensitivity to cancer treatment (Johnstone et al., 2002). There are potential benefits to targeting tumors at the level of their anti-apoptotic defenses. Direct inhibitors of anti-apoptotic defenses could bypass the need to inhibit multiple pathways by moving to a distal level at which multiple signals are integrated. Also, stimulators of apoptosis through specific signaling pathways that emerge during cancer development or are acquired during cancer chemotherapy could be targeted. Such an approach may be effective in the different mesothelioma subtypes, against a variety of apoptosis-inducing therapies, and without substantial injury to normal tissues where apoptosis signaling is not disturbed.

Cisplatin, most often in combination with other drugs is still the treatment of choice for mesothelioma. Cisplatin chemotherapy activates several signaling pathways and can cause cell cycle arrest, DNA repair and cell survival, and execution of cell death (Wang et al., 2004). Cisplatin kills cancer cells by inducing apoptosis (Chu, 1994) and specifically activates the mitochondrial signaling pathway of apoptosis, which is initiated by activation of BH3-only proteins i.e. pro-apoptotic members of the Bcl-2 family of proteins.

Targeting the anti-apoptotic Bcl-2 family of proteins, thus restoring apoptotic pathways, may overcome drug resistance to cancer chemotherapy. Down-regulation of Bcl-x_L or its cooperative Bcl-2 family member Mcl-1 expression or activity increases apoptosis *per se* as well as cisplatin sensitivity in MPM. The importance of these anti-apoptotic proteins in the protection against chemotherapy-induced apoptosis makes them obvious targets to (re-) chemosensitize malignant mesothelioma tumour cells (Varin et al., 2010).

Glycosylation defects seem universal in carcinogenesis. They may alter cell signalling, growth, adherence and motility. Essentially all experimental and human cancers have altered glycosphingolipid composition and metabolism (Hakomori & Zhong, 1997), and several tumour-associated antigens are indeed glycosphingolipids. The globotriaosylceramide membrane receptor (Gb3) is over-expressed in many human tumours and tumour cell lines including MPM with inherent or acquired MDR. Gb3 is co-expressed and interplays with the membrane efflux transporter P-gp encoded by the *MDR1* gene associated with multidrug resistance.

The bacterial toxin verotoxin-1 (VT-1) exerts its cytotoxicity by targeting Gb3. Recent work has shown that apoptosis and inherent or acquired multidrug resistance in Gb3-expressing MPM tumour cells could be affected by VT-1 holotoxin, a sub-toxic concentration of the holotoxin concomitant with chemotherapy or its Gb3-binding B-subunit coupled to cytotoxic or immuno-modulatory drug, as well as chemical manipulation of Gb3 expression (Johansson et al., 2010). The interplay between Gb3 and P-gp thus gives a possible physiological approach to augment the chemotherapeutic effect in multidrug resistant malignant mesothelioma.

We hereby summarize the possibility to target also Bcl-2 and Gb3 signalling as two novel treatment possibilities to overcome or re-sensitize resistant malignant pleural mesothelioma tumour cells to cisplatin.

2. Targeted chemotherapy of malignant pleural mesothelioma

Chemotherapy will continue to be important in the therapy of MPM. An increased understanding of the major molecular pathways of intrinsic and acquired resistance of MPM is needed to develop diagnostic, therapeutic, and prevention methods. Ideally, future MPM therapy should be guided by molecular characteristics of the tumour rather than clinical stage and patient features. Insights into the biological basis of MPM may lead to personalized treatment involving also early detection of poor prognostic indicators that will reduce the heterogeneity of the clinical response (Zucali et al., 2011).

None of the hitherto explored targeted treatments can currently be recommended as standard treatment in MPM. A much used combination of cisplatin and pemetrexed has yielded enhanced response rates. Most patients with MPM progress during or shortly after first-line treatment. Due to the limited efficacy of chemotherapy, new treatment options are clearly warranted and several targeted agents have thus been explored (Jakobsen & Sörensen, 2011).

Basic cancer research has given the insight that apoptosis and the genes that control it have a profound effect on the malignant phenotype. Most conventional treatments depend on an ability to induce apoptosis as a final common pathway (Zucali et al., 2011). The unresponsiveness of mesothelioma to most conventional agents may in part be explained by a resistance to the induction of apoptosis. The mutations that suppress apoptosis also reduce the sensitivity to cancer treatment (Johnstone et al., 2002). Most targeted therapies have focused on impairing signaling pathways on which cancers depend for survival.

There are potential benefits to targeting tumors at the level of their anti-apoptotic defenses. Direct inhibitors of anti-apoptotic defenses could bypass the need to inhibit multiple pathways by moving to a distal level at which multiple signals are integrated. Also, stimulators of apoptosis through specific signaling pathways that emerge during cancer development or are acquired during cancer therapy could be targeted. Such an approach may be effective in the different mesothelioma subtypes, against a variety of apoptosis-inducing therapies, and without substantial injury to normal tissues.

3. Cisplatin signal transduction during therapy and cisplatin resistance

3.1 Cisplatin therapy

Cisplatin kills cancer cells by inducing apoptosis (Chu, 1994). The pathways leading to cisplatin-induced apoptosis are subject of considerable current interest, hence yet not fully understood, but is known to involve the activation of the MAP kinases SAPK/JNK (stress-activated protein kinases/c-Jun-N-terminal kinases) and p38 kinases, leading to the induction of caspase activity and apoptosis (Mansouri et al., 2003; Brozovic & Osmak, 2007). The mitochondrial signaling pathway to apoptosis has recently attracted attention and an increasing number of articles on the effect of cisplatin action and cisplatin resistance involving the expression of Bcl-2 family proteins have been published.

3.2 Inherent and induced cisplatin resistance

Tolerance might occur to platinum, through decreased expression or loss of apoptotic signaling pathways (either the mitochondrial or death-receptor pathways) as mediated through various proteins such as p53, anti-apoptotic and pro-apoptotic members of the BCL-2 family, and JNK (Adducci et al., 2002).

The challenge is thus to determine the mechanism of why some tumours, and MPM in particular, are intrinsically resistant to cisplatin and how enhanced cisplatin resistance eventually is acquired during the course of therapy. The acquired resistance may not necessary be an enhancement of the tumours intrinsic resistance mechanisms. All alternations of signaling pathway that may lead to enhancement of apoptosis must thus be exploited.

Reduced cellular accumulation of platinum either by impaired uptake or increased efflux is often found in cells selected for cisplatin resistance, both *in vivo* and *in vitro*, and is generally considered as one of the most consistent characteristics of platinum resistant cells (Gately & Howell, 1993). Many papers have reported that the expression of the ATP-binding cassette (ABC) transport proteins renders tumor cells resistant to chemotherapeutic drugs that are substrates of these transporter proteins. The ABC transporter protein family includes multidrug resistance proteins (ABCB1), multidrug resistance-associated proteins (ABCC), and breast cancer resistance protein (ABCG2).

3.3 Cisplatin chemotherapy and apoptosis

The failure of drug-induced apoptosis is an underlying cause of drug resistance. Some studies have identified a number of key mediators of apoptosis that are altered in chemo-resistant cancer cells. Resistance to cisplatin might occur through decreased expression or loss of pro-apoptotic factors or increased expression of anti-apoptotic proteins (Brozovic & Osmak, 2007).

Apoptosis is initiated either by intrinsic death stimuli such as oncogene activation and DNA damage, or as response to extrinsic death stimuli such as binding to their cell surface receptors of the Fas or TNFα ligands as part of an immune response. Both apoptosis initiation signalling pathways meet at the mitochondrial outer membrane (MOM) where the Bcl-2 protein family members regulate apoptosis. Mitochondrial outer membrane permeabilization (MOMP), intermembrane space (IMS) protein release, activation of pro-apoptotic Bcl-2 and caspase family proteins have been identified as key events in the initiation, progression and execution of apoptosis. But, there is still much that we do not understand about how cell death signaling is fine-regulated, particularly how the signaling within a single cell is coordinated for its ultimate orchestration at the population level.

Apoptotic cysteine-aspartate proteases (caspases) are essential for the progression and execution of apoptosis, and detection of caspase fragmentation or activity is often used as markers of apoptosis. We compared a cisplatin-resistant pleural malignant mesothelioma cell line (P31res1.2) with its more cisplatin-sensitive parental cell line (P31) regarding the consequences of in vitro acquired cisplatin-resistance on basal and cisplatin-induced (equitoxic and equiapoptotic cisplatin concentrations) caspase-3, -8 and -9 fragmentation and proteolytic activity. Acquisition of cisplatin-resistance resulted in basal fragmentation of caspase-8 and -9 without a concomitant increase in proteolytic activity, and there was an increased basal caspase-3/7 activity. In P31s, we found that cisplatin exposure resulted in caspase-9-mediated caspase-3/7 activation, but in the induced cisplatin-resistant sub-line, P31res1.2, cisplatin-induced caspase-3/7 activation occurred before caspase-8 or -9 activation. We concluded that in vitro acquisition of cisplatin-resistance rendered P31res1.2 cells resistant to caspase-8 and caspase-9 fragments and that cisplatin-induced, initiator-caspase independent caspase-3/7 activation was necessary to overcome this resistance (Janson et al., 2010).

4. The intrinsic apoptotic pathway in cancer: The Bcl-2 family

The Bcl-2 family consists of three groups of proteins, the anti-apoptotic proteins Bcl-2, Bcl-x_L, Bcl-w, Mcl-1 and A1, the pro-apoptotic proteins, Bax, Bak and Bok, and the pro-apoptotic BH3-only proteins members such as Bad, Bim, Bid and Noxa (Shamas-Din et al., 2011).

The pro-survival members act to preserve the mitochondrial outer membrane permeabilization through the sequestration of pro-apoptotic proteins that induce cell death by triggering the release of cytochrome c and the subsequent caspases and nucleases activation. The BH3-only proteins act as cellular guards that sense the apoptotic signal and modulate the function of the other pro-apoptotic Bcl-2 family members. BH3-only proteins inhibit the anti-apoptotic proteins and activate the pro-apoptotic proteins to cause MOM permeabilisation (MOMP) leading to release of cytochrome c and SMAC into the cytoplasm where they activate caspases leading to apoptosis and elimination of the cell. MOMP is regarded as the 'point-of-no-return' for a cell (Varin et al., 2010).

The intricate balance between antagonistic anti- and pro-apoptotic Bcl-2 family proteins may thus have a deciding huge role on the susceptibility of cells to apoptosis. Studies of the mechanisms of activation or inhibition of the MOMP proteins Bax and Bak and the activator BH3-only proteins with the aim of modifying these processes is an important therapeutic goal in order to restore the three possible blocks that cancer cells can exploit: loss of BH3-only proteins (or inhibition of their activation), a reduction or elimination of multi-region pro-apoptotic proteins, and increased expression of an apoptosis inhibitor such as Bcl-2 or Mcl-1 (Deng et al., 2007).

The most common block noted in human cancers is the over-expression of anti-apoptotic proteins. Tumours are often dependent on the presence of one or more anti-apoptotic protein for survival. Being able to abolish Bcl-2 anti-apoptotic signalling would therefore represent a form of synthetic lethality that would kill predominantly cancer cells rather than normal cells that do not automatically engage apoptotic machinery. In tumours with the loss or inhibition of BH3-only proteins, BH3 mimetics replace the need to induce expression or activate BH3-only proteins to initiate death. On the other hand, in cancers over-expressing anti-apoptotic Bcl-2 family proteins, BH3 mimetics can compete with endogenous activator BH3-only proteins for binding to anti-apoptotic proteins (Leber et al., 2010).

Over-expression of *BCL-2* and *BCL-XL* genes contribute to apoptotic inhibition and the development of the multidrug resistance of human cancers. Directly inhibiting the interaction between the anti-apoptotic proteins and BH3 proteins would lead to apoptosis of multi-drug resistant tumour cells (Shamas-Din et al., 2011).

The BH3 mimetic ABT-737 binds to Bcl-x_L and Bcl-2 but not to Mcl-1 (Oltersdorf et al., 2005). ABT-737 displaces Bad and Bim from the binding pocket of Bcl-2 stimulating apoptosis. Cancer cells with higher levels of Bcl-2 and Bcl-x_L, but lower levels of Mcl-1 are therefore sensitive to ABT-737 (Del Gaizo Moore et al., 2007). Mcl-1 expression (maintaining anti-apoptotic function) is the determinant of resistance to ABT-737 (Deng et al., 2007).

Because resistance can be reversed by reducing Mcl-1 levels, combination with an inhibitor of Mcl-1 will permit a selective kill of a wide variety of tumours. Obatoclax is a derivate that in addition binds also to Mcl-1, and may overcome tumour cell resistance to ABT-737. BH3-mimetics that selectively antagonize the anti-apoptotic proteins may prove to be successful in cancer therapy (Shamas-Din et al., 2011).

5. Signal transduction to apoptosis in malignant pleural mesothelioma. Role of Bcl-2 family proteins

Apoptosis is an uncommon event in mesothelioma and low mean cleaved caspase-3 index has been demonstrated (Jin et al., 2010). Over-expression of anti-apoptotic proteins have been implicated in MPM resistance to therapy (O'Kane et al., 2006).

5.1 Apoptosis related to p53 inactivation

The tumour suppressor p53 is referred to as the guardian of the genome. It is mutated in a wide variety of human cancers. A key function is to induce growth arrest or apoptosis following stress. The apoptotic pathways regulated by p53 involve the Bcl-2 family of pro - and anti-apoptotic regulators. The p53 tumour suppressor transcriptionally regulates the expression of pro-apoptotic Bcl-2 members Bax, Noxa and Puma, which stimulate mitochondria-mediated apoptosis. Inactivating the apoptotic pathways regulated by p53 is crucial for emerging tumour cells and is most often accomplished by inactivation of p53 itself. Some tumours however retain wild type p53 expression but apoptotic suppression is instead performed by deregulating Bcl-2 family members such as Bcl-2 and Bcl-x_L (Yip & Reed, 2008).

Genetic inactivation of p53 by alteration of *TP53* is rare in MPM. Targets of the tumour suppressing microRNA miR-34b/c include down-regulation of Bcl-2. miR-34b/c is frequently down-regulated by aberrant methylation in MPM, resulting in the loss of tumor-suppressive p53 function. Epigenetic silencing of miR-34b/c might explain why p53 functions are impaired in MPM despite the presence of intact p53 in the majority of MPM. Normalization of miRNA expression could be a potential method of therapeutic intervention. As miR-34b/c acts as a tumor suppressor, its expression should be restored in targeted tumor cells by the delivery (Kubo et al., 2011).

5.2 MAP kinases activate cisplatin-induced apoptosis in malignant pleural mesothelioma

Mitogen-activated protein kinases (MAPKs) are activated in cisplatin-induced apoptosis in most investigated cell systems and induced cisplatin resistance is also associated with reduced activation of MAPKs. The mitogen activated protein kinase (MAPK) family of proteins (extracellular signal-regulated kinase (Erk) which are activated by growth hormone receptors via a Ras/Raf pathway and the c-Jun N-terminal kinase (Jnk) and p38 kinase are via Mkk4/Mkk7 and Mkk3/Mkk6 pathways, respectively, sequentially activated and regulate a number of cellular functions, including survival, growth, differentiation and apoptosis. The Erk pathway together with the PI3K/Akt pathway, are important mediators of cell growth, survival and differentiation i.e. pro-survival. The Jnk and p38 pathways are particularly associated with diverse apoptotic paradigms, mediated by transcription dependent and independent mechanisms (Brozovic & Osmak, 2007).

In pleural mesothelioma, p38 MAPKs have been suggested to play a major role in carcinogenesis and aggressiveness of tumours. The Erk1/2 and p38 MAPK signalling pathways can stimulate the expression of heat-shock-proteins (Hsp), Hsp27, Hsp40, and Hsp70 which can rescue tumour cells from cell death. Hsp70 increases the resistance of MPM cells to chemotherapeutic drugs. Intracellular Hsp has been implicated in the protection of tumour cells from apoptosis of other tumour types, while secreted Hsp stimulate the immune system to attack tumour cells (Roth et al., 2009).

The constitutively active p38 MAPK by MPM cells was essential for the expression of Hsp40 and Hsp70, while Erk1/2 MAPK seemed to play less important role. The p38 MAPK was constitutively activated and needed the interaction with Erk1/2 MAPK to increase Hsp expression. This constitutively active p38 MAPK together with Erk1/2 MAPK are central for

MPM cell proliferation. In contrast to other tumour types a central role of Hsp70 in heat stress survival is indicated for MPM. It might be more effective to suppress both Hsp40 and Hsp70 to sensitize MPM cells to heat. Therefore the inhibition of Hsp40/Hsp70 or Erk1/2 MAPK might present a new option to increase the success of hyperthermia in mesothelioma (Zhong et al., 2011).

5.3 Bcl-2 family member protein expression in MPM

Whereas expression of anti-apoptotic *BCL2* is rare, elevated levels of Bcl-x$_L$ mRNA and protein have been detected in all mesothelioma cell lines and tumour samples examined (Hopkins-Donaldson et al., 2003). Pro-apoptotic Bax is also expressed in mesothelioma cell lines, including those that are highly resistant to pro-apoptotic stimuli, suggesting that over-expression of Bcl-x$_L$ may be necessary to counteract the pro-apoptotic effect of Bax (Narasimhan et al., 1998).

Much less is known about pro-apoptotic Bcl-2 family proteins in human MPM. Pro-apoptotic BH3-only proteins (e.g. Bim EL, L and S; Pumaα and β; Bid; Bad; Bmf, Bik) bind to the pro-survival proteins and cause the release of pro-apoptotic Bax-like proteins (e.g. Bax, Bak) that mediate mitochondrial membrane permeabilisation (Willis et al., 2007). Loss of expression of Bad, Bid and Bim is described in human MPM samples (O'Kane et al., 2006).

During a 6-h exposure to a LD$_{50}$ concentration of cisplatin we found a transient increase in BH3-only proteins in the cisplatin-sensitive MPM parental cell line P31 whereas in the induced cisplatin resistant sub-line P31res1.2 most of the proteins were un-responsive or decreased. This indicates that BH3 mimetics could sensitize MPM cells to cisplatin exposure. The P31res1.2 cells had essentially unchanged Bcl-x$_L$ expression, but interestingly increased Bcl-2 expression and increased phosphorylation of Bcl-2 at ser70 which is necessary for Bcl-2 pro-survival function. We however found also a decrease of potent pro-apoptotic proteins and an increase of the expression of the weak pro-apoptotic proteins that were increased in the P31res1.2 cells. This could contribute to the resistance, as both Bcl-2 and Bcl-x$_L$ must be inhibited in the P31res1.2 cells, and activation of one or two weak pro-apoptotic proteins is insufficient for an optimal inhibition of these pro-survival proteins (Janson et al., 2011, unpublished results).

Targeting the anti-apoptotic Bcl-2 family of proteins, thus restoring apoptotic pathways, may overcome drug resistance to cancer chemotherapy (Letai et al., 2008). Studies have shown that the down-regulation of Bcl-x$_L$ expression (using antisense strategies) (Smythe et al., 2002) or activity (Cao et al., 2007) increases both apoptosis *per se* and drug sensitivity in MPM. Furthermore, it was shown that a reduction of Bcl-x$_L$ in human mesothelioma cell lines in combination with cisplatin causes reduction of tumor growth *in vivo* as well as increases survival in mouse models (Littlejohn et al., 2008). These studies underline the importance of this protein in the protection against chemotherapy-induced apoptosis and emphasize it as a pertinent target to chemosensitize malignant mesothelioma cells (Varin et al., 2010).

Bcl-x$_L$ regulation is not entirely understood. In some cell lines phosphorylation of Bcl-x$_L$ at serine 62 by stress response Jun kinase has been demonstrated to oppose the anti-apoptotic function of Bcl-x$_L$ permitting cells to die by apoptosis by inhibiting its ability to bind to Bax.

Also caspase-3/CPP32-like proteases have been observed to cleave Bcl-x_L protein resulting in accelerated apoptotic cell death (Katz et al., 2009).

2-methoxy antimycin A3 induces apoptosis by neutralizing protective effects of Bcl-2/Bcl-x_L. Most tumour cells have acquired multiple defects in cell cycle and other checkpoints, and are, therefore, highly dependent on the anti-apoptosis function of Bcl-2/Bcl-x_L for survival. Any approach to alter this delicate anti- and pro- apoptosis balance will lead to apoptosis. Because the threshold of apoptosis is much lower in tumour cells than normal, Bcl-2/Bcl-x_L inhibitor could selectively induce apoptosis in tumour and spare normal cells at certain doses. Bcl-2/Bcl-x_L inhibitors could become promising single cancer therapeutic agents and also render tumour cells more sensitive to conventional chemotherapeutic agents

Potential drug resistance mechanisms against Bcl-2/Bcl-x_L inhibitors pose particular problems. Due to the redundancy function of anti-apoptosis Bcl-2 family genes, it should be no surprise to find that over-expressed Bcl-2 family genes such as Mcl-1, Bcl-w or A1 will compensate the loss of anti-apoptosis function due to Bcl-2/ Bcl-x_L inhibition. Generating Bcl-2/ Bcl-x_L resistant cell lines will be important for future studies (Cao et al., 2007).

Interestingly, mesothelioma cells cultured as spheroids 3D acquired resistance to bortezomib by failing to up-regulate Noxa, a pro-apoptotic sensitizer BH3-only protein that acts by displacing Bim, a pro-apoptotic Bax/Bak-activator protein, thereby acquiring both apoptotic resistance and sensitivity to Bcl-2 blockade. Immunocytochemistry of 48 mesotheliomas, demonstrated accordingly that 69% expressed elevated Bim. Therefore, mesothelioma, a highly resistant tumour, may have an intrinsic sensitivity to Bcl-2 blockade that can be exploited therapeutically. Tumors identified as 'primed for death' may respond to inhibition of the anti-apoptotic defenses with small molecules such as ABT-737, an inhibitor of Bcl-2/Bcl-x_L. Bim was essential for the response to ABT-737, and the level of Bim correlated with sensitivity to ABT-737 indicating that Bim may be a predictive biomarker for the response of mesothelioma to ABT-737 together with bortezomib. Bim over-expression was frequent (90%) in the more chemosensitive epithelioid MPM subtype and uncommon (20%) in the more chemoresistant sarcomatoid subtype (Barbone et al., 2011).

As indicated above, Mcl-1 might cooperate with Bcl-x_L for protection against cell death. Using RNA interference, Bcl-x_L depletion sensitized two highly chemoresistant mesothelioma cell lines to cisplatin. Inhibition of Mcl-1 by cisplatin may contribute to the induction of cell death observed after Bcl-x_L down-regulation. Additionally, Mcl-1 has also been found to be over-expressed in most malignant mesothelioma cell lines and tumor tissues. Down-regulation of Mcl-1 was also observed in response to cisplatin in two MPM cell lines. These observations thus suggest that resistance to apoptosis in MPM could be rather related to Bcl-x_L and/or Mcl-1 than to Bcl-2. After concomitant siRNA down-regulation of Bcl-x_L and Mcl-1, the proportion of viable mesothelioma cells was dramatically reduced. None or little cell death was induced after transfection with single siRNA. Combination of both siRNAs with a low cisplatin concentration led to a nearly complete annihilation of tumor cells whereas normal mesothelial cells were marginally affected. The development of BH3-mimetic small-molecule inhibitors together with siRNA for gene silencing in cancer, may yield effective targeted strategy within short (Varin et al., 2010).

It has been shown that the BimEL/Mcl-1 and BimEL/ Bcl-x$_L$ complexes can be rapidly dissociated following activation of Erk1/2 by survival factors thus allowing Bax and Bak binding to Mcl-1 and Bcl-x$_L$ and thus inhibiting apoptosis (Ewing et al., 2007).

6. Glycosphingolipids in cancer development and chemotherapy resistance

6.1 Glycosphingolipids and globotriasosylceramide (Gb3)

Glycosphingolipids (GSLs) are components of all vertebrate cells and play a fundamental role during development and cell differentiation (Erdmann et al., 2006). GSLs are involved in cellular growth, signal transduction and cell-cell interaction (Lahiri & Futerman, 2007). GSL profiling indicate that neutral globo series GSLs, including the neutral glycosphingolipid cell verotoxin-1 (VT-1) surface receptor globotriaosylceramide (Gb3), have important roles in mediating *MDR1* transactivation and expression (Liu et al., 2010).

The expression and metabolism of cell surface glycolipids is changed during oncogenic transformation and altered glycosylation patterns affect tumour invasion and metastasis (Hakomori & Zhang, 1997). Gb$_3$ is expressed in several human malignancies such as breast cancer (Johansson et al., 2009). Gb$_3$ expression in colorectal cancer correlates with invasiveness and metastatic potential. Elevated levels of Gb3 have also been seen in drug-resistant cancers and cell lines and a functional interplay between membrane Gb3 and MDR1 has been suggested (Mattocks et al., 2006; De Rosa et al., 2008). Deletion of Gb$_3$ synthase needed for Gb3 synthesis renders mice completely resistant to verotoxins (Okuda et al., 2006). GSLs are the only functional VT-1 receptors (Lingwood et al., 2010). These findings suggest that the Gb3-binding specificity of VT-1 could be used to target tumours for the toxin in the receptive cancer cells.

GSLs in cells are clustered and assembled with specific membrane proteins and signal transducers to form GSL-enriched microdomains or lipid rafts. Rafts are rich in GSLs, cholesterol, lipid-modified- and transmembrane proteins. The length of the fatty acyl chain of Gb3 influences its receptor function, intracellular sorting and retro-translocation of VT-1 to the cytosol (Lingwood, 1996). Binding of VT-1 B-subunit with clustered raft-localized Gb3 receptors is a requirement for the retrograde transport (Falguieres et al., 2008) and for a cytotoxic effect in the ER (Smith et al., 2006). For cells with Gb$_3$ present in the non-raft plasma membrane fraction, the toxin receptor complex is internalized and trafficked to lysosomes where the toxin is degraded leading to VT-1 resistant cells. Furthermore, VT-1 B subunit binding to Gb3 induces lipid reorganization of the cell membrane leading to enhancement of VT-1 uptake into the cell (Römer et al., 2007). The membrane organization of the glycosphingolipid receptor is the main discriminator for pathology *in vivo* (Lingwood et al., 2010).

6.2 Multidrug resistance to cancer chemotherapy

Tumour over-expression of the membrane efflux transporter P-glycoprotein (P-gp) is a common alteration in drug resistance (Gottesman, 2002). P-gp, encoded by the *MDR1* gene (Ueda et al., 1986), was the first ABC protein demonstrated to confer resistance to cancer chemotherapeutics (Gottesman et al., 1996). Other transporter proteins such as multidrug resistance protein (MRP1) and breast cancer resistance protein (BCRP) have also been described. P-gp plays roles in the absorption, distribution and excretion of compounds in normal tissues. Over-expression of *MDR1* in tumours results in active efflux of several types of anticancer agents. P-gp is expressed by many types of primary solid tumours, as well as haematological malignancies (Sandor et al., 1998).

Exposure to chemotherapy can up-regulate tumour P-gp expression, which occurs in acquired drug resistance and severely limits the success of chemotherapy. MDR1 inhibitors have been clinically tested in order to block drug efflux. Specific modulators or inhibitors such as GG918 and LY335979 have overcome the toxic adverse effects noted in first generation modulators but still have minor effect when co-administrated with chemotherapeutics in trials in part due to *MDR1* polymorphisms (Liu et al., 2010).

6.3 Globotriasosylceramide (Gb3) and MDR1 expression

Little is known about the molecular mechanism underlying *MDR1* over-expression and how it interacts with other genes to impart drug-resistance. Over-expression of glucosylceramide synthase (GCS), the first enzyme of GSL synthesis, can result in multidrug resistance. Many cells expressing MDR1 show elevated levels of glucosylceramide (GlcCer) (Morjani et al., 2001) and inhibitors of GCS kill MDR cells (Nicholson et al., 1999). MDR1 can translocate glucosylceramide into the Golgi apparatus for neutral GSL synthesis, including Gb3. P-gp has been proposed as a Golgi glucosylceramide flippase that enhances neutral GSL synthesis as transfection of MDR1 increases, and inhibition of P-gp decreases neutral GSL biosynthesis in cells (De Rosa et al., 2004). GCS up-regulates *MDR1* expression and modulates drug resistance of cancer.

Partial MDR1 and Gb_3 cell surface co-localization has been observed and inhibition of GSL biosynthesis depletes cell surface MDR1. MDR1 may therefore interact with Gb_3. A significant fraction of surface MDR1 is not co-localized with Gb_3, and could therefore be VT-1-insensitive. MDR1 can be expressed in cells lacking Gb_3. However, drug-resistant metastatic ovarian tumour cells have a particularly high Gb_3 content and Gb_3 is highly expressed in metastatic colon carcinoma (Arab et al., 1997; Kovbasnjuk et al., 2005).

The water-soluble Gb_3 mimic adamantylGb$_3$, but not other GSL analogues, reversed MDR1-MDCK cell drug resistance (DeRosa et al., 2004). Verotoxin-mediated Gb_3 endocytosis also up-regulated total MDR1 and inhibited drug efflux (Pastan et al., 1988).

The Gb3 content, which is regulated by the expression of Gb3 synthase, determines the sensitivity of HeLa cells toward VT-1. We recently demonstrated extensive variability in breast cancer cell lines for apoptosis induction by VT-1. Sensitivity was correlated with Gb3 expression, and use of the drug PPMP, which down-regulates glucosylceramide production, inhibited VT-1-mediated apoptosis (Johansson et al., 2009).

7. Verotoxin-1

7.1 Verotoxin-1 structure and induction of apoptosis

VT-1 consists of one A and five B subunits. After B subunit binding to Gb3 (Wadell et al., 1990), it is endocytosed and follows the retrograde pathway to the endoplasmic reticulum where the A-subunit is translocated to the cytosol and inhibits protein synthesis (Raa et al., 2009).

Importantly, VT-1 also induces apoptosis through sequential activation of caspases, leading to nuclear changes, such as chromatin condensation and DNA fragmentation. VT-1-induced apoptosis in monocytic THP1 cells requires retrograde transport through the Golgi apparatus to the ER and the activation of caspase-3, the executioner caspase (Kojio et al., 2000). Similar apoptotic signalling pathways are triggered by Shiga toxins in different cell lines.

VT-1 induces a prominent ribotoxic stress signalling response leading to disrupted ribosomal RNA (rRNA) functions, protein synthesis inhibition and altered mitogen-activated protein kinase (MAPK) pathway signalling (Johannes & Römer, 2010). The anti-apoptotic function of Bcl-2 requires Jnk-mediated phosphorylation of Bcl-2. Alternative Bcl-2 phosphorylation reactions, including p38 MAPK-directed phosphorylation of Bcl-2, inhibit Bcl-2 function. Bcl-2 was differentially phosphorylated by VT-1 treatment of monocyte- *vs.* macrophage-like THP-1 cells. Levels of anti-apoptotic phospho-Bcl-2 molecules were transiently increased in macrophage-like cells, while levels declined in monocyte-like cells. Thus, the ribotoxic stress response induced by VT-1 may regulate the activation of the Bcl-2 family of proteins that, in turn, control apoptosis (Tesh, 2011).

7.2 Effect of cisplatin and verotoxin-1 on malignant pleural mesothelioma cells

We found that Mkk3/6 and Jnk was phosphorylated after cisplatin treatment in the cisplatin-sensitive MPM P31 cells, but not in the corresponding P31res1.2 sub-line with acquired-cisplatin resistance. VT-1 induced phosphorylation of Mkk3/6, which was enhanced when VT-1 was combined with cisplatin (Johansson et al., 2010). Mkk3/6 is known to activate P38 (Derijard et al., 1995; Han et al., 1996). P38 as well as Jnk has been shown to promote apoptosis in response to cellular stress (Kim et al., 2006). Treatment of cells with chemical inhibitors or siRNA targeting P38 was recently shown to specifically inhibit VT-1 transport to the Golgi apparatus complex and reduce VT-1 toxicity (Walchli et al., 2008), and VT-1 prolonged Jnk and P38 MAPK activation of macrophage-like cells (Lee et al., 2007). We have previously demonstrated Jnk phosphorylation in response to VT-1 treatment also in glioma and breast cancer cell lines (Johansson et al., 2006; 2009).

Apoptosis induced by VT-1 was associated with enhanced expression of the pro-apoptotic protein Bax (Jones et al., 2000) and over-expression of Bcl-2 protects cells against VT-1-induced cell death (Suzuki et al., 2000). Shiga toxins also inhibit the expression of the anti-apoptotic Bcl-2 family member Mcl-1 (Erwert et al., 2003). Interestingly, acquisition of cisplatin resistance in MPM cells increased cisplatin activation also of weak proapoptotic proteins of the Bcl-2 family of proteins but apparently not enough to counteract the increased expression of also of anti-apoptotis proteins (Janson et al., 2011, unpublished results).

8. Globotriasosylceramide, verotoxin-1 and cisplatin in targeting of resistant mesotheliomas

The possibility that VT-1 through the A-subunit could cause protein synthesis inhibition and induce apoptosis in normal cells constitutes a concern for the use of the holotoxin as an anticancer agent. The non-toxic VT-1 B subunit is stable at extreme pH, resist proteases, cross tissue barriers, distribute in the organism and generally resist extra- and intracellular inactivation (Johannes & Decaudin, 2005). The receptor selectivity of the B subunit has therefore been used to couple it to cytotoxic compounds such as the topoisomerase I inhibitor SN38 (El Alaoui et al., 2007) or induce an immune response (Vingert et al., 2006) with preferential effects on cancer cells.

Of primary cultures of gastrointestinal tumours, 80% were found to bind the VT-1 B subunit and could be detected on tumour cells after 5 days. The stable association of VT-1 B subunit with cells might be a useful property for diagnostic or therapeutic delivery strategies. This subunit has little immunologic properties (Bast et al., 1997) and is well tolerated in a mouse model (Smith et al., 2006).

An apparent treatment possibility to reverse MDR is to inhibit GSL biosynthesis by inhibiting GCS or Gb3 synthase enzyme expression and/or activity, or use Gb3 mimics like adamantylGb3 (Arab et al., 1997).

The treatment obstacle of acquired-cisplatin resistance in MPM and other cancers makes it necessary to find new strategies to overcome resistance. We showed that cisplatin can up-regulate Gb3 expression in MPM and NSCLC cells and thus sensitize the cells to VT-1-induced cytotoxicity. The increased proportion of Gb3-expressing cells after cisplatin treatment (Fig. 1) suggests that cisplatin induces Gb3 expression in cancer cells, that

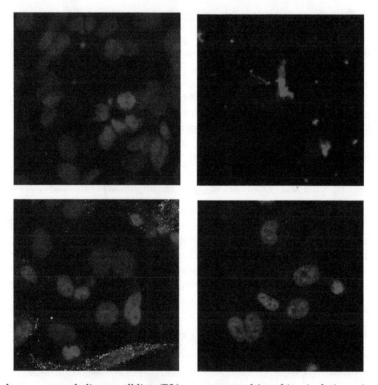

Fig. 1. The human mesothelioma cell line (P31 – upper panels) and its cisplatin-resistant sub-line (P31res1.2 – lower panels) were grown to confluence on glass cover-slips without (left panels) or with 15 μmol/L PPMP (right panels) for 72 h, then fixed with paraformaldehyde and stained for 1 h with rat primary IgM antibodies against globotriasosylceramide (Gb3). Secondary goat anti-rat IgM antibodies labeled with Alexa Fluor® 488 Dye were added for 1 h. Nuclei were visualized with DAPI staining DNA and visualizing cell nuclei. Images were captured on a Zeiss upright confocal microscope and analyzed using Zeiss ZEN 2010 software.

cisplatin preferentially eradicates cell with low Gb3 expression and that Gb3 expression is linked to acquired cisplatin-resistance (Johansson et al., 2010). We could also correlate increased expression of Gb3 in cisplatin-resistant MPM (P31res1.2) cells to increased expression of MDR1/PgP. This is important since MDR1/PgP generally is not over-expressed in MPM but expression could possibly occur following chemotherapy. This needs to be investigated further. PPMP reduced Gb3 expression in the resistant sub-line cells (Fig. 1) and particularly of the Gb3-expressing fraction that was induced when the mother cell line was made cisplatin-resistant. A strong super-additive effect of combined cisplatin and a sub-toxic concentration of VT-1 in cisplatin-resistant MPM cells were observed, indicating a new potential clinical treatment approach (Johansson et al., 2010).

The MAPK pathway is involved in proapoptotic signalling of VT-1 in stressed cell systems and the pathway is also involved in cisplatin-induced apoptosis and induced cisplatin resistance (Salhia et al., 2002; Johansson et al., 2010). Targeting the MAPK signalling pathway could, therefore, be an additional way to reduce cisplatin-induced tumour cells resistance.

The partial cell surface co-localization of Gb3/MDR1, the modulation of MDR1 cell surface expression by GSL and chemotherapy and the possibility to inhibit MDR1 expression by VT-1/VT-1 B-sub-unit, all indicate a functional link between Gb3 and MDR1. Targeting the physiological regulation of MDR1 could be an efficient way not only to prevent the development of drug resistance during cancer chemotherapy but also to reverse inherent and acquired drug resistance of MPM.

9. Conclusion

Improving our knowledge of the molecular alterations and signaling pathways specific to MPM should help in the identification of biomarkers useful novel treatment approaches. Such treatments might include targeted agents in combination with effective chemotherapeutic regimes. Personalized treatments based on the biological characteristics that follow that of the tumour will offer better future outcomes for MPM patients.

10. Acknowledgements

We would like to thank the Lions foundation, the Swedish Cancer Society, the County Council, and the Faculty of Medicine, Umea University, for funding.

11. References

Adducci, A., Cosio, S., Muraca, S. & Genazzani, A. R. (2002). Molecular mechanisms of apoptosis and chemosensitivity to platinum and paclitaxel in ovarian cancer: biological data and clinical implications. *Eur. J. Gynaecol. Oncol.* 23: 390–396.

Arab, S., Russel, E., Chapman, W.B., Rosen, B. & Lingwood, C.A. (1997). Expression of the verotoxin receptor glycolipid, globotriaosylceramide, in ovarian hyperplasias. *Oncol. Res.* 9: 553–563.

Barbone, D., Ryan, J.A., Kolhatkar, N., Chacko, A.D., Jablons, D.M., Sugarbaker, D.J., Bueno, R., Letai, A.G., Coussens, L.M., Fennell, D.A. & Broaddus, V.C. (2011). The Bcl-2 repertoire of mesothelioma spheroids underlies acquired apoptotic multicellular resistance. *Cell Death Dis.* 23: e174.

Bast, D.J., Sandhu, J., Hozumi, N., Barber, B. & Brunton, J. (1997). Murine antibody responses to the verotoxin 1 B subunit: demonstration of major histocompatibility complex dependence and an immunodominant epitope involving phenylalanine 30. *Infect. Immun.* 65: 2978-2982.

Bridda, A., Padoan, I., Mencarelli, R. & Frego, M. (2007). Peritoneal mesothelioma: a review. *Med. Gen. Med.* 9: 32.

Brozovic, A. & Osmak, M. (2007). Activation of mitogen-activated protein kinases by cisplatin and their role in cisplatin-resistance. *Cancer Lett.* 251: 1-16.

Cao, X,. Rodarte, C., Zhang, L., Morgan, C.D., Littlejohn, J. & Smythe WR. (2007). Bcl2/bcl-xL inhibitor engenders apoptosis and increases chemosensitivity in mesothelioma. *Cancer Biol. Ther.* 6: 246–252.

Chu, G. (1994). Cellular-responses to cisplatin – the roles of DNA-binding proteins and DNA-repair. *J. Biol. Chem.*, 269: 787–790.

Del Gaizo Moore, V., Brown, J.R., Certo, M., Love, T.M., Novina, C.D. & Letai, A. (2007). Chronic lymphocytic leukemia requires BCL2 to sequester prodeath BIM, explaining sensitivity to BCL2 antagonist ABT-737. *J. Clin. Invest.* 117: 112–121.

Deng, N., Carlson, K., Takeyama, P., Dal Cin, M., Shipp & Letai, A. (2007). BH3 profiling identifies three distinct classes of apoptotic blocks to predict response to ABT-737 and conventional chemotherapeutic agents. *Cancer Cell* 12: 171–185.

Derijard, B., Raingeaud, J., Barrett, T., Wu, I.H., Han, J., Ulevitch, R.J. & Davis, R.J. (1995) Independent human MAP-kinase signal transduction pathways defined by MEK and MKK isoforms. *Science* 267: 682-685

De Rosa, M.F., Ackerley, C., Wang, B., Ito, S., Clarke, D.M. & Lingwood, C. (2008). Inhibition of multidrug resistance by adamantylgb3, a globotriaosylceramide analog. *J. Biol. Chem.* 22: 4501-4511.

De Rosa, M.F., Sillence, D., Ackerley, C. & Lingwood, C. (2004). Role of multiple drug resistance protein 1 in neutral but not acidic glycosphingolipid biosynthesis. *J. Biol. Chem.* 279: 7867-7876.

El Alaoui, A., Schmidt, F., Amessou, M., Sarr, M., Decaudin, D., Florent, J.C. & Johannes, L. (2007). Shiga toxin-mediated retrograde delivery of a topoisomerase I inhibitor prodrug. *Angew. Chem. Int. Ed. Engl.* 46: 6469-6472.

Erdmann, M., Wipfler, D., Merling, A., Cao, Y., Claus, C., Kniep, B., Sadick. H., Bergler, W., Vlasak, R. & Schwartz-Albiez, R. (2006). Differential surface expression and possible function of 9-O- and 7-O-acetylated GD3 (CD60 b and c) during activation and apoptosis of human tonsillar B and T lymphocytes. *Glycoconj. J.* 23: 627–638.

Erwert, R.D, Eiting, K.T., Tupper, J.C., Winn, R.K., Harlan, J.M. & Bannerman, D.D. (2003). Shiga toxin induces decreased expression of the anti-apoptotic protein Mcl-1 concomitant with the onset of endothelial apoptosis. *Microb. Pathog.* 35: 87–93.

Ewings, K.E., Hadfield-Moorhouse, K., Wiggins, C.M., Wickenden, J.A., Balmanno, K., Gilley, R., Degenhardt, K., White, E. & Cook, S.J. (2007). ERK1/2-dependent phosphorylation of BimEL promotes its rapid dissociation from Mcl-1 and BCL-XL. *EMBO J.* 26: 2856-2867.

Falguières, T., Maak, M., von Weyhern, C., Sarr, M., Sastre, X., Poupon, M.-F., Robine, S., Johannes, L. & Janssen, K.-P. (2008). Human colorectal tumors and metastases express Gb3 and can be targeted by an intestinal pathogen-based delivery tool. *Mol. Cancer Ther.* 7: 2498–2508.

Gately, D.P. & Howell, S.B. (1993). Cellular accumulation of the anticancer agent cisplatin: a review. *Br. J. Cancer* 67: 1171-6.

Gottesman, M.M. (2002). Mechanisms of cancer drug resistance. *Annu. Rev. Med.* 53: 615-627.

Gottesman, M.M., Pastan, I. & Ambudkar, S.-V. (1996). P-glycoprotein and multidrug resistance. *Curr. Opin. Genet. Dev.* 6: 610-617.

Hakomori, S. & Zhang, Y. (1997). Glycosphingolipid antigens and cancer therapy. *Chem. Biol.* 4: 97-104.

Han, J., Lee, J.D., Jiang, Y., Li, Z., Feng, L. & Ulevitch, R.J. (1996). Characterization of the structure and function of a novel MAP kinase kinase (MKK6). *J. Biol. Chem.* 271: 2886-2891.

Jakobsen, J.N. & Sørensen, J.B. (2011). Review on clinical trials of targeted treatments in malignant mesothelioma. *Cancer Chemother. Pharmacol.* 68: 1-15.

Janson, V., Johansson, A. & Grankvist K. (2010). Resistance to caspase-8 and -9 fragments in a malignant pleural mesothelioma cell line with acquired cosplatin-resistance. *Cell Death Dis.* 1: e78.

Janson, V., Tyler, A., Behnam-Motlagh, P. & Grankvist, K. (2011). Acquisition of cisplatin-resistance in malignant mesothelioma cells deregulates pro-apoptotic BH3-only proteins. Manuscript.

Jin, L., Amatya, V.J., Takeshima, Y., Shrestha, L., Kushitani, K. & Inai, K. (2010). Evaluation of apoptosis and immunohistochemical expression of the apoptosis-related proteins in mesothelioma. *Hiroshima J. Med. Sci.* 59: 27-33.

Johannes, L. & Römer, W. (2010). Shiga toxins--from cell biology to biomedical applications. *Nat. Rev. Microbiol.* 8: 105-116.

Johansson, D., Andersson, C., Moharer, J., Johansson, A. & Behnam-Motlagh, P. (2010). Cisplatin-induced expression of Gb3 enables verotoxin-1 treatment of cisplatin resistance in malignant pleural mesothelioma cells. *Br. J. Cancer* 19: 383-391.

Johansson, D., Johansson, A., Grankvist, K., Andersson, U., Henriksson, R., Bergström, P., Brännström, T. & Behnam-Motlagh, P. (2006). Verotoxin-1 induction of apoptosis in Gb3-expressing human glioma cell lines. *Cancer Biol. Ther.* 5: 1211-1217.

Johansson., D., Kosovac, E., Moharer, J., Ljuslinder, I., Brännström, T., Johansson, A. & Behnam-Motlagh, P. (2009). Expression of verotoxin-1 receptor Gb3 in breast cancer tissue and verotoxin-1 signal transduction to apoptosis. *BMC Cancer* 9: 67.

Johnstone, R.W., Ruefli, A.A. & Lowe, S.W. (2002). Apoptosis: a link between cancer genetics and chemotherapy. *Cell* 108: 153-164.

Jones, N.L., Islur, A., Haq, R., Mascarenhas, M., Karmali, M.A., Perdue, M.H., Zanke, B.W. & Sherman, P.M. (2000). *Escherichia coli* Shiga toxins induce apoptosis in epithelial cells that is regulated by the Bcl-2 family. *Am. J. Physiol. Gastrointest. Liver Physiol.* 278: G811-G819.

Katz, S.I., Zhou, L., Chao, G., Smith, C.D., Ferrara, T., Wang, W., Dicker, D.T. & El-Deiry, W.S. (2009). Sorafenib inhibits ERK1/2 and MCL-1(L) phosphorylation levels resulting in caspase-independent cell death in malignant pleural mesothelioma. *Cancer Biol. Ther.* 8: 2406-2416.

Kim, B.J., Ryu, SW. & Song, B.J. (2006). JNK- and p38 kinase-mediated phosphorylation of Bax leads to its activation and mitochondrial translocation and to apoptosis of human hepatoma HepG2 cells. *J. Biol. Chem.* 281: 21256-21265.

Kojio, S., Zhang, H., Ohmura, M., Gondaira, F., Kobayashi, N. & Yamamoto, T. (2000). Caspase-3 activation and apoptosis induction coupled with the retrograde transport of Shiga toxin: inhibition by brefeldin A. *FEMS Immunol. Med. Microbiol.* 29: 275–281.

Kovbasnjuk, O., Mourtazina, R., Baibakov, B., Wang, T., Elowsky, C., Choti, M.A., Kane, A. & Donowitz, M. (2005). The glycosphingolipid globotriaosylceramide in the metastatic transformation of colon cancer. *Proc. Natl. Acad. Sci. USA.* 102: 19087–19092.

Kubo, T., Toyooka, S., Tsukuda, K., Sakaguchi, M., Fukazawa, T., Soh, J., Asano, H., Ueno, T., Muraoka, T., Yamamoto, H., Nasu, Y., Kishimoto, T., Pass, H.I., Matsui, H., Huh, N.H. & Miyoshi, S. (2011). Epigenetic silencing of microRNA-34b/c Plays an important role in the pathogenesis of malignant pleural mesothelioma. *Clin. Cancer Res.* 17: 4965-4974.

Lahiri, S. & Futerman, A.H. (2007). The metabolism and function of sphingolipids and glycosphingolipids. *Cell Mol. Life Sci.* 64: 2270–2284.

Leber, B, Geng, F., Kale, J. & Andrews, D.W. (2010). Drugs targeting Bcl-2 family members as an emerging strategy in cancer. *Expert. Rev. Mol. Med.* 12: e28.

Lee, S.Y., Cherla, R.P. & Tesh, V.L. (2007). Simultaneous induction of apoptotic and survival signaling pathways in macrophage-like THP-1 cells by Shiga toxin 1. *Infect. Immun.* 75: 1291-1302.

Letai, A.G. (2008). Diagnosing and exploiting cancer's addiction to blocks in apoptosis. *Nat. Rev. Cancer* 8: 121–132.

Lingwood, C.A., Binnington, B., Manis, A. & Branch, D.R. (2010). Globotriaosyl ceramide receptor function - where membrane structure and pathology intersect. *FEBS Lett.* 3: 1879-1886.

Lingwood, C.A. (1996). Aglycone modulation of glycolipid receptor function. *Glycoconj. J.* 13: 495–503.

Littlejohn, J.E., Cao, X., Miller, S.D., Ozvaran, M.K., Jupiter, D., Zhang, L., Rodarte, C. & Smythe, W.R. (2008). Bcl-xL antisense oligonucleotide and cisplatin combination therapy extends survival in SCID mice with established mesothelioma xenografts. *Int. J. Cancer* 123: 202–208.

Liu, Y.Y., Gupta, V., Patwardhan, G.A., Bhinge, K., Zhao, Y., Bao, J., Mehendale, H., Cabot, M.C., Li, Y.T. & Jazwinski, S.M. (2010). Glucosylceramide synthase upregulate Glucosylceramide synthase upregulates MDR1 expression in the regulation of cancer drug resistance through cSrc and beta-catenin signaling. *Mol. Cancer* 11: 145.

Mansouri, A., Ridgway, L.D., Korapati, A.L., Zhang, Q.,Tian, L., Wang,Y., Siddik, Z.H., Mills, G.B. & Claret, F.X. (2003). Sustained activation of JNK/p38 MAPK pathways in response to cisplatin leads to Fas ligand induction and cell death in ovarian carcinoma cells. *J. Biol. Chem.* 278: 19245-19256.

Mattocks, M., Bagovich, M., De Rosa, M., Bond, S., Binnington, B., Rasaiah, VI., Medin, J. & Lingwood, C. (2006). Treatment of neutral glycosphingolipid lysosomal storage diseases via inhibition of the ABC drug transporter, MDR1. Cyclosporin A can lower serum and liver globotriaosyl ceramide levels in the Fabry mouse model. *FEBS J.* 2739: 2064-2075.

Morjani, H., Aouali, N., Belhoussine, R., Veldman, R.J., Levade, T. & Manfait, M. (2001). *Int. J. Cancer* 94: 157–165.

Narasimhan, S.R., Yang, L., Gerwin, B.I. & Broaddus, V.C. (1998). Resistance of pleural mesothelioma cell lines to apoptosis: relation to expression of bcl-2 and bax. *Am. J. Physiol.* 275: L165–L171.

Nicholson, K., Quinn, D., Kellett, G. & Warr, J. (1999). Preferential killing of multidrug-resistant KB cells by inhibitors of glucosylceramide synthase. *Br. J. Cancer* 81: 423–430.

O'Kane, S.L., Pound, R.J., Campbell, A., Chaudhuri, N., Lind, M.J. & Cawkwell, L. (2006). Expression of bcl-2 family members in malignant pleural mesothelioma. *Acta Oncol.* 45: 449-453.

Okuda, T., Tokuda, N., Numata, S., Ito, M., Ohta, M., Kawamura, K., Wiels, J., Urano, T., Tajima, O., Furukawa, K. & Furukawa, K. (2006). Targeted disruption of Gb3/CD77 synthase gene resulted in the complete deletion of globo-series glycosphingolipids and loss of sensitivity to verotoxins. *J. Biol. Chem.* 281: 10230–10235.

Oltersdorf, T., Elmore, S.W., Shoemaker, A.R., Armstrong, R.C., Augeri, D.J., Belli, B.A., Bruncko, M., Deckwerth, T.L., Dinges, J., Hajduk, P.J., Joseph, M.K., Kitada, S., Korsmeyer, S.J., Kunzer, A.R., Letai, A., Li, C., Mitten, M.J., Nettesheim, D.G., Ng, S., Nimmer, P.M., O'Connor, J.M., Oleksijew, A., Petros, A.M., Reed, J.C., Shen, W. Tahir, S.K., Thompson, C.B., Tomaselli, K.J., Wang, B., Wendt, M.D., Zhang, H., Fesik, S.W. & Rosenberg, S.H. (2005). An inhibitor of Bcl-2 family proteins induces regression of solid tumours. *Nature* 435 (7042): 677-681.

Pastan, I., Gottesman, M., Ueda, K., Lovelace, E., Rutherford, A. & Willingham, M. (1988). *Proc. Natl. Acad. Sci. USA.* 85: 4486–4490.

Raa, H., Grimmer, S., Schwudke, D., Bergan, J., Walchli, S., Skotland, T., Shevchenko, A. & Sandvig, K. (2009). Glycosphingolipid requirements for endosome-to-Golgi transport of Shiga toxin. *Traffic* 10: 868–882.

Römer, W., Berland, L., Chambon, V., Gaus, K., Windschiegl, B., Tenza, D., Aly, M.R., Fraisier, V., Florent, J.C., Perrais, D., Lamaze ,C., Raposo, G., Steinem, C., Sens, P., Bassereau, P. & Johannes, L. (2007). Shiga toxin induces tubular membrane invaginations for its uptake into cells. *Nature* 450: 670-675.

Roth, M., Zhong, J., Tamm, M. & Szilard, J. (2009). Mesothelioma cells escape heat stress by upregulating Hsp40/Hsp70 expression via mitogen-activated protein kinases. *J. Biomed. Biotechnol.* 2009: 451084.

Salhia, B., Rutka, J.T., Lingwood, C., Nutikka, A. & Van Furth, W.R. (2002). The treatment of malignant meningioma with verotoxin. *Neoplasia* 4: 304–311.

Sandor, V., Fojo, T. & Bates, S.E. (1998). Future perspectives for the development of P-glycoprotein modulators. *Drug Resist. Updat.* 1: 190–200.

Shamas-Din, A., Brahmbhatt, H., Leber, B. & Andrews, D.W. (2011). BH3-only proteins: Orchestrators of apoptosis. *Biochim. Biophys. Acta* 1813: 508-520.

Smith, D.C., Sillence, D.J., Falguieres, T., Jarvis, R.M., Johannes, L., Lord, J.M., Platt, F.M. & Roberts, L.M. (2006). The association of Shiga-like toxin with detergent-resistant membranes is modulated by glucosylceramide and is an essential requirement in the endoplasmic reticulum for a cytotoxic effect. *Mol. Biol. Cell* 17: 1375–1387.

Smythe,W.R., Mohuiddin, I., Ozveran, M. & Cao, X.X. (2002). Antisense therapy for malignant mesothelioma with oligonucleotides targeting the bcl-xl gene product. *J. Thorac. Cardiovasc. Surg.* 123: 1191–1198.

Suzuki, A., Doi, H., Matsuzawa, F., Aikawa, S., Takiguchi, K., Kawano, H., Hayashida, M. & Ohno, S. (2000). Bcl-2 antiapoptotic protein mediates verotoxin II-induced cell death: possible association between Bcl-2 and tissue failure by *E. coli* O157:H7. *Genes Dev.* 14: 1734-1740.

Tesh, V.L. Activation of cell stress response pathways by shiga toxins. (2011). *Cell Microbiol.* In press.

Ueda, K., Cornwell, M.M., Gottesman, M.M., Pastan, I., Roninson, I.B., Ling, V.& Riordan, JR. (1986). The mdr1 gene, responsible for multidrug-resistance, codes for P-glycoprotein. *Biochem. Biophys. Res. Commun.* 141: 956-962.

Varin, E., Denoyelle, C., Brotin, E., Meryet-Figuière, M., Giffard, F., Abeilard, E., Goux, D., Gauduchon, P., Icard, P. & Poulain L. (2010). Downregulation of Bcl-xL and Mcl-1 is sufficient to induce cell death in mesothelioma cells highly refractory to conventional chemotherapy. *Carcinogenesis* 31: 984-993.

Vingert, B., Adotevi, O., Patin, D., Jung, S., Shrikant, P., Freyburger, L., Eppolito, C., Sapoznikov, A., Amessou, M., Quintin-Colonna, F., Fridman, W.H., Johannes, L. & Tartour, E. (2006). The Shiga toxin B-subunit targets antigen in vivo to dendritic cells and elicits anti-tumor immunity. *Eur. J. Immunol.* 36: 1124-1135.

Waddell, T., Cohen, A. & Lingwood, C.A., (1990). Induction of verotoxin sensitivity in receptor-deficient cell lines using the receptor glycolipid globotriosylceramide. *Proc. Natl. Acad. Sci. USA* 87: 7898-7901.

Walchli, S., Skanland, S.S., Gregers, T.F., Lauvrak, S.U., Torgersen, M.L., Ying, M., Kuroda, S., Maturana, A. & Sandvig, K. (2008). The Mitogen-activated protein kinase p38 links Shiga Toxin-dependent signaling and trafficking. *Mol. Biol. Cell* 19: 95-104.

Wang, G., Reed, E. & Li, Q.Q. (2004). Molecular basis of cellular response to cisplatin chemotherapy in non-small cell lung cancer. *Oncol. Rep.* 12: 955-965.

Willis, S.N., Fletcher, J.I., Kaufmann, T, van Delft, M.F., Chen, L., Czabotar, P.E., Ierino, H., Lee, E.F., Fairlie, W.D., Bouillet, P., Strasser, A., Kluck, R.M., Adams, J.M. & Huang, D.C. (2007). Apoptosis initiated when BH3 ligands engage multiple Bcl-2 homologs, not Bax or Bak. *Science* 315: 856-859.

Yip, K.W. & Reed, J.C. (2008). Bcl-2 family proteins and cancer. *Oncogene* 27: 6398-6406.

Zhong, J., Lardinois, D., Szilard, J., Tamm, M. & Roth, M. (2011). Rat mesothelioma cell proliferation requires p38δ mitogen activated protein kinase and C/EBP-α. *Lung Cancer* 73: 166-170.

Zucali, P.A., Ceresoli, G.L., De Vincenzo, F., Simonelli, M., Lorenzi, E., Gianoncelli, L. & Santoro, A. (2011). Advances in the biology of malignant pleural mesothelioma. *Cancer Treat. Rev.* 37: 543-558.

12

The Central Role of Survivin in Proliferation and Apoptosis of Malignant Pleural Mesothelioma

Julija Hmeljak and Andrej Cör
University of Primorska, Faculty of Health Sciences, Izola
Slovenia

1. Introduction

Malignant pleural mesothelioma is the most common mesothelial malignancy, which arises from the malignant transformation of mesothelial cells that line the pleural cavity. Malignant pleural mesothelioma is a highly invasive disease with a very long latency and treatment is rarely effective, since only few patients survive more than one year after diagnosis (Carbone et al., 2007). Asbestos, a fibrous mineral widely used throughout the 20th century, has been acknowledged to being the main causative agent (Wagner, 1979).

Although systemic chemotherapy with novel combinations of platinum-based drugs and antimetabolites showed some degree of success in selected patients, prognosis remains generally poor (Kindler, 2008;Robinson et al., 2005). The fact that the disease is often intrinsically resistant to treatment, combined with the notion that the majority of patients are elderly due to a long latency, and thus prone to complications and comorbidities, further limits treatment options (Ray, Kindler, 2009).

Malignant pleural mesothelioma is still regarded as a rare disease, despite the fact that its incidence has been steeply rising in the last decades and is not expected to level before the year 2020 (Robinson et al., 2005). Increased incidence and the fact that conventional antitumour treatment options are ineffective, highlight the need for novel therapies for MPM patients and underline the urgency for implementation of more effective diagnostic, prognostic, predictive and, nevertheless, therapeutic targets.

Thorough understanding of the differences between normal and malignant cells is crucial in the search and development of such targets. More comprehensive knowledge of tumour biology in general and malignant pleural mesothelioma in particular allows and facilitates the discovery and validation of novel potential markers. Several such potential markers can be found among proteins involved in the cellular pathways that mediate malignant transformation and, at least in part, constitute the so called hallmarks of cancer, e.g. cellular signalling, proliferation and apoptosis (Hanahan, Weinberg, 2000).

This chapter focuses on presenting survivin, a cancer-specific protein involved in both proliferation and apoptosis regulation. Furthermore, the aim of this review is to explore survivin's potential as a prognostic and therapeutic target for MPM.

2. Survivin as an interloper between apoptosis and proliferation

Hanahan and Weinberg described ten so called hallmarks of cancer and defined them as features common to all malignancies. They consist of acquired phenotypic properties, rooted in the defects of key regulatory mechanisms of cells within a tissue, namely: unlimited replication potential, self-sufficiency in growth signals and their transduction, insensitivity to growth inhibitors, resistance to apoptosis, as well as sustained angiogenesis, adjacent and distal tissue invasion, abnormal metabolic pathways, genome instability, avoidance of the immune system and chronic inflammation (Hanahan, Weinberg, 2000;2011). Among the latter, apoptosis and proliferation deregulation are at the very core of malignant transformation and have thus been given special attention in the present paper.

Apoptosis is an evolutionary conserved ATP-dependent type of programmed cellular death, executed by caspases (cysteine proteases), which lead to a progressive disruption of the cell structures and formation of membrane-enclosed vesicles, named apoptotic bodies. Apoptosis can be triggered by either intrinsic or extrinsic death signals and is regulated by two gene families, Bcl_2 and IAP (Pizem, Cor, 2003). Survivin is a member of the IAP (Inhibitor of Apoptosis Protein) family and is thus an important antagonist of apoptosis, whose biology is discussed in more detail in the present paper.

The very fact that survivin is a member of the IAP family and is structurally similar to IAPs, such as ILP-2, livin and apollon, means that initial research on this protein was focused on its antiapoptotic role (Li et al., 1998;Salvesen, Duckett, 2002). Even though a substantial body of work has been invested in elucidating survivin's role as an apoptosis inhibitor, several issues are unclear and remain a subject of discussion.

Survivin's central role is believed to be suppression of apoptosis during embryogenesis (Adida et al., 1998). Survivin inhibits apoptosis on several levels. It binds and inactivates effector caspases 3 and 7 (Pizem, Cor, 2003). Moreover, survivin inhibits apoptosis by preventing mitochondrial export of the proapoptotic protein SMAC/Diablo (Lima et al., 2009). Furthermore, survivin binds and is stabilised by the aryl hydrocarbon receptor-binding protein (AIP), which enhances survivin's antiapoptotic functions and helps elevate a cell's antiapoptotic threshold (Kang, Altieri, 2006). Another antiapoptotic function of survivin is directly connected to its promitotic functions, since the binding of survivin to mitotic spindle microtubuli inhibits a default intrinsic triggering of cellular death during mitosis (Li et al., 1998). Notably, survivin expression in cancer cells helps them overcome intrinsic and extrinsic death signals.

Following the discoveries of survivin's antiapoptotic and cytoprotective functions, it was subsequently discovered that survivin has several other functions and is actively involved in cellular proliferation (Lens et al., 2003), microtubule dynamics and cellular stress response (Fortugno et al., 2003). Survivin is thus now regarded as a multifunctional, nodal protein.

Although cellular death and cellular division seem to be directly opposite processes, they are indeed intimately related. And that relation makes perfect sense when tissue homeostasis is taken into account. Redundant, damaged or infected cells need to be removed by apoptosis, which does not damage adjacent cells, and substituted with new, well performing ones by mitosis. Progression through the cell cycle, which allows for the production of new cells, and programmed cellular death, which causes loss of cells within tissues, share a number of control mechanisms that need to be strongly interlinked in order to assure normal tissue development and homeostasis. Several proteins are involved in the regulation of both processes. Disruption of the balance between proliferation and apoptosis is an important feature of malignant tumours and further underlines the importance of cell cycle/apoptosis regulation proteins in tumourigenesis (Hanahan, Weinberg, 2011).

Cellular proliferation, like apoptosis, is a tightly regulated process. Survivin promotes proliferation by direct binding and stabilisation of mitotic spindle microtubuli during the initial stages of mitosis (Altieri, 2010) and by regulation of chromosome segregation. Additionally, survivin is an important part of the chromosome passenger protein complex (CPP) and interacts with several CPP components, assuring their stability (Fortugno et al., 2002). In fact, Li et al. demonstrated that disruption of the survivin-mitotic spindle microtubuli interaction results in the loss of survivin's antiapoptotic function and an increase in Caspase 3 activity, a mechanism of inter-mitotic apoptosis induction (Li et al., 1998). The latter suggests, as mentioned previously, that survivin functions as an inhibitor of a default triggering of apoptosis during the G2/M phase of the cell cycle and might explain why survivin expression peaks at the transition from phase G2 to M (Beardmore et al., 2004). This means that survivin overexpression allows malignant cells to overcome proapoptotic checkpoints and favours aberrant progression through mitosis, regardless of critical genome defects, absence of growth signals or stress.

Additionally to its promitotic and antiapoptotic functions, survivin has also been demonstrated to be involved in cellular stress response pathways, interacting with the molecular chaperone Hsp90. Hsp90 is a central stress response chaperone, which helps cells to adapt to stress. Fortugno et al. demonstrated that Hsp90 binds survivin and stabilises it, meaning that the formation of such Hsp90-survivin complexes efficiently prevents apoptosis and mediates cellular proliferation, overcoming the environmental stress. Since both Hsp90 and survivin are often overexpressed in cancer, such interaction mechanisms are often exploited by cancer cells, allowing them to retain their proliferative potential, despite unfavourable environmental conditions (Altieri, 2004;Fortugno et al., 2003).

Despite the fact that new pathways involving survivin are constantly being discovered, it is fairly clear that survivin is a very important cancer gene that adjuvates the accumulation of malignant phenotype features. In sharp contrast with its vast array of functions, survivin (**B**aculoviral **IAP** **R**epeat **C**ontaining 5; BIRC5) is a rather small protein of 16.5 kDa (142 amino acids) and is the smallest member of the IAP family (Pizem, Cor, 2003).

Unlike other IAP family members, survivin has only one BIR domain (Figure 1), which is essential for its antiapoptotic function (Ambrosini et al., 1997). Survivin spontaneously forms antiparallelic dimers *in vitro*, but novel data suggest that a monomeric form is required for its proper functioning (Altieri, 2008b). Within the cell, survivin can be present in the nucleus, cytosol and mitochondria (Mahotka et al., 2002). Its expression levels are cell-cycle dependent, with a peak expression at the transition from phase G2 to M, which means that survivin expression reaches its highest point at the initial stage of cellular division (Beardmore et al., 2004).

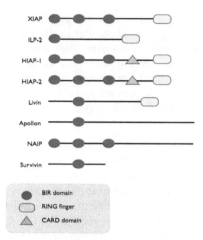

Fig. 1. Structures of IAP family proteins, adapted from (Salvesen, Duckett, 2002).

Survivin is encoded by the *BIRC5* gene, located on chromosome 17q25 in the human genome and is composed of four exons and three intons (Reed, 2001). Posttranscriptional modifications, namely alternative intron splicing, are responsible for the formation of alternative survivin isoforms (Noton et al., 2006), which are described in Table 1. The exact meaning of alternative *BIRC5* splicing is yet to be elucidated.

BIRC5 gene expression is controlled by a TATA-less inducible promoter with a canonical CpG domain and three cell cycle dependent elements (CDE) (Li, Altieri, 1999). Single nucleotide polymorphisms in the *BIRC5* promoter region and methylation of CpG domains have been demonstrated to affect *BIRC5* expression levels (Li, Altieri, 1999;Ma et al., 2010;Ma et al., 2011). The exact signals that trigger promoter activity and activate the expression of *BIRC5* are not completely understood. It is possible that tumour suppressors repress *BIRC5* expression, whereas oncogenes activate the promoter and trigger expression. Mirza et al. confirmed that wild-type p53, a crucial tumour suppressor, suppresses survivin expression (Mirza et al., 2002).

Isoform	Modification (relative to WT)
survivin-2A	none; wild type survivin isoform
survivin-2B	alternative exon 2
survivin-deltaEx-3	deletion of exon 3
survivin-3B	alternative exon 3

Table 1. Survivin isoforms, summarised from (Noton et al., 2006)

As mentioned previously, survivin is present in both the nucleus and cytoplasm. Its various subcellular localisations are inevitably linked to its distinct functions. Nuclear survivin is thought to be involved in proliferation regulation, whereas cytoplasmic survivin has an anti-apoptotic role (Stauber et al., 2007). It is believed that both survivin isoform and phosphorylation status dictate its subcellular localisation and function, but this theory has not been thoroughly researched yet (Altieri, 2010;Mahotka et al., 2002).

It should thus be noted that survivin has a unique role in the cell, providing an interplaying link between cellular death and cellular division. Both apoptosis and cellular proliferation are often deregulated in cancer and components of both pathways could be used as potential anticancer therapeutic targets.

3. Survivin in cancer

Very few potential anticancer therapeutic targets have boosted as much promise as survivin. In fact, one of survivin's most prominent features is its interesting expression pattern. Survivin is expressed in embryonal tissue and malignant cells, but is virtually absent from terminally differentiated tissues, with very limited exceptions, such as thymocytes, endothelial cells and bone marrow cells (Altieri, 2003a;Pizem, Cor, 2003;Sah et al., 2006). The almost exclusive tumour-specific expression pattern undoubtedly means that survivin has an important role in the development and progression of cancer (Altieri, 2008a). Survivin expression has been demonstrated in several types of human malignancies (Figure 2), such as medulloblastoma (Pizem et al., 2005), colorectal carcinoma (Sarela et al., 2000), lymphoma (Ambrosini et al., 1997) and many others (Nachmias et al., 2004). Klabatsa et al. demonstrated that survivin is also expressed in malignant pleural mesothelioma (Klabatsa et al., 2005).

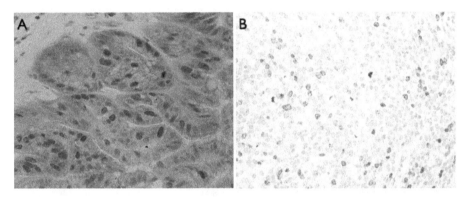

Fig. 2. Survivin expression in cancer. A: Gallbladder adenocarcinoma. B: Medulloblastoma (immunohistochemistry, 400x magnification).

Additionally to assessing survivin's presence, retrospective analyses demonstrated that survivin expression levels are linked to tumour progression and patient survival. Survivin over-expression proved to be a negative prognostic marker in several types of cancer, like colorectal (Sarela et al., 2001) and hepatocellular (Ikeguchi et al., 2002) carcinoma. On the other hand, Kennedy et al. confirmed that survivin expression is a positive prognostic marker for breast cancer (Kennedy et al., 2003). In fact, increased survivin expression correlated with more pronounced disease progression and a more aggressive phenotype, poorer response to treatment and shortened patient survival (Sah et al., 2006).

It is now generally accepted that survivin is both a negative prognostic marker and a positive predictive marker, since its expression reliably predicts response to treatment and disease progression (Kato et al., 2001). Moreover, it is possible that an increase in survivin expression might improve a tumour's response to therapy, since high-survivin tumors tend to be more aggressive and proliferative and thus more likely to respond to cytostatic treatment (Petrarca et al., 2011; Span et al., 2006).

Besides survivin's role in cancer progression, its sharp tumour-specific expression pattern means that survivin is a promising potential therapeutic target for many types of cancer. Several preclinical and early-stage clinical studies have indeed demonstrated the feasibility and effectiveness of survivin-based anticancer treatments (Altieri, 2003b).

4. The role of survivin in malignant pleural mesothelioma

4.1 Prognostic role

As mentioned previously, a straightforward negative prognostic value for survivin has been confirmed for several types of cancer throughout a vast array of retrospective studies. But very few studies on survivin's prognostic and predictive role in malignant pleural mesothelioma have been published so far (summarised in Table 2).

Unfortunately, as Table 2 indicates, results of those studies are still conflicting. Nevertheless, it appears that survivin has a negative impact on survival of malignant pleural mesothelioma patients, although the numbers of patients included in the studies were generally low. Notwithstanding the latter, it is important to note that those studies unanimously confirmed that survivin indeed is extensively expressed in malignant pleural mesothelioma (Figure 3).

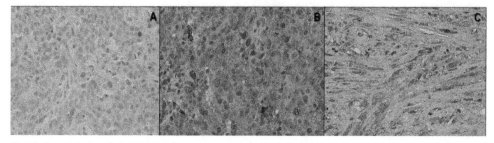

Fig. 3. Survivin expression in different histological types of malignant pleural mesothelioma. A: epitheloid histological type, B: biphasic histological type, C: sarcomatoid histological type (immunohistochemistry, 400x magnification).

As for those studies, differences in survivin detection and expression quantification methods might complicate any attempts at data comparison. But when the immunohistochemistry-based studies from Table 2 are selected and compared, striking differences are observed in the numbers of patients with survivin-positive tumours. Gordon et al. detected 76 % of survivin positive malignant pleural mesotheliomas (Gordon et al., 2007), which is in concordance with the 77 % of survivin positive malignant pleural mesotheliomas detected by (Klabatsa et al., 2005), whereas Kleinberg et al. demonstrated survivin expression in 64 % of malignant pleural mesothelioma patients included in their study (Kleinberg et al., 2007). In comparison, in our recently published paper, all (100 %) of the malignant pleural mesothelioma specimens from 101 patients analysed were survivin positive, with a median level of 67 % of survivin positive tumour cell nuclei (Hmeljak et al., 2011).

Those results, although very broad-range and seemingly inconsistent, underline a very important point: survivin is present and actively expressed in malignant pleural mesothelioma.

Authors	Year	Patients	*Methods	Correlation with survival	Reference
Klabatsa et al.	2005	32	immunohistochemistry	positive	(Klabatsa et al., 2005)
Gordon et al.	2007	66	immunohistochemistry, qRT-PCR	negative	(Gordon et al., 2007)
Kleinberg et al.	2007	77	immunohistochemistry, western blot	non significant	(Kleinberg et al., 2007)
Lan et al.	2010	44	immunocytochemistry, qRT-PCR	negative	(Lan et al., 2010)
Hmeljak et al.	2011	101	immunohistochemistry	non significant	(Hmeljak et al., 2011)

*Only patients with malignant pleural mesothelioma are included, although some of the studies comprised malignant peritoneal mesothelioma and reactive pleuritis patients.

Table 2. Overview of studies on the prognostic role of survivin in malignant pleural mesothelioma

And although its prognostic value in malignant pleural mesothelioma has not been conclusively assessed yet, survivin's role as a potential therapeutic target should not be dismissed.

4.2 Therapeutic role

Currently, malignant pleural mesothelioma treatment is consisted of platinum-based systemic chemotherapy with several additional combinations. One of the most successful approaches is combined systemic chemotherapy with cisplatin and pemetrexed (Belli et al., 2009). Surgical resection of the tumour is possible only in selected cases, which are rare, due to the fact that most patients are diagnosed at an advanced stage of the disease, when debulking surgery becomes too dangerous (Kindler, 2008). Another important obstacle of present therapies is the fact that malignant pleural mesothelioma often develops resistance to therapeutic approaches, rendering them ineffective.

Since conventional therapies regularly fail, a surprisingly high number of novel therapeutic approaches have been recently (and are being currently) explored. Such intensive research is motivated by increasing numbers of patients and the absence of current effective therapies (Ray, Kindler, 2009). It is a pleasant surprise that such an investment is being made in the treatment of a fairly rare disease. Among those novel strategies, special attention has been devoted to antisurvivin therapies, which have been extensively tested in the preclinical setting. Survivin inhibition resulted in decreased survival of malignant pleural mesothelioma cells (Xia et al., 2002) and increased sensitivity to radiotherapy (Kim et al., 2007). Data from those studies indicate that posttranscriptional targeting of survivin increases the rates of both spontaneous and radiation-induced apoptosis and highlight the central role of survivin in maintainig apoptosis resistance and mitotic potential of malignant pleural mesothelioma cells. Moreover, use of conditionally replicative adenoviruses containing the *BIRC5* promoter increased apoptosis in both *in vitro* and *in vivo* models of malignant pleural mesothelioma (Zhu et al., 2006).

Antisurvivin treatment approaches include not only posttranscriptional knockdown with antisense oligonucleotides or siRNA molecules. Low molecular weight chemical inhibitors, such as YM155 (Nakahara et al., 2007), and immunogenic peptides, such as survivin-2B80-88 (Tsuruma et al., 2004) are being tested in the preclinical and early-phase clinical setting for breast, lung and colorectal cancer. Promising results of such antisurvivin therapies, applied to other cancer types (Hansen et al., 2008; Olie et al., 2000;Tsuruma et al., 2008), further confirm the feasibility and effectiveness of antisurvivin therapeutic approaches for the treatment of malignant pleural mesothelioma patients.

Our group recently performed a pilot *in vitro* experiment, in which a combination of survivin knockdown by siRNA (Stealth® siRNA BIRC5HSS179403; Invitrogen, Carlsbad, CA, USA) and hypotonic chemotherapy with cisplatin (*cis*-diamminedichloroplatinum, CDDP) dissolved in ultrapure water, has been administered to mesothelioma cell line MSTO-211H. The survival of treated cells was assessed by the clonogenic assay (Figure 4). We found that the combination of survivin silencing and administration of a hypotonic solution of cisplatin very effectively reduced survival of MSTO-211H cells compared to survivin silencing only (p<0.001) and also compared to survivin silencing and application of isotonic cisplatin dissolved in phosphate buffered saline (p=0.005). Our preliminary results suggest that inhibition of survivin effectively reduces the survival of malignant pleural mesothelioma cells. Moreover, the effect is substantially amplified when a combined approach of gene therapy and chemotherapy with cisplatin is applied. The exact nature of the observed combined antitumour effect (whether it is additive or synergistic) was not determined in the present phase of experiments, but it should undoubtedly be interesting to assess.

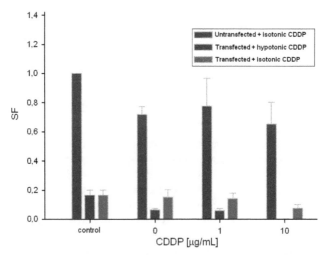

Fig. 4. Survival fractions of MSTO-211H cells after transfection with Stealth® siRNA BIRC5HSS179403 and subsequent chemotherapy with cisplatin.

Nowadays, malignant pleural mesothelioma rarely responds to conventional treatment and prognosis remains poor, despite extensive preclinical research and improvement in diagnosis. Novel, locally administered targeted therapies are promising, since pleural mesothelioma has some features that indicate the feasibility of such therapies. Surface accessibility of the tumour and predominantly local spread of the disease are characteristics that would allow successful local gene-therapy-based treatment (Albelda et al., 2009), such as antisurvivin siRNAs or antisense oligonucleotides.

Preclinical research on therapeutic targeting of survivin in malignant pleural mesothelioma has confirmed the effectiveness and feasibility of such approaches, especially when combined with existing conventional therapies and has laid a strong foundation for translation into the clinic.

4.3 Biological and ethiological role

Notwithstanding the widely acknowledged and studied presence of survivin in malignant pleural mesothelioma or its potential therapeutic value, very little is known about the actual mechanisms of activation of the *BIRC5* gene during malignant transformation of mesothelial cells. It has been suggested that activated oncogenes might trigger *BIRC5* expression, since Falleni et al. demonstrated a gradual increase in survivin mRNA from normal mesothelial cells through inflammatory pleuritis and malignant mesothelioma (Falleni et al., 2005). The latter indicates that survivin expression increases during the phases of malignant transformation and is correlated with a progressively increasing malignant phenotype. It has not, however, been elucidated, whether increased survivin expression is a cause or a consequence of malignant transformation. And even though thorough retrospective research might not manage to elucidate the value of survivin expression levels as a malignant pleural mesothelioma prognostic marker, survivin will still remain an intriguing and promising potential therapeutic target.

5. The role of survivin in malignant peritoneal mesothelioma

Although the primary focus of the present text is malignant pleural mesothelioma, the latter is not the only form of mesothelial malignancy. Malignant peritoneal mesothelioma (MePM) is a much rarer manifestation of mesothelial malignancies, accounting for 20 - 33 % of all malignant mesotheliomas (Bridda et al., 2007). Although the biology of malignant peritoneal mesothelioma remains largely unclear, this form of mesothelioma is known to arise from and spreads along the peritoneal mesothelium, remaining confined to the peritoneal cavity for most of its natural history (Deraco et al., 1999). Similarly to pleural mesothelioma, malignant peritoneal mesothelioma is characterised by a poor prognosis and poor response to treatment. Conversely, the importance of novel potential prognostic and therapeutic targets is just as urgent as in pleural mesothelioma. Zaffaroni et al. demonstrated that survivin is expressed in malignant peritoneal mesothelioma and its expression is a negative prognostic marker. Moreover, the same study confirmed that survivin knockdown using RNA interference markedly decreased MPeM cell survival *in vitro* (Zaffaroni et al., 2007).

6. Conclusions

The aim of modern anticancer treatment strategies is a "clean" removal of malignant cells with limited or, preferably, no damage to adjacent normal tissues. Despite recent advances in anticancer treatment, malignant pleural mesothelioma remains a fatal disease with an extremely poor prognosis. Several retrospective studies confirmed high levels of survivin expression in malignant pleural mesothelioma, but failed to conclusively assess its prognostic significance. On the other hand, survivin targeting proved to be an effective approach for malignant pleural mesothelioma treatment. Unfortunately, several important pieces of the survivin-mesothelioma story are still missing and a lot of research is still awaiting.

The present review only briefly explored the issue and we hope it helped pinpoint some of the missing bits of information that need to be clarified for a thorough understanding of the matter. It is our firm belief that combining survivin targeting with local or systemic conventional therapies would be a valuable therapeutic strategy for mesothelioma patients. Current preclinical data are extensive and incouraging and we can only hope that translation in the clinical setting will be prompt and successful. Malignant pleural mesothelioma is, in fact, a deadly disease and still has one of the worst prognoses among all malignancies. Research and validation of novel targets can bring new hope to patients, who often find themselves frustrated by the lack of effective treatment options. And in the case of malignant pleural mesothelioma, the numbers of those patients are increasing steeply at this very moment.

7. Acknowledgements

The present work was financially supported by Slovenian Research Agency (ARRS) grant no. P3-0003.

8. References

Adida C., Crotty P. L., McGrath J., Berrebi D., Diebold J., Altieri D. C. (1998). Developmentally regulated expression of the novel cancer anti-apoptosis gene survivin in human and mouse differentiation. *American Journal of Pathology*. 152: 1, 43-9, 0002-9440 (Print)

Albelda S. M., Vachani A., Haas A., Sterman D. H. (2009). Gene therapy/immunotherapy and mesothelioma: where are we? *Journal of Thoracic Oncology*. 4: 9, S73-S4, 1556-0864

Altieri D. C. (2003a). Survivin in apoptosis control and cell cycle regulation in cancer. *Prog Cell Cycle Res*. 5: 447-52, 1087-2957 (Print)

Altieri D. C. (2003b). Validating survivin as a cancer therapeutic target. *Nat Rev Cancer*. 3: 1, 46-54, 1474-175X (Print)

Altieri D. C. (2004). Coupling apoptosis resistance to the cellular stress response: the IAP-Hsp90 connection in cancer. *Cell Cycle*. 3: 3, 255-6, 1538-4101 (Print)

Altieri D. C. (2008a). Survivin, cancer networks and pathway-directed drug discovery. *Nat Rev Cancer*. 8: 1, 61-70, 1474-1768 (Electronic)

Altieri D. C. (2008b). New wirings in the survivin networks. *Oncogene*. 27: 48, 6276-84, 0950-9232

Altieri D. C. (2010). Survivin and IAP proteins in cell-death mechanisms. *Biochemical Journal*. 430: 199-205, 0264-6021

Ambrosini G., Adida C., Altieri D. C. (1997). A novel anti-apoptosis gene, survivin, expressed in cancer and lymphoma. *Nat Med.* 3: 8, 917-21, 1078-8956 (Print)

Beardmore V. A., Ahonen L. J., Gorbsky G. J., Kallio M. J. (2004). Survivin dynamics increases at centromeres during G2/M phase transition and is regulated by microtubule-attachment and Aurora B kinase activity. *J Cell Sci.* 117: Pt 18, 4033-42, 0021-9533 (Print)

Belli C., Fennell D., Giovannini M., Gaudino G., Mutti L. (2009). Malignant pleural mesothelioma: current treatments and emerging drugs. *Expert Opinion on Emerging Drugs.* 14: 3, 423-37, 1472-8214

Bridda A., Padoan I., Mencarelli R., Frego M. (2007). Peritoneal mesothelioma: a review. *MedGenMed.* 9: 2, 32, 1531-0132 (Electronic)

Carbone M., Albelda S. M., Broaddus V. C., Flores R. M., Hillerdal G., Jaurand M. C., Kjaerheim K., Pass H. I., Robinson B., Tsao A. (2007). Eighth International Mesothelioma Interest Group. *Oncogene.* 26: 49, 6959-67, 0950-9232

Deraco M., Santoro N., Carraro O., Inglese M. G., Rebuffoni G., Guadagni S., Somers D. C., Vaglini M. (1999). Peritoneal carcinomatosis: feature of dissemination. A review. *Tumori.* 85: 1, 1-5, 0300-8916 (Print)

Falleni M., Pellegrini C., Marchetti A., Roncalli M., Nosotti M. N., Palleschi A., Santambrogio L., Coggi G., Bosari S. (2005). Quantitative evaluation of the apoptosis regulating genes Survivin, Bcl-2 and Bax in inflammatory and malignant pleural lesions. *Lung Cancer.* 48: 2, 211-6, 0169-5002

Fortugno P., Beltrami E., Plescia J., Fontana J., Pradhan D., Marchisio P. C., Sessa W. C., Altieri D. C. (2003). Regulation of survivin function by Hsp90. *Proc Natl Acad Sci U S A.* 100: 24, 13791-6, 0027-8424 (Print)

Fortugno P., Wall N. R., Giodini A., O'Connor D. S., Plescia J., Padgett K. M., Tognin S., Marchisio P. C., Altieri D. C. (2002). Survivin exists in immunochemically distinct subcellular pools and is involved in spindle microtubule function. *J Cell Sci.* 115: Pt 3, 575-85, 0021-9533 (Print)

Gordon G. J., Mani M., Mukhopadhyay L., Dong L., Edenfield H. R., Glickman J. N., Yeap B. Y., Sugarbaker D. J., Bueno R. (2007). Expression patterns of inhibitor of apoptosis proteins in malignant pleural mesothelioma. *Journal of Pathology.* 211: 4, 447-54, 0022-3417 (Print)

Hanahan D., Weinberg R. A. (2000). The hallmarks of cancer. *Cell.* 100: 1, 57-70, 0092-8674

Hanahan D., Weinberg R. A. (2011). Hallmarks of cancer: the next generation. *Cell.* 144: 5, 646-74, 1097-4172 (Electronic)

Hansen J. B., Fisker N., Westergaard M., Kjaerulff L. S., Hansen H. F., Thrue C. A., Rosenbohm C., Wissenbach M., Orum H., Koch T. (2008). SPC3042: a proapoptotic survivin inhibitor. *Mol Cancer Ther.* 7: 9, 2736-45, 1535-7163 (Print)

Hmeljak J., Erculj N., Dolzan V., Kern I., Cor A. (2011). BIRC5 promoter SNPs do not affect nuclear survivin expression and survival of malignant pleural mesothelioma patients. *J Cancer Res Clin Oncol.* 137 (11): 1641-1651 (Electronic)

Ikeguchi M., Hirooka Y., Kaibara N. (2002). Quantitative analysis of apoptosis-related gene expression in hepatocellular carcinoma. *Cancer.* 95: 9, 1938-45, 0008-543X

Kang B. H., Altieri D. C. (2006). Regulation of survivin stability by the aryl hydrocarbon receptor-interacting protein. *J Biol Chem.* 281: 34, 24721-7, 0021-9258 (Print)

Kato J., Kuwabara Y., Mitani M., Shinoda N., Sato A., Toyama T., Mitsui A., Nishiwaki T., Moriyama S., Kudo J., Fujii Y. (2001). Expression of survivin in esophageal cancer: correlation with the prognosis and response to chemotherapy. *International Journal of Cancer.* 95: 2, 92-5, 0020-7136 (Print)

Kennedy S. M., O'Driscoll L., Purcell R., Fitz-simons N., McDermott E. W., Hill A. D., O'Higgins N. J., Parkinson M., Linehan R., Clynes M. (2003). Prognostic importance of survivin in breast cancer. *British Journal of Cancer.* 88: 7, 1077-83, 0007-0920

Kim K. W., Mutter R. W., Willey C. D., Subhawong T. K., Shinohara E. T., Albert J. M., Ling G., Cao C., Gi Y. J., Lu B. (2007). Inhibition of survivin and aurora B kinase sensitizes mesothelioma cells by enhancing mitotic arrests. *International Journal of Radiation Oncology Biology Physics.* 67: 5, 1519-25, 0360-3016

Kindler H. L. (2008). Systemic treatments for mesothelioma: standard and novel. *Curr Treat Options Oncol.* 9: 2-3, 171-9, 1534-6277 (Electronic)

Klabatsa A., Steele J., Fenneil D., Evans M., Rudd R., Sheaff M. (2005). Survivin and survival in malignant pleural mesothelioma. *Lung Cancer.* 49: S222-S, 0169-5002

Kleinberg L., Lie A. K., Florenes V. A., Nesland J. M., Davidson B. (2007). Expression of inhibitor-of-apoptosis protein family members in malignant mesothelioma. *Human Pathology.* 38: 7, 986-94, 0046-8177

Lan C. C., Wu Y. K., Lee C. H., Huang Y. C., Huang C. Y., Tsai Y. H., Huang S. F., Tsao T. C. Y. (2010). Increased Survivin mRNA in Malignant Pleural Effusion is Significantly Correlated with Survival. *Japanese Journal of Clinical Oncology.* 40: 3, 234-40, 0368-2811

Lens S. M., Wolthuis R. M., Klompmaker R., Kauw J., Agami R., Brummelkamp T., Kops G., Medema R. H. (2003). Survivin is required for a sustained spindle checkpoint arrest in response to lack of tension. *EMBO J.* 22: 12, 2934-47, 0261-4189 (Print)

Li F. Z., Altieri D. C. (1999). Transcriptional analysis of human survivin gene expression. *Biochemical Journal.* 344: 305-11, 0264-6021

Li F. Z., Ambrosini G., Chu E. Y., Plescia J., Tognin S., Marchisio P. C., Altieri D. C. (1998). Control of apoptosis and mitotic spindle checkpoint by survivin. *Nature.* 396: 6711, 580-4, 0028-0836

Lima F. D., Costa H. D., Barrezueta L. F. M., Oshima C. T. F., Silva J. A., Gomes T. S., Pinheiro N., Neto R. A., Franco M. (2009). Immunoexpression of inhibitors of apoptosis proteins and their antagonist SMAC/DIABLO in colorectal carcinoma: Correlation with apoptotic index, cellular proliferation and prognosis. *Oncology Reports.* 22: 2, 295-303, 1021-335X

Ma A. N., Huang W. L., Wu Z. N., Hu J. F., Li T., Zhou X. J., Wang Y. X. (2010). Induced epigenetic modifications of the promoter chromatin silence survivin and inhibit tumor growth. *Biochemical and Biophysical Research Communications.* 393: 4, 592-7, 0006-291X

Ma A. N., Lu J., Zhou X. J., Wang Y. X. (2011). Histone deacetylation directs DNA methylation in survivin gene silencing. *Biochem Biophys Res Commun.* 404: 1, 268-72, 1090-2104 (Electronic)

Mahotka C., Liebmann J., Wenzel M., Suschek C. V., Schmitt M., Gabbert H. E., Gerharz C. D. (2002). Differential subcellular localization of functionally divergent survivin splice variants. *Cell Death Differ.* 9: 12, 1334-42, 1350-9047 (Print) 1350-9047 (Linking)

Mirza A., McGuirk M., Hockenberry T. N., Wu Q., Ashar H., Black S., Wen S. F., Wang L., Kirschmeier P., Bishop W. R., Nielsen L. L., Pickett C. B., Liu S. (2002). Human survivin is negatively regulated by wild-type p53 and participates in p53-dependent apoptotic pathway. *Oncogene*. 21: 17, 2613-22, 0950-9232 (Print)

Nachmias B., Ashhab Y., Ben-Yehuda D. (2004). The inhibitor of apoptosis protein family (IAPs): an emerging therapeutic target in cancer. *Seminars in Cancer Biology*. 14: 4, 231-43, 1044-579X

Nakahara T., Takeuchi M., Kinoyama I., Minematsu T., Shirasuna K., Matsuhisa A., Kita A., Tominaga F., Yamanaka K., Kudoh M., Sasamata M. (2007). YM155, a novel small-molecule survivin suppressant, induces regression of established human hormone-refractory prostate tumor xenografts. *Cancer Research*. 67: 17, 8014-21, 0008-5472 (Print)

Noton E. A., Colnaghi R., Tate S., Starck C., Carvalho A., Ko Ferrigno P., Wheatley S. P. (2006). Molecular analysis of survivin isoforms: evidence that alternatively spliced variants do not play a role in mitosis. *J Biol Chem*. 281: 2, 1286-95, 0021-9258 (Print)

Olie R. A., Simoes-Wust A. P., Baumann B., Leech S. H., Fabbro D., Stahel R. A., Zangemeister-Wittke U. (2000). A novel antisense oligonucleotide targeting survivin expression induces apoptosis and sensitizes lung cancer cells to chemotherapy. *Cancer Research*. 60: 11, 2805-9, 0008-5472 (Print)

Petrarca C. R., Brunetto A. T., Duval V., Brondani A., Carvalho G. P., Garicochea B. (2011). Survivin as a predictive biomarker of complete pathologic response to neoadjuvant chemotherapy in patients with stage II and stage III breast cancer. *Clin Breast Cancer*. 11: 2, 129-34, 1938-0666 (Electronic)

Pizem J., Cor A. (2003). Survivin - an inhibitor of apoptosis and a new target in cancer. *Radiology and Oncology*. 37: 3,

Pizem J., Cor A., Zadravec-Zaletel L., Popovic M. (2005). Survivin is a negative prognostic marker in medulloblastoma. *Neuropathology and Applied Neurobiology*. 31: 4, 422-8, 0305-1846

Ray M., Kindler H. L. (2009). Malignant Pleural Mesothelioma An Update on Biomarkers and Treatment. *Chest*. 136: 3, 888-96, 0012-3692

Reed J. C. (2001). The Survivin saga goes in vivo. *Journal of Clinical Investigation*. 108: 7, 965-9, 0021-9738

Robinson B. W. S., Musk A. W., Lake R. A. (2005). Malignant mesothelioma. *Lancet*. 366: 9483, 397-408, 0140-6736

Sah N. K., Khan Z., Khan G. J., Bisen P. S. (2006). Structural, functional and therapeutic biology of survivin. *Cancer Lett*. 244: 2, 164-71, 0304-3835 (Print)

Salvesen G. S., Duckett C. S. (2002). IAP proteins: blocking the road to death's door. *Nat Rev Mol Cell Biol*. 3: 6, 401-10, 1471-0072 (Print)

Sarela A. I., Macadam R. C., Farmery S. M., Markham A. F., Guillou P. J. (2000). Expression of the antiapoptosis gene, survivin, predicts death from recurrent colorectal carcinoma. *Gut*. 46: 5, 645-50, 0017-5749 (Print)

Sarela A. I., Scott N., Ramsdale J., Markham A. F., Guillou P. J. (2001). Immunohistochemical detection of the anti-apoptosis protein, survivin, predicts survival after curative resection of stage II colorectal carcinomas. *Ann Surg Oncol*. 8: 4, 305-10, 1068-9265 (Print)

Span P. N., Tjan-Heijnen V. C., Manders P., van Tienoven D., Lehr J., Sweep F. C. (2006). High survivin predicts a poor response to endocrine therapy, but a good response to chemotherapy in advanced breast cancer. *Breast Cancer Res Treat*. 98: 2, 223-30, 0167-6806 (Print)

Stauber R. H., Mann W., Knauer S. K. (2007). Nuclear and cytoplasmic survivin: Molecular mechanism, prognostic, and therapeutic potential. *Cancer Research*. 67: 13, 5999-6002, 0008-5472

Tsuruma T., Hata F., Torigoe T., Furuhata T., Idenoue S., Kurotaki T., Yamamoto M., Yagihashi A., Ohmura T., Yamaguchi K., Katsuramaki T., Yasoshima T., Sasaki K., Mizushima Y., Minamida H., Kimura H., Akiyama M., Hirohashi Y., Asanuma H., Tamura Y., Shimozawa K., Sato N., Hirata K. (2004). Phase I clinical study of anti-apoptosis protein, survivin-derived peptide vaccine therapy for patients with advanced or recurrent colorectal cancer. *J Transl Med*. 2: 1, 19, 1479-5876 (Electronic)

Tsuruma T., Iwayama Y., Ohmura T., Katsuramaki T., Hata F., Furuhata T., Yamaguchi K., Kimura Y., Torigoe T., Toyota N., Yagihashi A., Hirohashi Y., Asanuma H., Shimozawa K., Okazaki M., Mizushima Y., Nomura N., Sato N., Hirata K. (2008). Clinical and immunological evaluation of anti-apoptosis protein, survivin-derived peptide vaccine in phase I clinical study for patients with advanced or recurrent breast cancer. *J Transl Med*. 6: 24, 1479-5876 (Electronic)

Wagner J. C. (1979). Citation Classic - Diffuse Pleural Mesothelioma and Asbestos Exposure in the North-Western-Cape-Province. *Current Contents/Clinical Practice*. 32, C14-C, 0091-1704

Xia C., Xu Z., Yuan X., Uematsu K., You L., Li K., Li L., McCormick F., Jablons D. M. (2002). Induction of apoptosis in mesothelioma cells by antisurvivin oligonucleotides. *Mol Cancer Ther*. 1: 9, 687-94, 1535-7163 (Print)

Zaffaroni N., Costa A., Pennati M., De Marco C., Affini E., Madeo M., Erdas R., Cabras A., Kusamura S., Baratti D., Deraco M., Daidone M. G. (2007). Survivin is highly expressed and promotes cell survival in malignant peritoneal mesothelioma. *Cellular Oncology*. 29: 6, 453-66, 1570-5870 (Print)

Zhu Z. B., Makhija S. K., Lu B. G., Wang M. H., Wang S. Y., Takayama K., Siegal G. P., Reynolds P. N., Curiel D. T. (2006). Targeting mesothelioma using an infectivity enhanced survivin-conditionally replicative adenoviruses. *Journal of Thoracic Oncology*. 1: 7, 701-11, 1556-0864

The Impact of Extracellular Low pH on the Anti-Tumor Efficacy Against Mesothelioma

T. Fukamachi[1], H. Saito[1], M. Tagawa[2] and H. Kobayashi[1]
[1]Chiba University
[2]Chiba Cancer Center Research Institute
Japan

1. Introduction

Inflammation and tumors have been demonstrated to have several common characteristics in their microenvironments. Extracellular acidosis is frequently associated both with inflammation area and tumor growth. Measurements of pH in peripheral tissues during the development of inflammation have shown extracellular pH values as low as 5.5–7.0 while the pH values of normal tissues are usually maintained at pH 7.4-7.5 mainly via pulmonary respiration and kidney perfusion of protons (Edlow & Sheldon, 1971). Similary, the extracellular pH in the central regions of tumors decreases below 6.7 in several tumors as a consequence of lactate accumulation derived from a lack of sufficient vascularization or an increase in tumor specific glycolysis under aerobic conditions combined with impaired mitochondrial oxidative phosphorylation (Simmen, 1993; Vaupel, 1989; Warburg, 1956). These pH declines affect cellular or tissue functions because their features are determined mainly by a variety of enzymatic proteins, and all enzymatic activities have each optimal pH. We have previously reported that the low pH conditions alter signal transductions. (1) The phosphorylations of several proteins were upregulated at low pH in leukemia cells (Fukamachi et al., 2001; Hirara et al., 2008). (2) CTIB, an Ikappa B beta variant, regulates cellular survival and gene expression exclusively under acidic environments in Chinese Hamster Ovary cells (Lao et al., 2005, 2006). Furthermore, the gene expressions related with tumor malignancy were upregulated at low pH in several tumor cell lines (Rofstad et al., 2006). These different characteristics dependent on extracellular pH provided us with a perspective that the inhibitory effect of anti-tumor drugs or molecular targeted inhibitors would vary at tumor-specific low pH, and the development of anti-tumor medicines, which have medical properties especially in acidic conditions, would lead to curative therapies for cancers.

Malignant mesothelioma is an aggressive tumor developed from the pleura or other mesothelioma surface. No efficient method for treatment, including chemotherapy and radiotherapy, has yet been established for advanced stage mesothelioma (Zucali & Giaccone, 2006). However, the efficacies of anti-tumor agents against not only mesothelioma but other tumors under acidic conditions have not yet been investigated exhaustively. Only some attributive information has emphasized the possibility of alteration in anti-tumor efficacy by extracellular pH and other conditions. The cytotoxicity of mitoxantrone and topotecan was reduced at low extracellular pH in murine EMT6 and in human MGH-U1 cells (Vukovic & Tannock, 1977). The impaired efficacy of mitoxantrone by acidosis was confirmed in M1R rat mammary carcinoma cells (Jähde et al., 1990). MCF-7 human breast cancer cells in vitro were more susceptible to doxorubicin toxicity at pH 7.4 compared to pH 6.8, probably due to its weak base conformation (Raghunand et al., 1999). On the other hands, mitomycin C showed higher cytotoxicity at low pH condition against EMT6 tumor cells (Rockwell, 1986). The research on pH dependent inhibitory effects has accumulated gradually, however the exhaustive investigation of efficacy at low pH using anti-tumor agents and molecular targeted inhibitors against mesothelioma is urgent and important for combinational therapy of anti-tumor agents or development of new drugs.

The screening of molecular targeted inhibitors, which inhibit cell growth preferentially at low pH conditions, has the potential to produce new therapeutic agents with less adverse effect against normal tissues because the development of malignant mesothelioma is associated with inflammation derived from asbestos exposure and the insides of mesothelioma tissues are also acidificated due to the mechanisms described above (Jähde et al., 1992). In order to develop a new therapeutic modality, in this article we discuss the effects of tumor specific microenvironments, especially under low pH conditions, on the efficacy of classical anti-tumor drugs and molecular targeted inhibitors.

2. The SCADs inhibitor kits and experimental procedure

We previously compared the cytotoxic efficacies of 93 molecular targeted inhibitors in SCADs inhibitor kit 1 at pH 7.5 and pH 6.7 against HeLa cells (Fukamachi et al., 2010). The tumor characteristics, however, differ widely and, moreover, SCADs inhibitor kits 2 and 3 have a number of other inhibitors, so we examined the cytotoxic efficacies of 272 kinds of molecular targeted inhibitors using SCADs inhibitor kits 1, 2 and 3 under different pH conditions against mesothelioma cells.

The inhibitory effects of chemical compounds in the SCADs inhibitor kits at different pH conditions were estimated by WST assay, a modified procedure of the MTT assay, as described in our previous reports (Fukamachi et al., 2010). Human pleural mesothelioma cell line NCI-H2052 was cultured in RPMI-1640 medium. To maintain medium pH for the comparison of inhibitory effects under different pH conditions, our group has added Good's buffer to media instead of sodium bicarbonate and found that all tumor cell lines we tested can proliferated both at pH 7.5 and 6.7 without sodium bicarbonate although the proliferation at pH 6.7 was slower than that at pH 7.5. The alteration of medium pH was not significant at pH 6.7 whereas the pH of alkaline medium declined to 7.4 after proliferation for 5 days (Fukamachi et al., 2001; Lao et al., 2005, 2006).

3. The effect of extracellular pH on classical anti-tumor agents against mesothelioma

SCADs inhibitor kits include 17 anti-tumor medicines those have already been prescribed for treatment of cancers. As shown in Table 1, none of the classical anti-tumor agents achieved better results against mesothelioma under acidic conditions. Cisplatin, mitomycin C, daunorubicin, aclarubicin, vinblastine sulfate, doxorubicin and cytochalasin D showed less cytotoxicity under acidic conditions. No pH dependency was seen with bleomycin sulfate, paclitaxel, actinomycin D, camptothecin or etoposide (Table 1, Fig.1). The remaining 6 medicines did not reduce cellular survival independently from medium pH at 2 microM.

Cytotoxicity at different pH	
higher cytotoxicity at low pH	—
lower cytotoxicity at low pH	Cisplatin, Mitomycin C, Daunorubicin/HCl, Doxorubicin/HCl Vinblastine sulfate, Aclarubicin, Cytochalasin D
no different cytotoxicity between pH 6.7 and 7.5	Bleomycin sulfate, Paclitaxel, Actinomycin D, Camptothecin Etoposide
no cytotoxicity under 2 micro M	5-FU, Bestatin, Methotrexate, Flutamide, Tamoxifen/citrate

Table 1. Cytotoxicity of classical anti-tumor drug at different pH conditions.

3.1 Cisplatin

The cytotoxicity of cisplatin has been reported previously to show high sensitivity at low pH in EMT mouse tumor or leukemia (Laurencot & Kennedy, 1995). However, the cytotoxicity against NCI-H2052 mesothelioma was impaired at pH 6.7 as shown in Table.1 and Fig.1. We suppose that this difference was derived from the alteration of intracellular pH value dependent on extracellular pH value and the composition of nutrients. In previous experiments, the medium pH values were set at pH 6.0 as acidic conditions in contrast to the pH value 6.7 in our reports. We confirmed that the intracellular pH values are maintained at pH above 7.1 in cells incubated in the medium with 10% FBS at pH 6.7 (data not shown). In addition to our experiments, the maintenance of intracellular pH values in weak acidic conditions was again confirmed in other tumor cell lines (Gerweck & Seethaaraman, 1996; Owen et al., 1997). Extracellular pH lower than 6.5, however, markedly reduced intracellular pH values (Rockwells, 1986). This large reduction of intracellular pH values has been associated with apoptosis being independent of the presence of anti-tumor agents, so the enhanced effect of cisplatin under acidic conditions below pH 6.0 might be derived from another mechanism. Although the pH sensitive, anti-tumor bis (aminoalcohol) dichloroplatinum(II) has been developed, but its low pH dependent cytotoxicity appeared pH only below pH 6.0 (Zorbas-Seifriends et al., 2006). The extracellular pH values in mesothelioma, are usually over 6.7 (Jahde et al., 1992), so we presume that the cytotoxic potential of cisplatin is reduced around at pH 6.7 in mesothelioma.

The mechanism of resistance against cisplatin under low pH conditions is unknown. Cisplatin-resistance has been related with the activity of several proteins such as BRCA1, which plays multiple role in DNA repair, or p21WAF1/CIP1 proteins (Alli et al., 2011; Wei et al., 2010). Although the activity of these proteins at pH 6.7 has not been investigated, acidosis affects several protein activity (Lao et al., 2006; Rofstad et al., 2006). So the alteration of these proteins' activity may contribute to the Cisplatin-resistance at low pH.

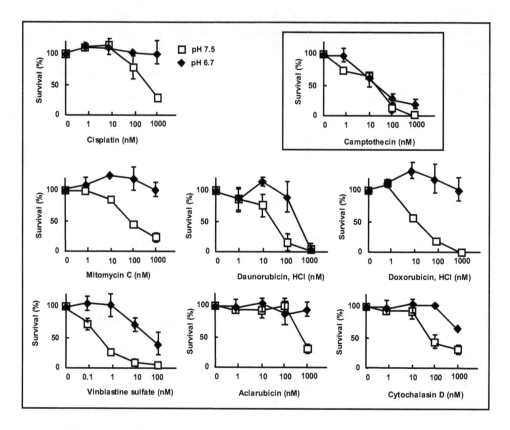

Fig. 1. pH-dependent cytotoxicity of classical anti-tumor drug.

3.2 Mitomycin C

Mitomycin C was reported to be potently its cytotoxic at low pH conditions against EMT6 tumor cells and this was associated with the upregulated binding of mitomycin C to DNA at low pH conditions (Rockwells, 1986). This result is different from our results, as shown in Table.1 and Fig.1. The medium pH values were at pH 5.7 in previous experiments, so probably the cytotoxicity of mitomycin C would be reduced at around pH 6.7. Resistance to mitomycin C by several cancers has been reported and related with glutathion S-transferase activity (Ruiz-Gomez et al., 2000). So the quantification of the expression or activity of glutathion S-transferase under acidic conditions may be important. Although the treatment against mesothelioma using mitomycin C has been investigated, its efficacy was less than those of cisplatin (Fennell et al., 2007) or oxalipalatin (Routh et al., 2011). In contrast, Co-treatment with mitomycin C, vinblastin and cisplatin achieved the improvement of symptoms including cough, dyspnoea and pains (Andreopoulou et al., 2004). So treatment with mitomycin C might be limited to improving the quality of life.

3.3 Doxorubicin and daunorubicin

The therapeutic effects of doxorubicin and daunorubicin against mesothelioma have been linked with the tumor-resistance mechanism of mesothelioma. Single treatment with doxorubicin and daunorubicin showed no significant anti-tumor activity (Harvey et al.,1984; Steele et al., 2001). Although this combination with cisplatin achieved some slight improvement, a high dose of doxorubicin was needed and this showed a toxic rather than curative effect (Stewart et al., 1994). These impaired efficacies of doxorubicin in mesothelioma have been thought to be due to upregulation of p-glycoprotein mediated drug efflux (Isobe et al., 1994) or multi drug associated protein (Kato et al., 1998). The expression of p-glycoprotein was up-regulated at low pH conditions in EMT6 cells and prostate cancer cells (Thews et al., 2006). This upregulation of p-glycoprotein is partially dependent on HIF-1 (Riganti et al., 2008) and extracellular low pH has been reported to induce HIF-1 (Mekhall et al., 2004). So, this mechanism might contribute to the pH-dependent loss of cytotoxicity as shown in Fig.1, in addition to the possibility derived from its weakly basic conformation (Raghunand et al., 1999). Drug resistance is also influenced by the activity of ROS scavengers. Most mesotheliomas express relatively large amount of manganese superoxide dismutase, catalase and cell surface NADH oxidase, and the cytotoxicitic function of ROS derived from doxorubicin were impaired in mesothelioma (Hedges et al., 2003; Kahlos et al., 1998).

3.4 Vinblastine sulfate, aclarubicin and cytochalasin D

These three agents has not been investigated at low pH conditions yet. So our experiment shown in Fig.1 was the first to show less cytotoxicity under acidic conditions. The reduced cytotoxicity of these three drugs, however, might be explained by the pH-dependent upregulation of p-glycoprotein as well as doxorubicin because vinblastine is also a p-glycoprotein substance (Gertner et al., 1998). Recent data indicated that the use of vinblastine should be limited to the improvement of symptoms as described above for mitomycin C (Andreopuoulou et al., 2004). It has been reported that the anti-tumor activity of aclarubicin is related to the production of ROS (Rogalska et al., 2008). So the mesothelioma cell, which expresses elevated amounts of ROS scavengers, may be resistant to aclarubicin.

The effects of cytochalasin D are derived from the breaking of actin filaments (Schiliwa, 1982). Human actin-depolymerizing factor and cofilin have been reported to be pH-sensitive (Pope et al., 2004). So this mechanism is likely to be associated with our results shown in Fig.1.

3.5 The pH dependency of other anti-tumor agents

Bleomycin was reported to show pH dependency in restricted conditions. The combination of high temperature and low pH enhanced the efficacy of bleomycin and 1,3-bis(2-chloroethyl)-1-nitrosourea but not methotrexate against Chinese hamster ovary, while there was no effect of pH at normal tissue temperature (Hahn & Shiu, 1983). The efficiency of bleomycin at low pH and high temperature has not been estimated against mesothelioma yet in vitro and vivo. Hyperthermia with bleomycin, however, may be worthwhile to examine against mesothelioma.

Although 5-Fluorouracil (5-FU) did not show cytotoxicity under both pH conditions as shown in Fig.1, high dose 5-FU previously showed the potential for pH dependent mesothelioma suppression (Nissen & Tanneberg, 1981). 5-FU inhibited the 3H-uridine incorporation preferentially at pH 7.4 compared to that at pH 6.8 at concentrations above 100 microM, so the comparison at each pH with higher doses of 5-FU is needed.

4. The effect of extracellular pH on molecular targeted inhibitors

As shown in Table 2, only four molecular targeted inhibitors, lovastatin, manumycin A, FTI-276 and cantharidin, showed higher cytotoxicity at low pH conditions in our exhaustively investigation against mesothelioma at different pH conditions using SCADs inhibitor kit. The inhibitory effect of aphidicolin, bisindolymaleimide I, N1,N12-diethylspermine, PKR inhibitor were impaired at low pH (Table 2, Fig.2).

Cytotoxicity at different pH	
higher cytotoxicity at low pH	Manumycin A, FTI-276, Cantharidin, Lovastatin
lower cytotoxicity at low pH	Aphidicolin, Bisindolymaleimide I/HCl, N1,N12-Diethylspermine PKR inhibitor
no different cytotoxicity between pH 6.7 and 7.5	Scriptaid, Trichostatin A, Cycloheximide, Radicicol, 17-AAG, Cucurbitacin PD 98059, MG-132, Lactacystin, Oligomycin, Bafilomycin A1, SB 225002 Monensin, Ouabain, Sanguinarine, Valinomycin, Nigericin, A23187 Ionomycin, Thapsigargin, Rotenone, Leptomycin B*, LY 83583, Chetomin α-Amanitin, MST-312, Akt Inhibitor IV, ATM kinase inhibitor Cdk2/9 inhibitor, AGL 2263, IKK-2 inhibitor VI, JAK Inhibitor I, PP2 SU11652, PDGF receptor tyrosine kinase inhibitor IV, LY-294002 Wortmannin, Go7874, KT5823, ZM 336372, SU1498 VEGFR receptor tyrosine kinase inhibitor III VEGF recptor 2 kinase inhibitor

Table 2. Cytotoxicity of molecular targeted inhibitor at different pH conditions.

4.1 Statin

4.1.1 The therapeutic capacity of statins against cancers

The pH-dependent cytotoxicity of lovastatin was observed previously in HeLa cells, mesothelioma cell line H2452 cells, pancreatic tumor cell line, BxPC-3 and Panc-1. Moreover, simvastatin, another lipophilic statin, inhibited cellular survival of HeLa cells as well as lovastatin (Fukamachi et al., 2010). These results indicated that pH-dependent cytotoxicity of lovastatin is common to several tumors and that other statins have similar properties. Statins (3-Hydroxy-3-methylglutaryl coenzyme A reductase inhibitors) block the *de novo* synthesis of cholesterol, resulting in lower plasma cholesterol levels. Although myopathy or its more severe form rhabdomyolysis is a significant adverse effect of statin treatment, the incidence is typically less than 0.1% (Ballantyne et al., 2003). Other adverse effects including hyperplasia of the liver, squamous epithelial hyperplasia of cataracts and vascular lesions in the central nervous system have lower incidences or need extreme inhibition of the enzyme with high doses of statins (Gerson et al., 1989). Due to its active effect against cholesterol synthesis and relatively safe features, lovastatin and other statins have been prescribed for treatment of hypercholesterolaemia since the late 1980s (Tobert, 2003). Furthermore, statins might have potential for other coronary artery diseases. In patients without established cardiovascular disease but with cardiovascular risk factors, statin use was associated with significantly improved survival and large reductions in the risk of major cardiovascular events (Bruqts et al., 2009).

In addition to its great curative effect for vascular disease, the relationship of statin with cancer treatments has been discussed, including mesothelioma. Lovastatin inhibited the growth of T cell leukemia (Newman et al., 1994), pancreatic tumor (Muller et al., 1998), glioma (Jones et al., 1994), lung cancer (Maksimova et al., 2008) and prostate cancer (Hoque et al., 2008). Other statins as well as lovastatin showed cytotoxicity against tumor cell lines. Simvastatin against HT29 human colon cancer cells (Cho et al., 2008), glioma (Wu et al., 2009), pravastatin against hepatoma (Kawata et al., 1992) have been reported. Moreover, several statins reduced the migration of human pancreatic tumors and mouse melanoma (Kusama et al., 2002). In addition to the cytotoxicity and suppression of invasion against tumor cell lines, statins' curative effect against several cancers was confirmed in patients. Conventional chemotherapy using simvastatin with irinotecan, 5-FU and leucovorin (FOLFIRI) was a feasible regimen with promising anti-tumor activity against metastatic colorectal cancers (Lee et al., 2009). Fluvastatin reduces proliferation and increases apoptosis in women with high grade breast cancer (Garwood et al., 2010). These results indicated that statins inhibit tumor proliferation and have the potential to be applied for cancer treatments.

4.1.2 The mechanism of statins cytotoxicity; cholesterol and protein prenylation

The mechanism underlying statins' pH-dependent cytotoxicity is unclear. Statins inhibit HMG-CoA reductase that converts HMG-CoA to mevalonate, resulting in the reduction of farnesyl pyrophosphate, a substance of cholesterol. The important feature of cholesterol is that cholesterol is critical substance in plasma and vesicle membranes, so the inhibition of cholesterol synthesis by statins reduces mitochondrial membrane potential and induces the release of pro-apoptotic factors including cytochrome c, resulting in the apoptosis or the increase of doxorubicin sensitivity in hepatocellular carcinoma (Montero et al., 2008). The amount of cholesterol also contributed to the tumor cell migration (Sekine et al., 2010). These contribution of cholesterol to tumor movement were impaired by the reduction of cholesterol by statins (Murai et al., 2011).

Another cascade downstream of the mevalonate pathway might be important to influence cellular function or tumor survival. Farnesyl pyrophosphate is converted into geranylgeranyl pyrophosphate and both phosphates are substances of protein prenylation. Proteins acquire lipophilicity with prenylation by farnesyl transferase or geranylgeranyl transeferase and bind to membrane or hydrophobic grooves on the surface of soluble protein factors (Gelb et al., 2006). In association with tumors, the prenylation of low molecular mass G protein has been examined, because their membrane association is induced by prenylation (Finegold et al., 1990). Lovastatin inhibits the prenylation of G proteins and alters their localization (Girgelt et al., 1994; Muller et al., 1998). Simvastatin interfered with angiogenesis via inhibition of the geranylgeranylation and membrane localization of RhoA (Park et al., 2002). RhoA activity and JNK, downstream of RhoA, were also inhibited by atorvastatin, resulting in the suppression of osteosacroma invasion (Fromigue et al., 2008). In addition, Rab protein, which was recently reported to be involved in protein transport across the secretory, was geranylgeranylated by Rab geranylgeranyl transferase, and mediated cancer invasion (Leung et al., 2006).

4.1.3 The mechanism of statins cytotoxicity; downstream of G protein

In the downstream of these low molecular mass G protein prenylations, statins induced an mTOR-dependent Ser166 phosphorylation of Mdm2, and this effect may attenuate the duration and intensity of the p53 response to DNA damage in hepatocytes (Paajarvi et al., 2005). Atorvastatins induce autophagy and autophagy-associated cell death in PC3 cells, likely through inhibition of geranylgeranylation (Parikh et al., 2010). GGTI-286, an inhibitor of geranylgeranyl transeferase, induced G0/G1 arrest and p21 resulting in tumor suppression (Vogt et al., 1997). These effects derived from p21 were related with the inhibition of histone deacetylase activity and release of promoter-associated HDAC1/2(Lin et al., 2008). Lovastatin induced U87 glioblastoma cell death in correlation with significantly increased levels of the BH3-only protein and the activation of MAPK. All of these alterations were prevented by geranylgeranyl pyrophosphate (Jiang et al., 2004). Statins have the potential to regulate gene expression related with cancer progression. MMP-9 reduction by lovastatin resulted in the suppression of invasion (Wang et al., 2000). Pitavastatin at low dose inhibits NF-kappaB activation and decreases IL-6 production induced by TNF-alpha (Wang & Kitajima, 2007). Atorvastatin inhibits inflammatory angiogenesis in mice through down-regulation of VEGF, TNF-alpha, and TGF-beta1 (Araujo et al., 2010). These reports suggest that several cancers are sensitive to statins and the inhibitors of protein prenylation.

4.1.4 The effect of statins against mesothelioma under acidic conditions

In contrast to statins' inhibitory effect against several cancers, little has been reported about the treatment of mesothelioma with statins or prenylation inhibitors. A few previous reports and our results, however, stress the possibility of mesothelioma treatment by statins. Lovastatin reduced malignant mesothelioma viability with altering the membrane association of Ras, and this cytotoxic effect was impaired by addition of mevalonate (Rubins et al., 1998). It is still unclear whether the cytotoxicity was dependent on the reduction of cholesterol or on the prenylation of proteins. In regard to the doxorubicin sensitivity of mesothelioma up-regulated by statins, the inhibition of protein prenylation was thought to potentiate the cytotoxicity of doxorubicin (Riganti et al., 2006). Both mevastatin and simvastatin increased the doxorubicin sensitivity via the increase of NO, and this effect was mimicked by GGTI-286 and Y-27632, an inhibitor of ROCK which is a downstream protein of Rho GTPase. Although, there has been no discussion about the contribution of the decreased cholesterol, the decline of cholesterol level would reduce the mitochondrial membrane potential, resulting in the release of pro-apoptotic protein. So both mechanisms are thought to contribute to the up-regulation of doxorubicin sensitivity.

Our resent results indicated that mesothelioma cells can proliferate under acidic conditions, and the pH-dependent cytotoxicity was due to the pH-dependent activity of prenylated proteins or the pH-dependent alteration of protein prenylation because manumycin A, an inhibitor of farnesyl and geranylgeranyl transferase, showed pH-dependent cytotoxicity as well as statins while no pH-dependent cytotoxicity appeared with YM-53601, an inhibitor of squalene synthase (Fukamachi et al., 2010). This importance of protein prenylation was reinforced by our result that three out of the only four inhibitors including FTI-276, an inhibitor of farnesyl transferase, are related with protein prenylation as shown in Table 2. It is not clear which protein's prenylation or activity is important in mesothelioma cells under acidic conditions. The signal transductions under acidic environments are different from those at normal tissue pH. The phosphorylation of p38 was increased at low pH (Hirata et al., 2008). The activity of the Erk/Ap-1 pathway is also activated at low pH in melanoma cells (Kato et al., 2005). These results indicate that the upstream proteins of MAPK are likely to be important at low pH. In fact, the activity of ERK in cardiac myocytes at low pH was related with Ras activation (Haworth et al., 2006). The morphological changes under acidic conditions were associated with Rho kinase (Hyvelin et al., 2004). Rab11b and its mediator Rip11 regulate V-ATPase traffic elevated at low pH in duct cells (Oehike et al., 2011). These results suggested that low molecular mass G protein might be important in tumor proliferation under acidic conditions. It remains unclear yet why statins inhibit cellular proliferation preferentially in tumor growth. Recently, a novel approach to identify geranylgeranylated protein was developed using azide binding geranylgeraniol which converted to geranylgeranyl pyrophosphate in cytosol (Chan et al., 2009). So the proteins, which play a critical role for mesothelioma proliferation at low pH, will be identified soon.

4.2 Cantharidin

4.2.1 The mechanism of cantharidin to suppress tumor growth

Cantharidin, a natural compound isolated from beetles, has the inhibitory activity of protein phosphatase (PP2A or PP1). Cantharidin was first found to be effective against various warts (Cusack et al., 2008). Cantharidine has also been traditionally used as an anti-cancer agent in China (Pang et al., 2007). The mechanism against cancer via the inhibition of protein phosphatase is poorly understood except for a few reports regarding to apoptosis and signal pathways. Cantharidin caused G2/M arrest through inhibition of CDK1 activity (Huang et al., 2011) and apoptosis via mitochondrial pathways including Bax, Bcl-2, Bcl-xl resulting in caspase activation (Kok et al., 2005). Cantharidin was recently shown to have passive cytotoxicity against tumor cells via the JAK/STAT pathway (Sagawa et al., 2008) and the involvement of NF-kB pathways in cantharidin-induced apoptosis was also reported (Li et al., 2011).

4.2.2 The problem with cantharidin and derivatives of cantharidin

Although these features of cantharidin are important for anti-tumor activity, the clinical application of cantharidin is limited due to its severe side-effects and highly toxic nature. The protein phosphatase-inhibitory toxins have been shown to induce hyper-phosphorylation of cytoskeletal proteins like keratin in isolated rat hepatocytes, and to cause disruption of the intracellular network of keratin intermediate filaments (Blankson et al., 1995). The toxins also inhibit hepatocellular processes like autophagy, endocytosis, and protein synthesis and elicit apoptotic cell death when administered to hepatocytes in culture (Blankson et al., 2000).

Therefore, the development of more selective and effective analogs of cantharidin with less toxicity has become a challenge for cancer treatment. LB1.2, a synthesized cantharidin derivative, showed significant enhancement of cancer chemotherapy on glioblastoma and neuroblastoma cancer cells with no acute or chronic toxicity. This tumor-suppressive effect was derived from the quiescent cells cycle and caused by blocking other replication checkpoints triggered by DNA damage through the significant inhibition effect of PP2A (Rajski & Williams., 1998). Norcantharidin (NCTD) is another demethylated derivative of cantharidin possessing anti-cancer activity less toxic to normal cells, and has been used to gastric cancer (McCluskey., 2002). NCTD inhibited the activity of PP2A, and was able to promote the cell cycle from G1 to S phase with subsequent G2/M arrest (Yu et al., 2006). In addition to this phosphatase inhibitory effect, recent studies have demonstrated that cantharidin and NCTD can cause DNA damage, which may be the main contributory factor in the cytotoxicity of NCTD and cantharidin (Efferth et al., 2005). NCTD-induced caspase-dependent apoptosis was accompanied by an increase in ROS production, loss of mitochondrial membrane potential with release of cytochrome c from the mitochondria to the cytosol, and down-regulation of anti-apoptotic protein Bcl-2 (Chang et al., 2010).

4.2.3 The therapeutic capacity of cantharidin against mesothelioma

Combinational therapy with these new cantharidin derivatives may be used for treatment of mesothelioma. In combinational treatment with doxorubicin and LB1, the effectiveness of doxorubicin was greatly enhanced by the LB1 in the xenograft growth inhibition and lung metastases prevention of an aggressive sarcoma derived from transformed mesenchymal stem cells in syngeneic rats with little side toxicity (Zhang et al., 2010). Meanwhile, there have been several reports to show that cantharidin and its derivatives are relatively ineffective as an anti-cancer agent (Jiang et al., 1983). The contradiction may be related to cantharidin being less effective at alkaline pH but more active at acidic pH (Fukamachi et al., 2010)

It remains unclear why cantharidin inhibits more strongly at acidic pH and which pathways are inhibited by cantharidin under acidic environments. The protein phosphatase, which has been related with mesothelioma proliferation, is mainly PTEN (phosphatase and tensin homologue deleted from chromosome 10). The activity of PTEN was suppressed in mesothelioma (Opitz et al., 2008), and the elevated PI3K/Akt pathway, which is the target pathway of PTEN, was repeatedly confirmed and related with mesothelioma proliferation (Altomare et al., 2005). So the inhibition of PTEN by cantharidin is not likely to lead to mesothelioma death. In other cell tumors, cantharidin induced G2/M arrest through inhibition of CDK1 (Huang et al., 2011), and induced NF-kappaB activity via constitutive phosphorylation of IKK. So the sensitivity of these proteins, especially NF-kappaB, to low pH may be important because the translocation of NF-kappaB was altered dependent on extracellular pH in T cells (unpublished data). Taken together, the pharmacologic inhibition of PP2A with less-toxic cantharidin derivatives may be a useful strategy against mesothelioma as a single treatment or combined with other anti-tumor agents including doxorubicin.

4.3 The impaired effect of molecular targeted inhibitors

4.3.1 Aphidicolin

Aphidicolin is a specific inhibitor of DNA polymerase alpha and delta, resulting in DNA double-strand breaks leading to the activation of Ataxia-Telangiectasia Mutated: ATM (Ge & Blow, 2010), the inhibition of DNA replication and cell cycle arrest in G1/S phase (Dhillon et al., 2003). The impaired activity of aphidicolin at pH 6.7 shown in Table 2 and our previous result (Fukamachi et al., 2010) suggested that mesothelioma cells might have an acquired resistance to DNA double-strand breaks. Recently, an aphidicolin-resistant Chinese hamster V79 cell mutant had aphidicolin-resistant DNA polymerase that had an increased affinity for dNTP (Syljuasen et al., 2007). Furthermore, the checkpoint adaptation was observed in aphidicolin-treated Xenopus, and this system was expected to function in human cells (Herbst et al., 2003). The mechanism by which mesothelioma proliferates at pH 6.7 with aphidiconis is unclear yet. The most important point is that the ATM signal above has been thought to contribute to the exclusion of DNA mutated cells leading to tumorgenesis or tumor malignancy. Our result (Fig.2) may suggest that the extracellular acidosis influences tumor malignancy via impaired ATM signals.

4.3.2 Bisindolmaleimide

Bisindolmaleimide is a specific inhibitor of PKC (Toullec et al., 1991). PKC is a ubiquitous phospholipid-dependent serine/threonine kinase involved in major signaling events that regulate cellular growth, migration, apoptosis, and a wide variety of biological responses to stimuli (Sukumaran & Prasadarao, 2002). Several studies have indicated that the inhibition of PKC represses tumor proliferation although it depend on the PKC class (Hu et al., 2011; Toton et al., 2011). PKCbeta1 was expressed in the majority of MPM and the treatment of MPM cell lines with PKC inhibitor showed synergy when combined with cisplatin in vitro (Faoro et al., 2008). Moreover the inhibition of protein kinase C prevents asbestos-induced *c-fos* and *c-jun* proto-oncogene expression in mesothelial cells (Fung et al., 1997). Despite these results relating tumor progression with PKC, our results showed less sensitivity to Bisindolmaleimide (Table 2 & Fig.2). The suppressive acitivity of PKC at low pH was demonstrated in prostate carcinoma (Thews et al., 2006). So the impaired activity of Bisindolmaleimide may be due to the decline of PKC activity under acidic conditions.

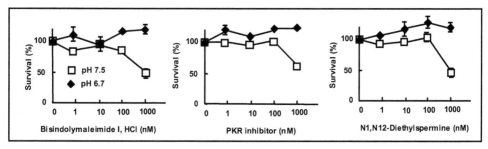

Fig. 2. pH dependency of molecular targeted inhibitors

4.3.3 PKR inhibitor

PKR, double-stranded RNA dependent protein kinase R, is activated by heme deficiency, the absence of amino acids, folded proteins accumulated in the ER, and dsRNA. The activated PKR phosphorylates eIF2α, and the phosphorylated eIF2α acts as a dominant inhibitor of the guanine exchange factor eIF2B, which prevents the recycling of eIF2 between succeeding rounds of protein synthesis and eventually leads to a global obstruction of mRNA translation initiation. This allows cells to adapt to stressful conditions by economizing on energy expended by protein synthesis (Wek et al., 2006). The adaptation process of eIF2α phoshorylation involves the selective translation of transcription factors such as activating transcription factor 4 (ATF4) (Vattem & Wek, 2004) and ATF5 (Zhou et al., 2008), which induce the expression of genes that facilitate adaptation. In cases of prolonged stress, the induction of eIF2α phosphorylation leads to cell death through the induction of apoptotic pathways (Wek et al., 2006). The results in Fig. 2 may suggest that the activity of PKR is less important in the proliferation of mesothelioma under acidic condition. Acidic conditions, in fact, enhanced the phosphorylation of eIF2, but this was confirmed at pH lower than 5.5 and not over 6.2 in a partially PKR-independent manner (Vantelon et al., 2007). So the phosphorylation of eIF2 without PKR at pH 6.7 might not cause this PKR independency at pH 6.7. Recently, there has been strong evidence to suggest that mammalian eIF2α kinases including PKR can also mediate activate glycogen synthase kinase 3 to promote the proteasomal degradation of p53 independently of eIF2α phosphorylation (Baltzis et al., 2007). So another mechanism may be critical in this reduced inhibitory effect at low pH.

4.3.4 The impaired effect of N1,N12-Diethylspermine

N1,N12-Diethylspermine lost its cytotoxic activity as shown in Table 2 and Fig. 2. N1, N12 - Diethylspermine (BESpm) caused a specific induction of spermidine/spermine N'-acetyltransferase (SSAT) activity, a cytosolic enzyme is induced in response to a variety of toxic agents, hormones and polyamine derivative (Casero et al., 1990). Polyamines are aliphatic cations present in all cells. SSAT is a rate-limiting step in polyamine catabolism, which catalyzes the transfer of the acetyl group from acetyl-CoA to the spermidine or spermine and has a predominant role in the regulation of intracellular polyamine concentrations in mammalian cells (Vujcic et al., 2000). Decreases in polyamines have been shown to promote decreased growth or apoptosis (Khan et al., 1992), depending on the cell type and the particular stimulus, suggesting a complex interaction between polyamines, cell growth, and cell death. Therefore, although polyamines are required for cell growth and differentiation, SSAT is thought to prevent overaccumulation of the higher polyamines from becoming toxic to the cell and may play a role in reducing the growth rate by decreasing intracellular polyamines. It has been shown that the regulation of SSAT by the natural polyamines and the anti-tumor polyamine analogues is through the polyamine response element (Wang et al., 1998). Furthermore, the superinduction of SSAT by polyamine analogues has been implicated in the cell type-specific cytotoxic response of several important human tumors including human lung cancer (Casero et al., 1990, 1992; Chang et al., 1992; Kim et al., 2005). Consistent with these previous reports, BESpm reduced cellular survival at pH 7.5 against mesothelioma as shown Fig. 2, probably via the inhibition of

SSAT by BESpm, leading to the disruption of polyamine regulation while no inhibitory effect was observed at pH 6.7. This result suggests that proliferation of mesothelioma cell line may be independent of the regulation of polyamine.

5. Novel anti-tumor therapy being dependent on pH

5.1 The effect of Alkylating drug

Some alkylating anti-tumor drugs including chlorambucil, carboquone and cyclophosphamide were reported to have higher cytotoxocity at low pH, probably because of their weak acid conformation or the decrease of drug resistance (Mikkelsen et al., 1985). It is difficult, however, to use them due to their causing the development of other tumors in common with alkyl agents (Rai et al., 2000).

5.2 Lowering the intracellular pH using nigericin

Low intracellular pH has been associated with enhanced cytotoxicity of anti-tumor drugs, so drugs to reduce intracellular pH have been investigated. The intracellular pH is higher than the extracellular pH, as mentioned above, so nigericin, an ionophore that acidifies the cytoplasm by exchanging cations with protons in cells placed in medium at low pH, was co-incubated with anti-tumor agents. Amiloride and 4,4'-diisothiocyanostilbene 2,2-disulfonic acid, inhibitors of the Na/H and HCO3/Cl exchangers, respectively, decreased intracellular pH in the presence of nigericin at low extracellular pH against Chinese hamster ovary and human bladder cancer MGH-U1 cells (Rotin et al., 1987).

5.3 The pH-dependent cytotoxicity of N-dodecylimidazole

N-dodecylimidazole is a compound, which acquires detergent properties under acidic conditions, and is thought to be useful for selectively killing cells under intratumor low pH environments. N-dodecylimidazole displayed pH-dependent cytotoxicity against EMT-6 and MGH-U1 cells. The cytotoxicity was enhanced 100-fold at pH 6.0 compared with pH 7.0 (Boyer et al., 1993). However, these liposomal formulations need to be optimized to achieve higher concentrations of pH-sensitive detergents within the endosome to facilitate efficient cytosolic release of liposome-entrapped contents (Chen et al., 2003). Various kinds of pH sensitive detergents have recently been developed to carry the anti-tumor drugs to the tumor nest, burst, and effuse the contents, dependent on the tumor pH. An acid-cleavable PEG lipid, 1'-(4'-cholesteryloxy-3'-butenyl)-omega-methoxy-polyethylene glycolate (CVEP), has been developed that produces stable liposomes when dispersed as a minor component (0.5-5 mol %) in 1,2-dioleoyl-sn-glycero-3-phosphoethanolamine (DOPE). Cleavage of CVEP at mildly acidic pH results in dePEGylation of the latently fusogenic DOPE liposomes, thereby triggering the onset of content release (Boomer et al., 2009). Physical and chemical instabilities have limited the use of these drug carriers as pharmaceutical products. Recently, however, the preparation of freeze-dried pharmaceuticals has proven to be a successful strategy implemented to improve the stability of these formulations. Long-circulating and pH-sensitive liposomes containing Cisplatin are now being applied in vivo experiments (Giuberti et al., 2010).

5.4 The pH dependent cytotoxicity of tirapazamine

Low pH can substantially potentiate the cytotoxic effect of the bioreductive drug tirapazamine in HT-29 human tumor cells (Skarsgard et al., 1993). Tirapazamine is the lead member of a class of bioreductive drugs and requires metabolic activation to give a cytotoxic free radical species via a variety of cellular reductases, including NADPH cytochrome c reductase (Chinje et al., 2003). Combination therapy with tirapazamine and cisplatin has shown increased treatment efficacy compared with cisplatin alone in malignant melanoma and non-small-cell lung cancer, and also may be of benefit when combined with both radiotherapy and cisplatin in head and neck cancer (Williams et al., 2001).

6. Conclusion

As discussed in this review, there are no classical anti-tumor drugs which show high cytotoxicity against mesothelioma at pH 6.7. So it might be much important to prescribe both drugs whose cytotoxicity is enhanced at low pH and drugs which induce cell death at normal tissue pH for mesothelioma treatment. Although classical anti-tumor medicines have potent tumor suppressive effects, they also have severe toxicities for normal tissues. So the therapeutic regimes with lesser amounts of classical anti-tumor agents are urgently required. To this end, drugs which show higher cytotoxicity at low pH, including statins and cantharidins would be conventional candidates for co-treatment of mesothelioma. In fact, the combination treatment of solid tumors with statins enhanced anti-tumor drugs in vivo (Agarwal et al., 1999; Gao et al., 2010; O'Brien et al. 2003; Zhao et al., 2010). So the development of new compounds with anti-tumor activity preferentially at low pH would be useful for chemotherapy of mesothelioma.

7. Acknowledgements

The authors would like to express thanks to Mr. Yusuke Mochizuki, Ms. Shoko Ikeda and Ms. Hiroe Wada for helping the experiments. We also would like to appreciate Screening Committee of Anticancer Drugs supported by Grant-in-Aid for Scientific Research on Priority Area "Cancer" from The Ministry of Education, Culture, Sports, Science and Technology, Japan for donating the inhibitor kit. This work was supported in part by Grants-in-Aid for Scientific research from the Hamaguchi Foundation for the Advancement of Biochemistry, and by Special Funds for Education and Research (Development of SPECT Probes for Pharmaceutical Innovation) from the Ministry of Education, Culture, Sports, Science and Technology of Japan.

8. References

Agarwal, B., Bhendwal, S., Halmos, B., Moss, F., Ramey, G. & Holt, R. (1999) Lovastatin augments apoptosis induced by chemotherapeutic agents in colon cancer cells. *Clin Cancer Res.* Vol.5, No.8, pp.2223, ISSN 1078-2432

Alli, E., Sharma, B., Hartman, R., Lin, S.,McPherson, L. & Ford, M. (2011) Enhanced sensitivity to cisplatin and gemcitabine in Brca1-deficient murine mammary epithelial cells. *BMC Pharmacol.* Vol.11, pp.7, ISSN 1471-2210

Altomare, A., You, H., Xiao, H., Ramos-Nino, E., Skele, L., Rienzo, A., Jhanwar, C., Mossman, T., Kane, B. & Testa, R. (2005) Human and mouse mesotheliomas exhibit elevated AKT/PKB activity, which can be targeted pharmacologically to inhibit tumor cell growth. *Oncogene*. Vol.24, No.40, pp.6080, ISSN 0950-9232

Araújo, A., Rocha, A., Mendes, B. & Andrade, P. (2010) Atorvastatin inhibits inflammatory angiogenesis in mice through down regulation of VEGF, TNF-alpha and TGF-beta1. *Biomed Pharmacother*. Vol.64, No.1, pp.29, ISSN 0753-3322

Ardizzoni, A., Rosso, R., Salvati, F., Fusco, V., Cinquegrana, A., De Palma, M., Serrano, J., Pennucci, MC., Soresi,, E. & Crippa, M., et al. (1991) Activity of doxorubicin and cisplatin combination chemotherapy in patients with diffuse malignant pleural mesothelioma. An Italian Lung Cancer Task Force (FONICAP) Phase II study. *Cancer*. Vol.67, No.12, pp.2984, ISSN 1097-0142

Ballantyne, CM., Corsini, A., Davidson, MH., Holdaas, H., Jacobson, TA., Leitersdorf, E., März, W., Reckless, JP. & Stein, EA. (2003) Risk for myopathy with statin therapy in high-risk patients. *Arch Intern Med*. Vol.163, No.5, pp.553, ISSN 0003-9926

Baltzis, D., Pluquet, O., Papadakis, I., Kazemi, S., Qu, K. & Koromilas, E. (2007) The eIF2α kinases PERK and PKR activate glycogen synthase kinase 3 to promote the proteasomal degradation of p53. *J Biol Chem*. Vol.282, No.43, pp.31675, ISSN 0021-9528

Blankson, H., Holen, I., & Seglen, O. (1995) Disruption of the cytokeratin cytoskeleton and inhibition of hepatocytic autophagy by okadaic acid. *Exp. Cell Res*. Vol.218, pp522–530. ISSN 0014-4827

Blankson, H., Grotterød, M. & Seglen, O. (2000) Prevention of toxin-induced cytoskeletal disruption and apoptotic liver cell death by the grapefruit flavonoid, naringin. *Cell Death Differ*. Vol.7, pp. 739–746. ISSN 1350-9047

Boyer, J., Horn, I., Firestone, A., Steele-Norwood, D. & Tannock, F. (1993) pH dependent cytotoxicity of N-dodecylimidazole: a compound that acquires detergent properties under acidic conditions. *Br J Cancer*. Vol.67, No.1, pp.81, ISSN 0007-0920

Boomer, JA., Qualls, MM., Inerowicz, HD., Haynes, RH., Patri, VS., Kim, JM. & Thompson, DH. (2009) Cytoplasmic delivery of liposomal contents mediated by an acid-labile cholesterol-vinyl ether-PEG conjugate. *Bioconjug Chem*. Vol.20, No.1, pp47, ISSN 1043-1802

Brugts, J., Yetgin, T., Hoeks, E., Gotto, M., Shepherd, J., Westendorp, G., de Craen, J., Knopp, H., Nakamura, H., Ridker, P., Domburg, R. & Deckers, JW. (2009) The benefits of statins in people without established cardiovascular disease but with cardiovascular risk factors: meta-analysis of randomised controlled trials. *BMJ*. Vol.338, pp.2376, ISSN 1759-2151

Casero, A., Celano, P., Ervin, J., Wiest, L. & Pegg, E. (1990) High specific induction of spermidine/spermine N1-acetyltransferase in a human large cell lung carcinoma. *Biochem J*. Vol.270, No.3, pp.615, ISSN 0264-6021

Casero, A., Mank, R., Xiao, L., Smith, J., Bergeron, J., & Celano, P. (1992) Steady-state messenger RNA and activity correlates with sensitivity to N1,N12-bis(ethyl)spermine in human cell lines representing the major forms of lung cancer. *Cancer Res*. Vol.52, No.5359, pp.5363, ISSN 0008-5472

Chan, N., Hart, C., Guo, L., Nyberg, T., Davies, S., Fong, G., Young, G., Agnew, J. & Tamanoi, F. (2009) A novel approach to tag and identify geranylgeranylated proteins. *Electrophoresis*. Vol.30, No.20, pp.3598, ISSN 0173-0835

Chang, K., Bergeron, J., Porter, W., Vinson, R., Liang, Y., & Libby, R. (1992) Regulatory and antiproliferative effects of N-alkylated polyamine analogues in human and hamster pancreatic adenocarcinoma cell lines. *Cancer Chemother. Pharmacol.* Vol.30, No.183, pp.188, ISSN 0344-5704

Chang, C., Zhu, Q., Mei, J., Liu, Q. & Luo, J. (2010) Involvement of mitochondrial pathway in NCTD-induced cytotoxicity in human hepG2 cells. *J Exp Clin Cancer Res.* Vol.29, pp.145, ISSN 0392-9078

Chen, J., Asokan, A. & Cho, J. (2003) Cytosolic delivery of macromolecules: I. Synthesis and characterization of pH-sensitive acyloxyalkylimidazoles. *Biochim Biophys Acta.* Vol.1611, No.1-2, pp.140, ISSN 0006-3002

Chinje, C., Cowen, L., Feng, J., Sharma, P., Wind, S., Harris, L. & Stratford, J. (2003) Non-nuclear localized human NOSII enhances the bioactivation and toxicity of tirapazamine (SR4233) in vitro. *Mol Pharmacol.* Vol.63, No.6, pp.1248, ISSN 0026-895X

Cho, SJ., Kim, JS., Kim, JM., Lee, JY., Jung, HC. & Song, IS. (2008) Simvastatin induces apoptosis in human colon cancer cells and in tumor xenografts, and attenuates colitis-associated colon cancer in mice. *Int J Cancer.* Vol.123, No.4, pp.951, ISSN 0020-7136

Cusack, C., Fitzgerald, D., Clayton, TM. & Irvine, AD. (2008) Successful treatment of florid cutaneous warts with intravenous cidofovir in an 11-year-old girl. *Pediatr Dermatol.* Vol.25, No.3, pp.387, ISSN 0736-8046

Dhillon, S., Husain, A. & Ray, N. (2003) Expression of aphidicolin-induced fragile sites and their relationship between genetic susceptibility in breast cancer, ovarian cancer, and non-small-cell lung cancer patients. *Teratog Carcinog Mutagen.* Vol.1, pp.35, ISSN 0270-3211

Edlow, D. W., & Sheldon, W. H. (1971) The pH of inflammatory exudates. *Proc. Soc. Exp. Biol. Med.* Vol. 137, pp. 1328, ISSN 0037-9727

Efferth, T., Rauh, R., Kahl, S., Tomicic, M., Böchzelt, H., Tome, E., Briehl, M., Bauer, R. & Kaina, B. (2005) Molecular modes of action of cantharidin in tumor cells. *Biochem Pharmacol.* Vol.69, No.5, pp.811, ISSN 0006-2952

Elbling, L., Berger, W., Weiss, RM., Printz, D., Fritsch, G. & Micksche, M. (1998) A novel bioassay for P-glycoprotein functionality using cytochalasin D. *Cytometry.* Vol.31, No.3, pp.187, ISSN 1552-4922

Faoro, L., Loganathan, S., Westerhoff, M., Modi, R., Husain, N., Tretiakova, M., Seiwert, T., Kindler, L., Vokes, E. & Salgia, R. (2008) Protein kinase C beta in malignant pleural mesothelioma. *Anticancer Drugs.* Vol.19, No.9, pp.841, ISSN 0959-4973

Fennell, DA., Steele, JP., Shamash, J., Evans, MT., Wells, P., Sheaff, MT., Rudd, RM. & Stebbing, J. (2007) Efficacy and safety of first- or second-line irinotecan, cisplatin, and mitomycin in mesothelioma. *Cancer.* Vol.109, No.1, pp.93, ISSN 1097-0142

Finegold, A., Schafer, R., Rine, J., Whiteway, M. & Tamanoi, F. (1990) Common modifications of trimeric G proteins and ras protein: involvement of polyisoprenylation. *Science.* Vol.249, No.4965, pp.165, ISSN 0036-8075

Fukamachi, T., Saito, H., Kakegawa, T. & Kobayashi, H. (2002) Different proteins are phosphorylated under acidic environments in Jurkat cells. *Immunol Lett.* Vol.82, No.1-2, pp.155, ISSN 0165-2478

Fukamachi, T., Chiba, Y., Wang, X., Saito, H., Tagawa, M. & Kobayashi, H. (2010) Tumor specific low pH environments enhance the cytotoxicity of lovastatin and cantharidin. *Cancer Lett.* Vol.297, No.2, pp182, ISSN 0304-3835

Fung, H., Quinlan, R., Janssen, M., Timblin, R., Marsh, P., Heintz, H., Taatjes, J., Vacek, P., Jaken, S. & Mossman, T. (1997) Inhibition of protein kinase C prevents asbestos-induced c-fos and c-jun proto-oncogene expression in mesothelial cells. *Cancer Res.* Vol.57, No.15, pp.3101, ISSN 0008-5472

Fromigué, O., Hamidouche, Z. & Marie, J. (2008) Blockade of the RhoA-JNK-c-Jun-MMP2 cascade by atorvastatin reduces osteosarcoma cell invasion. *J Biol Chem.* Vol.283, No.45, pp.30549, ISSN 0021-9258

Gaertner, LS., Murray, CL. & Morris, CE. (1998) Transepithelial transport of nicotine and vinblastine in isolated malpighian tubules of the tobacco hornworm (Manduca sexta) suggests a P-glycoprotein-like mechanism. *Exp Biol.* Vol.201, No.18, pp.2637, ISSN 0176-8638

Gao, J., Jia, D., Li, S., Wang, W., Xu, L., Ma, L., Ge, S., Yu, H., Ren, H., Liu, B. & Zhang, H. (2010) Combined inhibitory effects of celecoxib and fluvastatin on the growth of human hepatocellular carcinoma xenografts in nude mice. *J Int Med Res.* Vol.38, No.4, pp.1413, ISSN 0300-0605

Garwood, R., Kumar, S., Baehner, L., Moore, H., Au, A., Hylton, N., Flowers, I., Garber, J., Lesnikoski, A., Hwang, S., Olopade, O., Port, R., Campbell, M. & Esserman, J. (2010) Fluvastatin reduces proliferation and increases apoptosis in women with high grade breast cancer. *Breast Cancer Res Treat.* Vol.119, No.1, pp.137, ISSN 0167-6806

Ge, Q. & Blow, J. (2010) Chk1 inhibits replication factory activation but allows dormant origin firing in existing factories. *J Cell Biol.* Vol.191, No.7, pp.1285, ISSN 0021-9525

Gelb, H., Brunsveld, L., Hrycyna, A., Michaelis, S., Tamanoi, F., Van, C. & Waldmann, H. (2006) Therapeutic intervention based on protein prenylation and associated modifications. *Nat Chem Biol.* Vol.2, No.10, pp.518, ISSN 1552-4469

Gerson, J., MacDonald, S., Alberts, W., Kornbrust, J., Majka, A., Stubbs, J., Bokelman, L. (1989) Animal safety and toxicology of simvastatin and related hydroxy-methylglutaryl-coenzyme A reductase inhibitors. *Am J Med.* Vol.87, No.4A, pp.28S, ISSN 0002-9343

Gerweck, LE., & Seetharaman, K. (1996) Cellular pH gradient in tumor versus normal tissue: potential exploitation for the treatment of cancer. *Cancer Res.* Vol.56. No.6, pp.1194, ISSN 0008-5472

Girgert, R., Marini, P., Janessa, A., Bruchelt, G., Treuner, J. & Schweizer, P. (1994) Inhibition of the membrane localization of p21 ras proteins by lovastatin in tumor cells possessing a mutated N-ras gene. *Oncology.* Vol.51, No.4, pp.320, ISSN 2156-6976

Giuberti, C., Reis, C., Rocha, G., Leite, A., Lacerda, G., Ramaldes, A. & Oliveira, C. (2011) Study of the pilot production process of long-circulating and pH-sensitive liposomes containing cisplatin. *J Liposome Res.* Vol.21, No.1, pp.60, ISSN 0898-2104

Hahn, GM. & Shiu, EC. (1983) Effect of pH and elevated temperatures on the cytotoxicity of some chemotherapeutic agents on Chinese hamster cells in vitro. *Cancer Res.* Vol.43, No.1, pp.5789, ISSN 0008-5472

Harvey, VJ., Slevin, ML., Ponder, BA., Blackshaw, AJ. & Wrigley, PF., (1984) Chemotherapy of diffuse malignant mesothelioma. Phase II trials of single-agent 5-fluorouracil and adriamycin. *Cancer.* Vol.54, No.6, pp.961, ISSN 1097-0142

Haworth, S., Dashnyam, S. & Avkiran, M. (2006) Ras triggers acidosis-induced activation of the extracellular-signal-regulated kinase pathway in cardiac myocytes. *Biochem J.* Vol.399, No.3, pp.493, ISSN 0264-6021

Hedges, KL., Morré, DM., Wu, LY. & Morre, DJ. (2003). Adriamycin tolerance in human mesothelioma lines and cell surface NADH oxidase. *Life Sci.* Vol.73, No.9, pp.1189, ISSN 0024-3205

Herbst, S. & Kies, S. (2003) Gefitinib: current and future status in cancer therapy. *Clin. Adv. Hematol. Oncol,* Vol.1, pp.466, ISSN 1543-0790

Hirata, S., Fukamachi, T., Sakano, H., Tarora, A., Saito, H. & Kobayashi, H. (2008) Extracellular acidic environments induce phosphorylation of ZAP-70 in Jurkat T cells. *Immunol Lett.* Vol.115, No.2, pp.105, ISSN 0165-2478

Hoque, A., Chen, H., Xu & XC. (2008) Statin induces apoptosis and cell growth arrest in prostate cancer cells. *Cancer Epidemiol Biomarkers Prev.* Vol.17, No.1, pp.88, ISSN 1055-9965

Hu, T., Wu, R., Cheng, C., Wang, S., Wang, T., Lee, C., Wang, J., Pan, M., Chang, Y. & Wu, S. (2011) Reactive oxygen species-mediated PKC and integrin signaling promotes tumor progression of human hepatoma HepG2. *Clin Exp Metastasis.* [Epub ahead of print] ISSN 0262-0898

Huang, WW., Ko, SW. & Tsai, HY., et al. (2011) Cantharidin induces G2/M phase arrest and apoptosis in human colorectal cancer colo 205 cells through inhibition of CDK1 activity and caspase-dependent signaling pathways. *Int J Oncol.* Vol.38, No.4, pp.1067, ISSN 0020-7136

Hyvelin, M., O'Connor, C. & McLoughlin, P. (2004) Effect of changes in pH on wall tension in isolated rat pulmonary artery: role of the RhoA/Rho-kinase pathway. *Am J Physiol Lung Cell Mol Physiol.* Vol.287, No.4, pp.L673, ISSN 1040-0605

Isobe, H., Wellham, L., Sauerteig, A., Sridhar, KS., Ramachandran, C. & Krishan, A. (1994) Doxorubicin retention and chemoresistance in human mesothelioma cell lines. *Int J Cancer.* Vol.57, No.4, pp.581, ISSN 0020-7136

Jähde, E., Glüsenkamp, KH. & Rajewsky, MF. (1990) Protection of cultured malignant cells from mitoxantrone cytotoxicity by low extracellular pH: a possible mechanism for chemoresistance in vivo. *Eur J Cancer.* Vol.26, No.26, pp.101, ISSN 0959-8049

Jähde, E., Volk, T., Atema, A., Smets, LA., Glüsenkamp, KH. & Rajewsky, MF. (1992) pH in human tumor xenografts and transplanted rat tumors: effect of insulin, inorganic phosphate, and m-iodobenzylguanidine. *Cancer Res.* Vol. 52, No. 22, pp.6209, ISSN 0008-5472

Jiang, L., Salmon, E. & Liu, M. (1983) Activity of camptothecin, harringtonin, cantharidin and curcumae in the human tumor stem cell assay. *Eur J Cancer Clin Oncol* Vol.19, No.2, pp.263, ISSN 0277-5379

Jiang, Z., Zheng, X., Lytle, A., Higashikubo, R. & Rich, M. (2004) Lovastatin-induced up-regulation of the BH3-only protein, Bim, and cell death in glioblastoma cells. *J Neurochem.* Vol.89, No.1, pp.168, ISSN 0022-3042

Jones, KD., Couldwell, WT., Hinton, DR., Su, Y., He, S., Anker, L. & Law, RE. (1994) Lovastatin induces growth inhibition and apoptosis in human malignant glioma cells. *Biochem Biophys Res Commun.* Vol.205, No.3, pp.1681, ISSN 0006-291X

Kahlos, K., Anttila, S., Asikainen, T., Kinnula, K., Raivio, KO., Mattson, K., Linnainmaa, K. & Kinnula, VL.(1998) Manganese superoxide dismutase in healthy human pleural mesothelium and in malignant pleural mesothelioma. *Am J Respir Cell Mol Biol.*Vol.18, No.4, pp.570, ISSN 1044-1549

Kato, Y., Lambert, CA., Colige, AC., Mineur, P., Noël, A., Frankenne, F., Foidart, JM., Baba, M., Hata, R., Miyazaki, K. & Tsukuda, M. (2005) Acidic extracellular pH induces matrix metalloproteinase-9 expression in mouse metastatic melanoma cells through the phospholipase D-mitogen-activated protein kinase signaling. *J Biol Chem.* Vol.280, No.12, pp10938, ISSN 0021-9258

Kawata, S., Kakimoto, H., Ishiguro, H., Yamasaki, E., Inui, Y. & Matsuzawa, Y. (1992) Effect of pravastatin, a potent 3-hydroxy-3-methylglutaryl-coenzyme A reductase inhibitor, on survival of AH130 hepatoma-bearing rats. *Jpn J Cancer Res.* Vol.83, No.11, pp.1120, ISSN 0910-5050

Khan, U., Mei, H. & Wilson, T. (1992) A proposed function for spermine and spermidine: protection of replicating DNA against damage by singlet oxygen. *Proc. Natl. Acad. Sci. U.S.A.* Vol.89, No.23, pp.11426, ISSN 0027-8424

Kim, K., Ryu, H., Park, W., Kim, S. & Chun, S. (2005) Induction of a SSAT isoform in response to hypoxia or iron deficiency and its protective effects on cell death. *Biochem.Biophys. Res. Commun.* Vol.331, No.7, pp85, ISSN 0006-291X

Kok, H., Cheng, J. & Hong, Y, et al. (2005) Norcantharidin-induced apoptosis in oral cancer cells is associated with an increase of proapoptotic to antiapoptotic protein ratio. *Cancer Lett.* Vol.217, No.1, pp.43, ISSN 0304-3835

Kusama, T., Mukai, M., Iwasaki, T., Tatsuta, M., Matsumoto, Y., Akedo, H., Inoue, M. & Nakamura, H. (2002) 3-hydroxy-3-methylglutaryl-coenzyme a reductase inhibitors reduce human pancreatic cancer cell invasion and metastasis. *Gastroenterology.* Vol.122, No.2, pp.308, ISSN 0016-5085

Lagadic-Gossmann, D., Huc, L. & Lecureur,.V. (2004) Alterations of intracellular pH homeostasis in apoptosis: origins and roles. *Cell Death Differ.* Vol.11, No.9, pp.953, ISSN 1350-9047

Lao, Q., Kuge, O., Fukamachi, T., Kakegawa, T., Saito, H., Nishijima, M. & Kobayashi, H. (2005) An IkappaB-beta COOH terminal region protein is essential for the proliferation of CHO cells under acidic stress. *J Cell Physiol.* Vol.203, NO.1, pp.186, ISSN 0021-9541

Lao, Q., Fukamachi, T., Saito, H., Kuge, O., Nishijima, M. & Kobayashi, H. (2006) Requirement of an IkappaB-beta COOH terminal region protein for acidic-adaptation in CHO cells. *J Cell Physiol.* Vol.207 NO.1, pp.238, ISSN 0021-9541

Laurencot, CM. & Kennedy, KA. (1995) Influence of pH on the cytotoxicity of cisplatin in EMT6 mouse mammary tumor cells. *Oncol Res.* Vol. 7-8, No., pp.371, ISSN 0965-0407

Lee, J., Jung, H., Park, S., Ahn, B., Shin, J., Im, A., Oh do, Y., Shin, B., Kim, W., Lee, N., Byun, H., Hong, S., Park, O., Park, H., Lim, Y. & Kang, K. (2009) Simvastatin plus irinotecan, 5-fluorouracil, and leucovorin (FOLFIRI) as first-line chemotherapy in metastatic colorectal patients: a multicenter phase II study. *Cancer Chemother Pharmacol.* Vol.64, No.4, pp.657, ISSN 0344-5704

Leung, F., Baron, R. & Seabra, C. (2006) Thematic review series: lipid posttranslational modifications. geranylgeranylation of Rab GTPases. *J Lipid Res.* Vol.47, No.3, pp.467, ISSN 0022-2275

Li, W., Chen, Z. & Zong, Y. (2011) PP2A inhibitors induce apoptosis in pancreatic cancer cell line PANC-1 through persistent phosphorylation of IKK and sustained activation of the NF-B pathway. *Cancer Lett.* Vol.304, No.2, pp.117, ISSN 0304-3835

Lin, C., Lin, H., Chou, W., Chang, F., Yeh, H. & Chen, C. (2008) Statins increase p21 through inhibition of histone deacetylase activity and release of promoter-associated HDAC1/2. *Cancer Res.* Vol.68, No.7, pp.2375, ISSN 0008-5472

Lu, J., Zhuang, Z., Song, DK., Mehta,GU., Ikejiri,B., Mushlin,H., Park,DM. &Lonser, RR. (2010) The effect of a PP2A inhibitor on the nuclear receptor corepressor pathway in glioma. *J Neurosurg.* Vol.113. No.2. pp225, ISSN 0022-3085

Maksimova, E., Yie, TA. & Rom, WN. (2008) In vitro mechanisms of lovastatin on lung cancer cell lines as a potential chemopreventive agent. *Lung.* Vol.186, No.1, pp.45, ISSN 0341-2040

McCluskey, A., Sim, T. & Sakoff, A. (2002) Serine-threonine protein phosphatase inhibitors: development of potential therapeutic strategies. *J Med Chem.* Vol.45, No.6, pp.1151, ISSN 0022-2623

Mekhail, K., Gunaratnam, L., Bonicalzi, ME. & Lee, S. (2004) HIF activation by pH-dependent nucleolar sequestration of VHL. *Nat Cell Biol.* Vol.6, No.7, pp.642, ISSN 1097-6256

Montero, J., Morales, A., Llacuna, L., Lluis, M., Terrones, O., Basañez, G., Antonsson, B., Prieto, J., García-Ruiz, C., Colell, A. & Fernández-Checa, C. (2008) Mitochondrial cholesterol contributes to chemotherapy resistance in hepatocellular carcinoma. *Cancer Res.* Vol.68, No.13, pp.5246, ISSN 0008-5472

Müller, C., Bockhorn, AG., Klusmeier, S., Kiehl, M., Roeder, C., Kalthoff, H. & Koch, OM. (1998) Lovastatin inhibits proliferation of pancreatic cancer cell lines with mutant as well as with wild-type K-ras oncogene but has different effects on protein phosphorylation and induction of apoptosis. *Int J Oncol.* Vol.12, No.3, pp.717, ISSN 1019-6439

Murai, T., Maruyama, Y., Mio, K., Nishiyama, H., Suga, M. & Sato, C. (2011) Low cholesterol triggers membrane microdomain-dependent CD44 shedding and suppresses tumor cell migration. *J Biol Chem.* Vol.286, No.3, pp.1999, ISSN 0021-9258

Newman, A., Clutterbuck, RD., Powles, RL. & Millar, JL. (1994) Selective inhibition of primary acute myeloid leukaemia cell growth by lovastatin. *Leukemia.* Vol.8, No.2, pp.274, ISSN 0887-6924

Nissen, E. & Tanneberger, S. (1981) Influence of pH and serum on the effectivity of antineoplastic agents in vitro. Arch Geschwulstforsch. Vol. 51, No. 1, pp152, ISSN 0003-911x

O'Brien, G., Meinhardt, P. & Bond, E., et al. (2003) Effects of imatinib mesylate (STI571, Glivec) on the pharmacokinetics of simvastatin, a cytochrome p450 3A4 substrate, in patients with chronic myeloidleukaemia. *Br J Cancer.* Vol89., No.10, pp.1855, ISSN 0007-0920

Oehlke, O., Martin, W., Osterberg, N., Roussa, E. (2011) Rab11b and its effector Rip11 regulate the acidosis-induced traffic of V-ATPase in salivary ducts. *J Cell Physiol.* Vol.226, No.3, pp.638, ISSN 0021-9541

Opitz, I., Soltermann, A., Abaecherli, M., Hinterberger, M., Probst-Hensch, N., Stahel, R., Moch, H. & Weder, W. (2008) PTEN expression is a strong predictor of survival in mesothelioma patients. *Eur J Cardiothorac Surg.* Vol.33, No.3, pp.502, ISSN 1010-7940

Owen, CS., Pooler, PM., Wahl, ML., Coss, RA. & Leeper, DB. (1997) Altered proton extrusion in cells adapted to growth at low extracellular pH. *J Cell Physiol.* Vol.173, No.3, pp.397, ISSN 0021-9541

Pääjärvi, G., Roudier, E., Crisby, M., Högberg, J. & Stenius, U. (2005) HMG-CoA reductase inhibitors, statins, induce phosphorylation of Mdm2 and attenuate the p53 response to DNA damage. *FASEB J.* Vol.19, No.3, pp.476, ISSN 0892-6638

Pang, K., Yu, W., Au-Yeung, C. & Ho, P. (2007) DNA damage induced by novel Demethylcantharidin – integrated platinum anticancer complexes. *Biochem Biophys Res Commun.* Vol.363, No.1, pp.235, ISSN 0006-291X

Parikh, A., Childress, C., Deitrick, K., Lin, Q., Rukstalis, D. & Yang, W. (2010) Statin-induced autophagy by inhibition of geranylgeranyl biosynthesis in prostate cancer PC3 cells. *Prostate.* Vol.70, No.9, pp.971, ISSN 0270-4137

Park, J., Kong, D., Iruela-Arispe, L., Begley, U., Tang, D. & Galper, B. (2002) 3-hydroxy-3-methylglutaryl coenzyme A reductase inhibitors interfere with angiogenesis by inhibiting the geranylgeranylation of RhoA. *Circ Res.* Vol.91, No.2, pp.143, ISSN 0009-7330

Pope, BJ., Zierler-Gould, KM., Kühne, R., Weeds, AG. & Ball, LJ. (2004) Solution structure of human cofilin: actin binding, pH sensitivity, and relationship to actin-depolymerizing fact0or. *J Biol Chem.* Vol.279, No.6, pp.4840, ISSN 0021-9528

Raghunand, N., He, X., van Sluis, R., Mahoney, B., Baggett, B., Taylor, CW., Paine-Murrieta, G., Roe, D., Bhujwalla, ZM. & Gillies RJ. (1999) Enhancement of chemotherapy by manipulation of tumour pH. *Br J Cancer* .Vol.80, No.7, pp.1005, ISSN 0007-0920

Rai, R., Peterson, L., Appelbaum, R., Kolitz, J., Elias, L., Shepherd, L., Hines, J., Threatte, A., Larson, A., Cheson, D. & Schiffer, A. (2000) Fludarabine compared with chlorambucil as primary therapy for chronic lymphocytic leukemia. *N Engl J Med.* Vol.343, No.24, pp.1750, ISSN 0028-4793

Rajski, R. & Williams, M. (1998) DNA Cross-Linking Agents as Antitumor Drugs. *Chem Rev.* Vol.98, No.8, pp.2723, ISSN 0009-2665

Riganti, C., Orecchia, S., Pescarmona, G., Betta, G., Ghigo, D. & Bosia, A. (2006) Statins revert doxorubicin resistance via nitric oxide in malignant mesothelioma. *int J Cancer.* Vol.119, No.1, pp.17, ISSN 0020-7136

Riganti, C., Doublier, S., Aldieri, E., Orecchia, S., Betta, PG., Gazzano, E., Ghigo, D. & Bosia, A. (2008) Asbestos induces doxorubicin resistance in MM98 mesothelioma cells via HIF-1alpha. *Eur Respir J.* Vol.32, No.2, pp.443, ISSN 0903-1936

Rockwells, S. (1986) Effect of some proliferative and environmental factors on the toxicity of mitomycin C to tumor cells in vitro. *Int J Cancer.* Vol.38, No.2, pp.229, ISSN 0020-7136

Rofstad, EK., Mathiesen, B., Kindem, K. & Galappathi, K. (2006) Acidic extracellular pH promotes experimental metastasis of human melanoma cells in athymic nude mice. *Cancer Res.* Vol.66, No.13, pp.6699, ISSN 0008-5472

Rogalska, A., Koceva-Chyła, A. & Jóźwiak, Z. (2008) Aclarubicin-induced ROS generation and collapse of mitochondrial membrane potential in human cancer cell lines. *Chem Biol Interact.* Vol.176, No.1, pp.58, ISSN 0009-2797

Rotin, D., Wan, P., Grinstein, S. & Tannock, I. (1987) Cytotoxicity of compounds that interfere with the regulation of intracellular pH: a potential new class of anticancer drugs. *Cancer Res.* Vol.47, No.6, pp.1497, ISSN 0008-5472

Rubins, B., Greatens, T., Kratzke, A., Tan, T., Polunovsky, A. & Bitterman, P. (1998) Lovastatin induces apoptosis in malignant mesothelioma cells. *Am J Respir Crit Care Med.* Vol.157, No.1, pp.1616, ISSN 1073-449X

Rueth, NM., Murray, SE., Huddleston, SJ., Abbott, AM., Greeno, EW., Kirstein, MN. & Tuttle, TM. (2011) Severe electrolyte disturbances after hyperthermic intraperitoneal chemotherapy: oxaliplatin versus mitomycin C. *Ann Surg Oncol.* Vol.18, No.1, pp.174, ISSN 1068-9265

Ruiz-Gómez, J., Souviron, A., Martínez-Morillo, M. & Gil, L. (2000) P-glycoprotein, glutathione and glutathione S-transferase increase in a colon carcinoma cell line by colchicine. *J Physiol Biochem.* Vol.56, No.4, pp.307, ISSN 1138-7548

Sagawa, M., Nakazato, T., Uchida, H., Ikeda, Y. & Kizaki, M. (2008) Cantharidin induces apoptosis of human multiple myeloma cells via inhibition of the JAK/STAT pathway. *Cancer Sci.* Vol.99, No.9, pp.1820, ISSN 1347-9032

Sauvant, C., Nowak, M., Wirth, C., Schneider, B., Riemann, A., Gekle, M. & Thews, O. (2008) Acidosis induces multi-drug resistance in rat prostate cancer cells (AT1) in vitro and in vivo by increasing the activity of the p-glycoprotein via activation of p38, *Int. J. Cancer.* Vol.123, pp.2532, ISSN 0020-7136

SCADs inhibitor kit 1, Available from: < http://scads.jfcr.or.jp/file/kit1ver-2.3.xls>

SCADs inhibitor kit 2, Available from: < http://scads.jfcr.or.jp/file/kit2.xls>

SCADs inhibitor kit 3, Available from: < http://scads.jfcr.or.jp/file/kit3-1.2.xls>

Sekine, Y., Demosky, J., Stonik, A, Furuya, Y., Koike, H., Suzuki, K. & Remaley, T. (2010) High-density lipoprotein induces proliferation and migration of human prostate androgen-independent cancer cells by an ABCA1-dependent mechanism. *Mol Cancer Res.* Vol.8, No.9, pp.1284, ISSN 1541-7786

Schliwa, M. (1982) Action of cytochalasin D on cytoskeletal networks. *J Cell Biol.* Vol.92, No.1, pp.79, ISSN 0021-9525

Shannon, HE., Martin, WR. & Silcox, D. (1978) Lack of antiemetic effects of delta9-tetrahydrocannabinol in apomorphine-induced emesis in the dog. *Life Sci.* Vol.23, No.1, pp.49, ISSN 0024-3205

Simmen, H. P. (1993) J. Blaser. Analysis of pH and pO_2 in abscesses, peritoneal fluid, and drainage fluid in the presence or absence of bacterial infection during and after abdominal surgery. *Am. J. Surg.* Vol.166, pp.24, ISSN 0147-5185

Skarsgard, D., Skwarchuk, W., Vinczan, A. & Chaplin, J. (1993) The effect of pH on the aerobic and hypoxic cytotoxicity of SR4233 in HT-29 cells. *Br J Cancer.* Vol.,68 No.4, pp.681, ISSN 0007-0920

322

2222

Steele, JP., O'Doherty, CA., Shamash, J., Evans, MT., Gower, NH., Tischkowitz, MD. & Rudd, RM. (2001) Phase II trial of liposomal daunorubicin in malignant pleural mesothelioma. *Ann Oncol.* Vol.12, No.4, pp.497, ISSN 0923-7534

Stewart, DJ., Gertler, SZ., Tomiak, A., Shamji, F., Goel, R. & Evans WK. (1994) High dose doxorubicin plus cisplatin in the treatment of unresectable mesotheliomas: report of four cases. *Lung Cancer.* Vol.11, No.3-4, pp.251, ISSN 0169-5002

Sukumaran, K. & Prasadarao, V. (2002) Regulation of protein kinase C in Escherichia coli K1 invasion of human brain microvascular endothelial cells. *J Biol Chem.* Vol.277, No.14, pp.12253, ISSN 0021-9258

Syljuåsen, R.G. (2007) Checkpoint adaptation in human cells. *Oncogene.* Vol.26, pp.5833, ISSN 0950-9232

Thews, O., Gassner, B., Kelleher, DK., Schwerdt, G. & Gekle, M. (2006) Impact of extracellular acidity on the activity of P-glycoprotein and the cytotoxicity of chemotherapeutic drugs. *Neoplasia.* Vol.8, No.2, pp.143, ISSN 1552-8002

Tobert, JA. (2003) Lovastatin and beyond: the history of the HMG-CoA reductase inhibitors. *Nat Rev Drug Discov.* Vol.2, No.7, pp.517, ISSN 1474-1776

Totoń, E., Ignatowicz, E., Skrzeczkowska, K. & Rybczyńska, M. (2011) Protein kinase Cε as a cancer marker and target for anticancer therapy. *Pharmacol Rep.* Vol.63, No.1, pp.19, ISSN 1734-1140

Toullec, D., Pianetti, P., Coste, H., Bellevergue, P., Grand-Perret, T., Ajakane, M., Baudet, V., Boissin, P., Boursier, E. & Loriolle, F., et al. (1991) The bisindolylmaleimide GF 109203X is a potent and selective inhibitor of protein kinase C. *J Biol Chem.* Vol.266, No.24, pp.15771, ISSN 0021-9258

Vantelon, N., Rioux-Bilan, A., Ingrand, S., Pain, S., Page, G., Guillard, O., Barrier, L., Piriou, A. & Fauconneau, B. (2007) Regulation of initiation factors controlling protein synthesis on cultured astrocytes in lactic acid-induced stress. *Eur J Neurosci.* Vol.26, No.3, pp.689, ISSN 0953-816X

Vattem, M. & Wek, C. (2004) Reinitiation involving upstream ORFs regulates ATF4 mRNA translation in mammalian cells. *Proc Natl Acad Sci U S A.* Vol.101, No.31 pp11269, pp.74, ISSN 0027-8424

Vaupel, P., Kallinowski, F. & Okunieff, P. (1989) Blood flow, oxygen and nutrient supply, and metabolic microenvironment of human tumors. *Cancer Res.* Vol.49, pp. 6449, ISSN 0008-5472

Vogt, A., Sun, J., Qian, Y., Hamilton, D. & Sebti, M. (1997) The geranylgeranyltransferase-I inhibitor GGTI-298 arrests human tumor cells in G0/G1 and induces p21(WAF1/CIP1/SDI1) in a p53-independent manner. *J Biol Chem.* Vol.272, No.43, pp.27224, ISSN 0021-9258

Vukovic, V. & Tannock, IF. (1997) Influence of low pH on cytotoxicity of paclitaxel, mitoxantrone and topotecan. *Br J Csancer.* Vol.75, No.8, pp.1167, ISSN 0007-0920

Vujcic, S., Halmekyto, M., Diegelman, P., Gan, G., Kramer, L., Janne, J. & Porter, W. (2000) Effects of conditional overexpression of spermidine/spermine N1-acetyltransferase on polyamine pool dynamics, cell growth, and sensitivity to polyamine analogs. *J. Biol. Chem.* Vol.275, No.49, pp.38319, ISSN 0021-9528

Wang, Y., Xiao, L., Thiagalingam, A., Nelkin, D. & Casero, A. (1998) The identification of a cis-element and a trans-acting factor involved in the response to polyamines and polyamine analogues in the regulation of the human spermidine/spermine N1-

acetyltransferase gene transcription. *J. Biol. Chem.* Vol.273, No.51, pp34623, ISSN 0021-9258

Wang, K., Lin-Shiau, Y. & Lin, K. (2000) Suppression of invasion and MMP-9 expression in NIH 3T3 and v-H-Ras 3T3 fibroblasts by lovastatin through inhibition of ras isoprenylation. *Oncology.* Vol.59, No.3, pp.245, 0030-2414

Wang, J., Kitajima, I. (2007) Pitavastatin inactivates NF-kappaB and decreases IL-6 production through Rho kinase pathway in MCF-7 cells. *Oncol Rep.* Vol.17, No.5, pp.1149, ISSN 1523-3790

Warburg,O. (1956) On the origin of cancer cells. *Science.* Vol. 123, pp. 309, ISSN 0036-8075

Wei, J., Zhao, J., Long, M., Han, Y., Wang, X., Lin, F., Ren, J., He, T. & Zhang H. (2010) p21WAF1/CIP1 gene transcriptional activation exerts cell growth inhibition and enhances chemosensitivity to cisplatin in lung carcinoma cell. *BMC Cancer.* Vol.10, pp.632, ISSN 1471-2407

Wek, C., Jiang, Y. & Anthony, G. (2006) Coping with stress: eIF2 kinases and translational control. *Biochem Soc Trans.* Vol.34, No.7, No.1, pp.11, ISSN 0300-5127

Williams, J., Cowen, L. & Stratford, J. (2001) Hypoxia and oxidative stress. Tumour hypoxia--therapeutic considerations. *Breast Cancer Res.* Vol.3, No.5, pp.328, ISSN 0167-6806

Wu, H., Jiang, H., Lu, D., Xiong, Y., Qu, C., Zhou, D., Mahmood, A. & Chopp, M. (2009) Effect of simvastatin on glioma cell proliferation, migration, and apoptosis. *Neurosurgery.* Vol.65, No.6, pp.1087, ISSN 0148-396X

Yu, W., Li, K., Pang, K., Au-Yeung, C. & Ho, P. (2006) Anticancer activity of a series of platinum complexes integrating demethylcantharidin with isomers of 1,2-diaminocyclohexane. *Bioorg Med Chem Lett.* Vol.16, No.6, pp.1686, ISSN 0960-894X

Zhang, C., Peng, Y., Wang, F., Tan, X., Liu, N., Fan, S., Wang, D., Zhang, L., Liu, D., Wang, T., Wang, S., Zhou, Y., Su, Y., Cheng, T., Zhuang, Z. & Shi, C. (2010) A synthetic cantharidin analog for the enhancement of doxorubicin suppression of stem cell-derived aggressive sarcoma. *Biomaterials.* Vol.31, No.36, pp.9535, ISSN 0142-9612

Zhao, TT., Trinh, D., Addison, CL. & Dimitroulakos, J. (2010) Lovastatin inhibits VEGFR and AKT activation: synergistic cytotoxicity in combination with VEGFR inhibitors. *PLoS One.* Vol.5, No.9, pp.e12563, ISSN 1932-6203

Zhou, D., Pallam, R., Jiang, L., Narasimhan, J., Staschke, A. & Wek, C. (2008) Phosphorylation of eIF2 directs ATF5 translational control in response to diverse stress conditions. *J Biol Chem.* Vol.283, No.11, pp7064, ISSN 0021-9258

Zorbas-Seifried, S., Hartinger, CG., Meelich, K., Galanski, M., Keppler, BK. & Zorbas, H. (2006) DNA interactions of pH-sensitive, antitumor bis (aminoalcohol) - dichloroplatinum(II) complexes. *Biochemistry.* Vol.45, No.49, pp.14817, ISSN 0006-2960

Zucali, P.A. & Giaccone, G. (2006) Biology and management of malignant pleural mesothelioma. *Eur. J. Cancer.* Vol. 42, pp.2706, ISSN 0959-8049

Why Anti-Energetic Agents Such as Citrate or 3-Bromopyruvate Should be Tested as Anti-Cancer Agents: Experimental *In Vitro* and *In Vivo* Studies

Philippe Icard[1,2], Xiao-Dong Zhang[2], Emilie Varin[2],
Stéphane Allouche[3], Antoine Coquerel[4], Maria Paciencia[5], Luc Joyeux[1],
Pascal Gauduchon[2], Hubert Lincet[2] and Laurent Poulain[2]
*[1]Department of Thoracic Surgery, University Hospital of Caen Basse-Normandie,
[2]Groupe Régional d'Etudes sur le Cancer (EA 1772), IFR 146 ICORE,
University of Caen Basse-Normandie,
[3]Department of Biochemistry, University Hospital of Caen Basse-Normandie,
[4]Department of Pharmacology, University Hospital of Caen Basse-Normandie,
[5]Department of Pathology, University Hospital of Caen Basse-Normandie,
Unité "Biologie et Thérapies Innovantes des Cancers Localement Agressifs",
and Centre de Lutte Contre le Cancer François Baclesse, Caen
France*

1. Introduction

1.1 The Warburg effect (Fig.1)

Cancer cells are eager to glucose and consume about 10 times more glucose than normal cells. Glucose transformation results in the formation of lactic acid, even in the presence of oxygen. This phenomenon named "aerobic glycolysis" was first observed by Otto Warburg in the 20s (Warburg, 1930), who considered later, it was the result of a defect of mitochondrial respiration, causing cancer (Warburg, 1956). The energy efficiency of aerobic glycolysis is low, since 2 ATP are produced, which represents eighteen times less than the complete degradation of glucose producing 36 ATP (Campbell & Smith, 2000; Lehninger 1975; Stryer, 1981). However, because cancer cells find all nutrients in abundance in their environment, they would focus more on promoting metabolic ways needed for biosynthesis, rather than would search the most efficient energetic way (Grüning, 2010; Israël, 2004, 2005; Vander Heiden, 2009). Cancer cells not only consume glucose in excess (a great part of it, is diverted towards ribose synthesis), but also amino acids, especially glutamine, derived from muscle proteolysis. Glutamine, which is the preferential mode of transportation of blood nitrogen, provides amine groups for several biosynthetic processes, such as purine and pyrimidine bases synthesis (DeBerardinis, 2008, 2010; Eagle, 1956; Reitzer, 1979). At the same time, cancer cells might burn fatty acid through the mitochondrial β-oxidation, a very energetic pathway producing ATP. From the intermediate molecules provided by enhanced glycolysis and glutaminolysis (and may be also by β-oxidation), cancer cells will synthesize most of the macromolecules required to duplicate their biomass and genome (proteins, nucleic acids, membrane lipids) (Grüning, 2010; Israël, 2004, 2005; Vander Heiden, 2009). Due to the frequent impairment of mitochondrial respiration resulting in a defective oxidative phosphorylation (OXPHOS), ATP production by mitochondria can be reduced. In that situation, glycolysis will provide a more significant part of ATP as OXPHOS will be defective (Lopez-Rios, 2007; Samudio, 2009; Simonnet, 2003; Xu, 2005). ATP, NAD^+ and $NADPH,H^+$ are required in large amounts in the cytoplasm of cancer cells. NAD^+ is not only necessary for the functioning of the increased glycolysis at the glyceraldehyde 3-phosphate dehydrogenase (G3PD) level, but also for the action of the Poly ADP-ribose polymerase (PARP), which participates to the enhanced nucleotides synthesis (Grüning, 2010). $NADPH,H^+$ is required for lipid synthesis and for the functioning of enzymes, such as the glutathione reductase, which reduce toxic reactive oxygen species (ROS) (3-7). LDH transforms pyruvate into lactate and regenerates NAD^+. As aforementioned, this cofactor is crucial for the functioning of glycolysis at the G3PD level (Campbell & Smith, 2000; Israël, 2004, 2005; Lehninger 1975; Stryer, 1981). To support a high glycolytic flux required to produce anabolic intermediates, the NAD^+ pool must be continuously regenerated in the cytoplasm by several dehydrogenases such as the LDH. Because there is a "bottle neck" at the end of glycolysis due to the low activity of the pyruvate kinase PKM2 (see below), it is likely than an important part of the pyruvate used by LDH might come from glutaminolysis and transamination of alanine, produced by muscular proteolysis which is particularly enhanced in cachectic patients (Israël, 2004, 2005) but also from cytosolic citrate (Icard & Lincet, 2012, in press). It has been shown that lactic acid, more than a waste product, can be taken up by oxygenated tumor cells to restore pyruvate, sparing glucose for most the hypoxic tumor cells (Feron, 2009). Like NAD^+, NADPH, H^+ must be also continuously regenerated, either through the pentose phosphate pathway (PPP) producing ribose and or by cytosolic enzymes, such as the malic enzyme, which converts malate into pyruvate. As seen later, malate is coming from oxaloacetate (OAA), and OAA results form the action of ATP-citrate lyase (ACLY) on citrate, giving acetyl-coA donor for the *de novo* fatty acid synthesis. Thus, citrate, coming from mitochondria, feeds fatty acid synthesis in one way, and the formation in pyruvate (and lactate) in another way. Finally, while reserves are normally used to produce nutrients, ketones bodies and glucose, cancer cells use these reserves for burning glucose and building new tumor substance. The eagerness of cancer tumors for glucose has been confirmed by PET scan, which is currently used to detect tumors and metastases (Caretta, 2000; Vander Heiden, 2009). The decrease in tracer uptake (2-deoxy-glucose-FD) is often considered as a good predictor of the effectiveness of chemotherapy (Eagle, 1956), while highly glycolytic tumors are generally considered as the most aggressive (proliferative and/or chemoresistant) ones (DeBerardinis, 2008, 2010; Eagle, 1956; Reitzer, 1979).

Because of the PKM2 bottle neck and the inactivation of pyruvate dehydrogenase, there is a disjunction between glycolysis and TCA cycle. Glycolysis serves to produce ribose for nucleotides synthesis, glycerol for lipid synthesis, whereas lactate is rejected. Proteolysis produces alanine which fed the LDH reaction whereas transaminations provide also aspartate serving to nucleotides synthesis. Glutaminolysis feeds the TCA cycle and results in the formation of OAA. Lipolysis produces acetyl-CoA (in place of glycolysis) which is condensed with OAA to form citrate through the action of the citrate synthase (CS). Then

Why Anti-Energetic Agents Such as Citrate or 3-Bromopyruvate Should be Tested as Anti-Cancer Agents: Experimental In Vitro and In Vivo Studies

227

citrate goes outside mitochondria to re-forms acetyl-CoA which is used for lipid synthesis whereas OAA is finally converted in pyruvate by malate dehydrogenase (MDH) and malic enzyme (ME). Finally proteolysis and lipolysis contribute to produce pyruvate in place of glycolysis, and this pyruvate is transformed in lactic acid, the LDH reaction forming NAD+ which is crucial for the functioning of glycolysis.

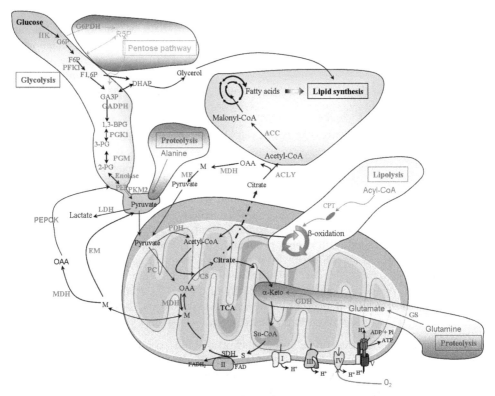

Fig. 1. Reorganization of catabolic and anabolic pathways in cancer cells.

ACC: acetyl-coA carboxylase, ACLY: ATP-citrate lyase, CPT: carnitine palmitoyl transferase, CS: citrate synthase, F1,6BPase: fructose 1,6 biphosphatase, F2,6BPase: fructose 2,6 biphosphatase, FAD: flavine adenine dinucleotide, FH: fumarate hydratase, GADPH: glyceraldehyde 3-phosphate dehydrogenase, GDH: glutamate dehydrogenase, GPD: glycerol 3-phosphate dehydrogenase, GS: glutamine synthetase, G6PDH: glucose 6-phosphate dehydrogenase, G6P: glucose 6-phosphate, G3P: glycerol 3-phosphate, HAT: histone acetyl transferase, HK: hexokinase, LDH: lacticodehydrogenase, MDH: malate dehydrogenase, ME: malic enzyme, NAD+: nicotinamide adenine dinucleotide, NADPH,H+: nicotinamide adenine dinucleotide phosphate, PC: pyruvate carboxylase, PDH: pyruvate dehydrogenase, PEPCK: phosphoenolpyruvate carboxykinase, PFK: phosphofructokinase, PGK: phosphoglycerate kinase, PGM: phosphoglucomutase, PKM2: embryonic isoform of pyruvate kinase, R5P: ribose 5-phosphate, SDH: succinate dehydrogenase.

1.2 The mechanisms involved in the Warburg effect are complex

The mechanisms involved in the Warburg effect generate an increasing interest (Bellance, 2009; Grüning, 2010; Israël, 2004, 2005; Kroemer & Pouyssegur, 2008; Vander Heiden, 2009). Briefly, glycolysis would be truncated at its end because pyruvate kinase (PK) of cancer cells would function at a low activity. Indeed, PK is re-expressed in cancer cells in its embryonic form, PKM2, which is less active than the adult form PKM1 (Christofk, 2008a, 2008b; Grüning, 2010; Israël, 2004, 2005; Kroemer & Pouyssegur, 2008; Mazurek, 2002; Vander Heiden, 2009). This event creates a block or " bottle neck" leading to the accumulation of intermediates upstream which are derived mainly towards the formation of ribose (through the PPP) and glycerol, respectively required for nucleotides and lipid biosynthesis. The reversion of PKM2 to PKM1 abrogates the Warburg effect (Christofk, 2008a, 2008b). As see above, others sources of pyruvate than glucose are stimulated, such as proteolysis providing alanine and glutaminolysis, which leads to the formation of acetyl-CoA furnishing citrate. Pyruvate feeds preferentially the LDH, because pyruvate dehydrogenase (PD) is blocked in cancer cells by pyruvate dehydrogenase kinase (PDK) (Kim, 2006). It is noteworthy that glycolysis, although poorly efficient in producing energy, might furnish an important part of ATP. It is a much faster way to product ATP than OXPHOS, which allows cells to adjust very quickly their consumption of glucose to their high energy requirement, like muscle during effort. Because several complexes of the respiratory chain could be defective in cancer cells, OXPHOS could be dysfunctional. In that case, glycolysis may become the principal mode, if not unique, of energy production (Lopez-Rios, 2007; Simonnet, 2003; Xu, 2005). These alterations might occur from complex I to complex V (Lopez-Rios, 2007; Samudio, 2009; Simonnet, 2003; Xu, 2005), creating a second "bottle neck", associated with ROS production. When the detoxification capacity of the cells is overwhelmed, ROS create mitochondrial and cellular damages, which aggravate in turn the cell and mitochondrial dysfunctions, leading to alterations in the first place of the respiratory chain and OXPHOS.

A reprogramming of the signaling pathways would conduct these biochemical rearrangements through translational and transcriptional mechanisms (Bellance, 2009; Grüning, 2010; Israël, 2004, 2005; Kroemer & Pouyssegur, 2008; Vander Heiden, 2009). The over expression of oncogenes (PI3K/AKT/mTOR pathway, c-Myc and particularly of the activation of the hypoxia inducible factor-1α (HIF-1α)) (Kim, 2006; Marin-Hernández, 2009), associated with mutation of suppressor genes (P53, P21, PTEN, PP2A, etc.) would support the special metabolism of cancer cells (Bellance, 2009; Grüning, 2010; Israël, 2004, 2005; Kroemer & Pouyssegur, 2008; Vander Heiden, 2009). For example, HIF-1α stimulates the overexpression of membrane glucose transporters (GLUT1, GLUT3) and of several enzymes of glycolysis (especially HK, PFK, PKM2, LDH) (Marin-Hernández, 2009), whereas it induces pyruvate dehydrogenase kinase (PDK) (Kim, 2006). This latter action counteracts the activity of pyruvate dehydrogenase (PDH), leading that pyruvate is preferentially derived to form lactic acid through the action of the LDH. This enzyme is not only induced by HIF-1α but also by a variety of oncogenes like c-Myc (Bellance, 2009; Feron, 2009; Grüning, 2010; Israël, 2004, 2005; Kroemer & Pouyssegur, 2008; Vander Heiden, 2009). LDH activation ensures a rapid consumption of pyruvate even when O_2 is available and continuously regenerates NAD+ which sustains enhanced glycolysis (Grüning, 2010; Israël, 2004, 2005; Vander Heiden, 2009). Through various mechanisms (decrease of the ratio cAMP / cGMP, increase of NO, etc.), the process of cancer would be enhanced with activation of mitosis, whereas the metabolic shift from OXPHOS to aerobic glycolysis (Warburg effect) would be promoted. It is likely that this special metabolism helps cancer cells to tolerate their hypoxic microenvironment, and contributes to viability, autonomous growth, migration and chemoresistance of cells, giving them also the ability to control ROS levels and to avoid apoptosis, all mechanisms which are hallmarks of cancer.

1.3 If do we block glycolysis, do we stop cancer cell proliferation?

Whatever are these complexes and intricate mechanisms supporting this reprogramming metabolism, if we block aerobic glycolysis, do we stop cell growth or kill cells?

With this hypothesis we worked within the Biology and Therapies for Locally Aggressive Cancer (Bioticla) of the Normandy Regional Study Group on Cancer (GRECAN), on cultured cells of human cancers and on nude mice bearing human mesothelioma. We chose to work preferentially on this cancer, because our region is particularly affected by this cancer due to local industries which have used largely asbestos since long date. We report herein a synthesis of various works that have been carried out at our laboratory, showing the interest of using anti-glycolytic molecules such as 2-deoxyglucose (2-DG), 3-bromopyruvate (3-BrPA) and citrate (Lu, 2011; Zhang, 2006, 2009a, 2009b). Because citrate have demonstrated several interesting anti-cancer actions, and because none toxicity have been reported about this physiologic molecule (Diaz, 1994; Vagianos, 1990), toxicity studies were performed about it and presented in this review.

2. Materials and methods

2.1 In vitro

12 lines of human cancers of various origins (liver, ovaries, brain, colon, head and neck, mesothelioma) were initially used to check the validity of our hypothesis, namely that the blocking of glycolysis led to the arrest of the growth or to the death of cancer cells. For that purpose, cells were exposed to 5mM of 2-deoxyglucose (2-DG), a glucose analogue that is not metabolized (Zhang, 2006). Then, we focused our work on malignant mesothelioma, studying two human cell lines (MSTO-211H and NCI-H28), which appeared representative of other lines tested in the laboratory (NCI-H2052, IST-Mes3). These lines were acquired from the American Type Culture Collection (ATCC). The doubling time of MSTO-211H was about 24 hours, whereas NCI-H28 cells proliferated more slowly. We observed that NCI-H28 cells were resistant to high dose (one injection at a dose of 20 µg per ml) of cisplatin, in contrast to MSTO-211H cells which were sensitive to this high dose, but resistant to a lower dose (5µg per ml). At such dose, MSTO-211H demonstrated only a transient slowing of their proliferation, the recovery of their growth being observed from the 5th day after the injection of cisplatin.

2.2 In vivo

We used Swiss mice/Nude CD1 females aging from 4 to 6 weeks, weighing about 25 g (Charles River France). These mice developed peritoneal carcinomatosis after receiving an intra-peritoneal (ip) injection of 2×10^7 MSTO-211H cells in 1 ml. This peritoneal carcinomatosis was visible from the 15th day, and caused death of animals in about 30 days. Using this method, the taking tumor was generally excellent, reaching 100 %. Peritoneal carcinomatosis was made of mesothelioma tumor nodules, which were confirmed by histological examination (Pr Françoise Galateau-Sallé, Department of Anatomical Pathology, CHU de Caen). We favored this model of peritoneal carcinomatosis because it was easier to reproduce than a pleural model and because it allowed repeated therapeutic injections, that were impossible or otherwise very difficult to realize with a pleural model, due to the risk of pneumothorax. Furthermore, involvement of the peritoneum is also a common feature either in the course of advanced pleural mesothelioma, or as primary localization (about 5 % of cases).

2.3 Anti-glycolytic agents

2-DG is an analog of glucose, described as an inhibitor of the first step of glycolysis, because it would be not metabolized.

3-BrPA is theoretically an inhibitor of all reactions involving pyruvate. Furthermore, it has been reported as an inhibitor of HK II (Danial, 2003; Pastorino, 2008; Pedersen, 2002), that demonstrated a very good efficacy in rabbits and mice bearing hepatocarcinoma (Geschwind, 2004; Ko, 2004).

Citrate is a well-known physiological inhibitor of phosphosfructokinase (PFK1), the key enzyme regulating glycolysis. Inhibition of PFK1 is total when citrate is abundant (Stryer, 1981). This allosteric enzyme, converts fructose 6-phosphate in fructose 1-6 bisphosphate, and acts as a true gauge of energy inside the cell. It is inhibited by ATP when it is in excess, whereas it is activated by ADP, when the cell lacks of energy. By this feedback, the flow of the glycolysis is adjusted to the ATP requirements (Campbell & Smith, 2000; Lehninger 1975; Stryer, 1981). The fact that PFK1 is also inhibited by citrate, which is produced by the first step of the tricarboxylic acid cycle (TCA cycle), adjusts very quickly the flow of glycolysis with that of the TCA cycle, because citrate diffuses rapidly outside the mitochondria, in contrast to ATP which necessitates a complex system carrier. Other actions of citrate will be presented in the discussion.

These agents were provided by Sigma Aldrich.

2.4 Toxicity studies about citrate

Acute and chronic toxicity (in various organs such as liver, heart, lung, kidney, etc.) were determined in mice after ip injection of sodium citrate. We chose to study primarily this way of administration, considering futures clinical applications. Experiments were performed in the Department of Clinical Pharmacology of the University Hospital of Caen (directed by Pr Antoine Coquerel). For determining acute toxicity, increasing doses of citrate buffer were administered by ip injections to mice (5 to 8 animals per group), since the dose of 50 mg per kg to the maximum dose of 12 g per kg. Chronic toxicity was studied on mice (10 animals per group) which received either 5 ip injections per week of 200 mg per kg of sodium citrate during 3 weeks, or 3 ip injections per week of 500 mg per kg of sodium citrate during 5 weeks. Several groups of mice received also daily oral administration of citrate (500 mg/kg 5 day/ 7). Clinical examinations were repeated until sacrifice (day 90) whereas organs (liver, kidneys, lungs and heart) were taken for histological analysis in the Pathological Department of the hospital (Dr Maria Paciencia) checking for histological signs of toxicity such as edema, necrosis, inflammation, fibrosis.

3. Results

Our works have resulted in several publications (Lu, 2011; Varin, 2010; Zhang, 2006, 2009a, 2009b):

- we observed first that inhibition of glycolysis by exposure of cells during 7 days to 5 mM of 2-DG, led to a clear inhibition of cancer growth cells (varying from 63.7% to 94.3%) of 12 different lines of various cancers we tested. Significant cell death apoptosis was observed in some strains (Zhang, 2006). This study showed the interest of counteracting cancer cells development by anti-glycolytic agents.

- focusing our studies on mesothelioma, we observed that ip injections of 2-DG had no effect on survival of nude mice bearing human mesothelioma. In contrast, survival of animals (12 animals per group) was very significantly lengthened (p <0.0001) when they were treated since day 21, with two series of four weekly ip injections of 3-Bromopyruvate (3-BrPA). This drug was administered at a dose of 2.67 mg per kg (0.8 ml to 500 microM) per day (4) (Fig. 2a). With our protocol (two series of injection), 17 % (2 / 12) of mice treated with 3-BrPA as the sole treatment demonstrated complete tumor response (Zhang, 2009). In contrast, a sole series of 4 ip injections of 3-BrPA or a sole ip injection of cisplatin at 21 days (at a dose of 4 mg per kg), had no effect. Interestingly, the association of drugs was very effective, leading to a highly significant prolongation of survival (p = 0.002) (Zhang, 2009b) (Fig. 2b).

- in cultured cells, a low dose of cisplatin (5 µg per ml), administered after three days of exposure to citrate 10 mM, led to complete death of MSTO-211H cells (Zhang, 2009a). This death involved the mitochondrial apoptotic pathway, and no secondary recurrence of proliferation was visible until the 14th day of culture. In contrast, exposure to citrate 10 mM alone had only a cytostatic effect, whereas exposition to cisplatin alone caused only a temporary slowing of the proliferation (Fig. 3 a and b).

- in MSTO-211H cells, we observed that citrate induced an early diminution of the expression of the anti-apoptotic protein Mcl-1 (Fig. 3 c), which is a protein member of the Bcl-2 family playing a key role, with Bcl-x_L, in the chemoresistance of malignant cancers, especially of mesothelioma, as we showed (Varin, 2010). Indeed, concomitant inhibition of these two anti-apoptotic proteins by specific siRNA (directed against Mcl-1 or Bcl-x_L) caused complete cell death of MSTO-211H cells, whereas inhibition of only one of these two anti-apoptotic molecules, even combined with cisplatin at a low dose (5 µg per ml), was not sufficient to eradicate cultured cells (34). This anti Mcl-1action of citrate was confirmed on two lines of gastric cancer, exposed for 3 days to 10 mM (Lu, 2011) and recently on several ovarian cancer lines (data not shown).

- For trying to better understand the different behavior of our two mesothelioma cell lines, we studied their mitochondrial respiration. MSTO-211H cells, which may undergo apoptosis, had a functional mitochondrial respiration, which was reactive to succinate, a substrate of the complex II of the respiratory chain (Zhang, 2009b). In contrast, the robust NCI-H28 cells, insensitive to high doses of cisplatin, seemed to be destroying only by a mechanism of necrosis death, when exposed to 3-BrPA or citrate at higher concentration, beyond 200 microM or 20 mM respectively (data not shown). We showed these cells have no functional mitochondrial respiration, insensible to succinate (28). Therefore, we wondered if they were able to undergo apoptosis? We showed they could, if they were treated by two specific siRNA directed against Mcl-1 or Bcl-x_L associated with a low dose of cisplatin (5µg per ml) (Varin, 2010).

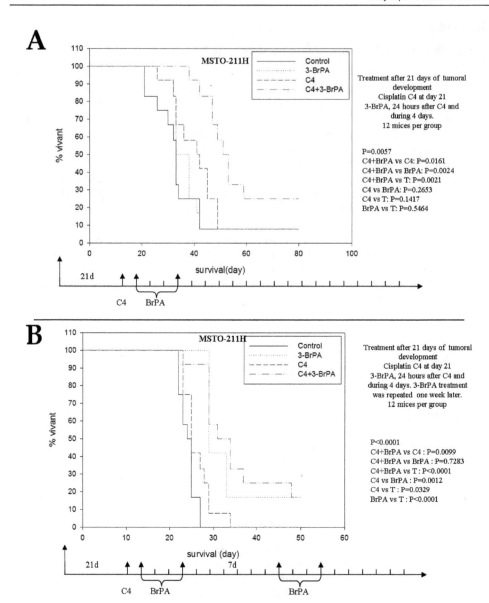

Fig. 2. Effect of 3-BrPA on survival of nude mice carrying a peritoneal carcinomatosis obtained by injection of human mesothelioma cells MSTO-211H.
A: This experiment showed the efficacy of the association of a cisplatin injection at 21, followed by a series of 4 intra-peritoneal injections of 3-BrPA. In contrast, these agents were inefficient when administrated alone.
B: This second experiment showed that the association of drugs was efficient, whereas cisplatin alone was inefficient in prolonging survival of mice. When a second series of 3-BrPA injections was performed, 3-BrPA alone was efficient in prolonging survival.

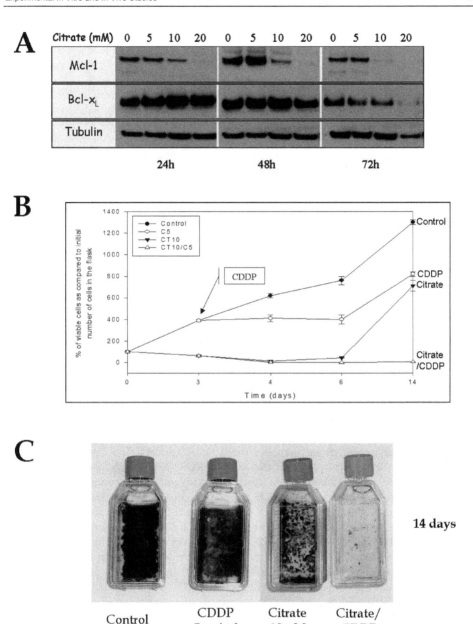

Fig. 3. Effect of citrate, cisplatin and combinaison of drugs on human MSTO-211H cells.
A: Western blot after 24h exposure to citrate (10mM) on anti-apoptotic proteins Mcl-1 and
Bcl-x$_L$. B: Kinetic evolution of cell viability (blue trypan exclusion test) in response to
continuous 72h initial exposure of citrate (10mM), cisplatin injection at day 3 (5µg/ml), and
combinaison of treatment on MSTO-211H cells. C : Aspect of cell flask cultures on day 14.

3.1 Acute and chronic toxicities of citrate

Citrate was toxic only at high doses: the 50 % lethal dose (LD) in mice was 4 g per kg, the minimum LD was 2 g per kg, whereas the mortality reached 100 % for 8 g per kg. At autopsy we observed an intra-abdominal bleeding and or the presence of ascite. We observed signs of clinical acute toxicity at doses > 500 mg / kg, which were in chronological order: immobility, tachypnea with cyanosis of the extremities, bristling hair, tremors and convulsions. The latter signs occurred within 3 to 8 minutes after the ip injection. The occurrence of convulsions in high doses of citrate and the known properties of calcium chelating of this acid led us to treat animals receiving lethal doses of citrate by calcium chloride, injected immediately after the ip injection of citrate, with an equivalent molar dose. All animals survived.

None chronic toxicity was observed with the protocol tested. All animals were in good health before sacrifice at day 90. Histological studies revealed none chronic signs of toxicity in the organs, except in the lungs where we observed diffuse or multifocal alveolar hemorrhage and bronchial lymphocytic infiltrate in all animals including in all controls.

4. Discussion

Chemoresistance made the seriousness of cancer, because in absence of an effective chemotherapy, others treatments (surgery, radiotherapy) are often doomed to failure. Even when tumors are diagnosed at an early stage, where surgical resection is feasible, survivals are generally less than 50% at 5 years for many solid cancers (lung, liver, pancreas, stomach, colon, ovaries, etc.). When metastases are present, survival does not exceed a few months in general, despite chemotherapy and/or radiotherapy treatments. For mesothelioma the survival is generally poor (the median duration of survival is often less than one year), due to its high resistance to chemotherapy. Therefore, it is fundamental to understand the mechanisms of drug resistance and to find new treatments overcoming such resistance.

Chemotherapy cause intracellular damages (such DNA adducts after cisplatin treatment blocking mitosis) and results in an overproduction of ROS (Reactive Oxygen Species) toxics for the cells. These damages lead to cell death apoptosis, when the capacities of cells for repairing damages and for detoxifying ROS are exceeded (Bellance, 2009; Gogvadze, 2009; Grüning, 2010; Israël, 2004, 2005; Kroemer & Pouyssegur, 2008; Olovnikov, 2009; Vander Heiden, 2009). Cells may also develop drug resistance by over expressing anti-apoptotic proteins (Burz, 2009; Green, 2004; Yip, 2008), or by over expressing the transporter P-glycoprotein 170, a protein which expels the chemotherapy drug outside at their membrane. This membrane carrier belongs to the family of the ATP transporters associated with the Multi Drug Resistance phenotype (MDR) (Comerford, 2002). All these mechanisms leading to drug resistance occur either primarily as it is usual for mesothelioma, or secondarily, as often see for ovarian cancer, a cancer disease actively studied in our laboratory.

When active, chemotherapies lead to apoptotic death of cancer cells (Burz, 2009; Green, 2004; Yip, 2008). Apoptosis is a physiological mechanism used for modeling the form of the embryo or for eliminating damaged or aged cells during life (Green, 2004). Apoptosis results from the leakage of the mitochondria outer membrane where pores open and release various molecules into the cytoplasm, such cytochrome c oxidized. Then caspases are activated in the cytosol. The activation of caspases (9 and 3 in particular) leads to fragmentation of the nucleus (as evidenced by the cleavage of PARP) and by the transformation of the cells into debris, which are eliminated by the macrophages. Apoptosis is controlled by genes that encode for pro-apoptotic (Bid, Bax, Bak, BH3-only...) and anti-apoptotic proteins (Bcl-2 type, Mcl-1, Bcl-x_L...). It ultimately results in the imbalance between these two kinds of proteins, all belonging to the Bcl-2 family (Burz, 2009; Green, 2004; Yip, 2008). It seems that pro-apoptotic proteins such as Bak and Bax need to trigger apoptosis, to be first translocated from the cytoplasm to the mitochondria. This translocation occur after these pro-apoptotic proteins have inhibited the anti-apoptotic proteins located on the surface of mitochondria either by direct contact or through indirect mechanisms involving the subfamily of pro-apoptotic proteins BH3-only, such as Noxa, Puma, Bad (Willis, 2005). As it was shown in our laboratory (Varin, 2010), concomitant inhibition by specific siRNA directed against Mcl-1 and Bcl-x_L proteins was sufficient to destroy all MSTO-211H cells in culture, whereas the robust NCI-H28 cells, were destroyed in the same way by the adjunction of a low dose of cisplatin. So, anti-apoptotic strategies are thought to play an important role in next future to overcome drug resistance of cancers (Burz, 2009).

Whatever the mechanisms involved in the drug resistance (MDR, resistance to apoptosis, enhancement of detoxification and of damage repairing process, etc.), all these processes require large amounts of ATP and cofactors such NAD^+ or NADPH, H^+. If the damages are significant, DNA repairing enzymes, like PARP, are highly activated, requiring large amounts of ATP and NAD^+. The functioning of the P-glycoprotein 170, associated with the MDR phenotype needs also great amounts of ATP to expulse drugs outside (Comerford, 2002). In definitive, ATP is required for all process of life, and higher level is required by cancer cells for surviving cellular damages caused by chemotherapy. Therefore, we may hypothesize that if we diminish the level of ATP and of the cofactors inside cells, we will facilitate the action of chemotherapy, cells lacking of ATP and cofactors necessary to repair. The intensity of the ATP depletion would result in cell death apoptosis which requires ATP, or in necrosis, when ATP depletion will be severe enough or brutal inside cells (Leist, 1997; Lelli, 1998).

Our results show that blocking glycolysis, can effectively trigger apoptosis or necrosis and sensitize cells to chemotherapy. The mechanism leading to cell death remains to be studied: energy depletion ?, blockade of ribose formation derived from glucose transformation ?, other actions?

We chose to work on mesothelioma, but we think any significant results obtain in this highly chemoresistant cancer, should be reasonably extrapolated for others solid cancers. Our results confirm the therapeutic benefit against cancer cells that could be taken when glycolysis is slowed down or blocked using anti-glycolytic agents (Geschwind, 2004; Ko, 2004; Xu, 2005). When death occurs, it happened either by apoptotic or by necrotic mechanisms, a type of death that could be related to the intensity of ATP depletion. When studying the effects of 3-BrPA and citrate, we observed that cell death effect was dose and time dependant. When the dose was high, necrosis was dominant. Our studies (Zhang, 2009b) confirm the anti-cancer action of 3-BrPA (Geschwind, 2004; Ko, 2004) and demonstrated *in vivo* the interest of this agent to sensitize cells to cisplatin, which has been observed *in vitro* (Ihrlund, 2008). We showed similar anti-cancer action of citrate which demonstrated also interesting anti-Mcl-1 properties (Zhang, 2009a; Lu, 2011). It is noteworthy that these anti-glycolytic molecules might have a crucial role for destroying robust cells like our chemoresistant NCI-H28 cells, which are presumably the most hypoxic ones, lacking functional mitochondrial respiration (Xu, 2005). Cells which cannot adapt such severe environmental conditions spontaneously died, forming necrosis, as it is often see in the core part of large tumors, such as non squamous lung cancers. For surviving these severe hypoxic conditions, cells should have necessarily adapt a robust defense system supported by an enhanced glycolysis providing ATP, in place of OXPHOS because of the lack of O_2. It is tempting to link the high chemoresistance of these cells to their altered mitochondrial respiration (Zhang, 2009a) and may be also to the overexpression of the anti-apoptotic molecules Mcl-1 and Bcl-x_L on the outer membrane of mitochondria as we showed (Varin, 2010). High concentrations of 3-BrPA or citrate were able to kill these cells by necrosis, which would occur when ATP depletion would be severe beyond a threshold (Leist, 1997; Lelli, 1998). Interestingly, we showed however that these NCI-H28 cells can undergo apoptosis, if both anti-apoptotic molecules Mcl-1 or Bcl-x_L are inhibited by specific siRNA. In that case, a small dose of cisplatin becomes efficient (Varin, 2010). Of particular interest also to overcome chemoresistance, should be the association of agents like 3-BrPA or citrate to cisplatin, as we observed either *in vitro* or *in vivo* studies (Zhang, 2009a, 2009b).

In contrast to NCI-211H, we may reasonably suppose that cells like MSTO-211H could be located in the well oxygenated peripheral part of tumors, where they proliferate rapidly. The sole inhibition of glycolysis by 3-BrPA or citrate 10 mM did not lead to complete destruction of cells, but only a slowdown or an arrest of the proliferation. This could be due to their functional mitochondrial respiration with an OXPHOS providing the most part of ATP. Therefore, the sole glycolysis inhibition is not sufficient to arrest the ATP production and to cell death. In such type of cells, 3-BrPA or citrate should be used primarily to sensitize cells to chemotherapy, as we observed *in vitro* and *in vivo* (Zhang, 2009a, 2009b). Our study confirms the anti-cancer action of 3-BrPA already reported (Geschwind, 2004; Ko, 2004), this molecule being able to sensitive cells to cisplatin (Ihrlund, 2008).

It should be tempting to inhibit concomitantly with glycolysis, glutaminolysis but also β-oxidation (Hatzivassiliou, 2005; Paumen, 1997; Wang, 2010).

The mechanisms of action of 3-BrPA and citrate remain largely hypothetical:

-   3-BrPA might inhibit glycolysis by interfering with all reactions involving pyruvate such LDH, PC, or PDH, and such inhibitions eventually lead to a blockage or a slowdown of the metabolism (pyruvate is at the crossroad of various metabolic pathways), resulting in a loss of ATP inside the cell and or in a blockage of molecules required for the proliferation. Furthermore 3-BrPA would also inhibit HK II resulting in apoptosis, because HK II is linked to the apoptotic pathway (Danial, 2003; Geschwind, 2004; Ko, 2004; Pastorino, 2008; Pedersen, 2002; Xu, 2005). HK II is located on the outer membrane of mitochondria, where glucose is converted in glucose 6-phosphate. HK II is associated with the VDAC (voltage dependent anion channel), and would be part of the PTP (permeability transitory pore) (Danial, 2003; Pastorino, 2008). The inhibition of HK II by 3-BrPA would lead to the release of HKII from the outer membrane, and would lead to the removal of the anti-apoptotic Bcl-2 proteins inhibition, leading to the channel opening and release of cytochrome c, activating caspases (Burz, 2009; Green, 2004; Yip, 2008). Moreover, 3-BrPA might also increase the production of ROS, toxic for the cell (Ihrlund, 2008). Recently, it has been shown that the main of action of 3-BrPA should be an alkylation of the GAPDH (Glyceraldehyde 3-phosphate dehydrogenase) (Ganapathy-Kanniappan, 2010).

- *Citrate* is a powerful indicator of energy production, which inhibits PFK1, the key enzyme regulating the entrance of glycolysis. This inhibition leads to an accumulation of glucose-6-phosphate upstream, which will inhibit HK II, by negative feedback, leading to apoptosis through the mechanism aforementioned (Danial, 2003; Pastorino, 2008; Pedersen, 2002). Citrate inhibits also PKF2 (Chesney, 2006), the powerful allosteric activator enzyme system of PFK1 (Campbell & Smith, 2000; Lehninger 1975; Stryer, 1981; Yalcin, 2009). PKF2 produces fructose 2-6 bisphosphate (F2,6P), which physiologically may override the inhibition of PFK1 by ATP when glucose is abundant. This is the case in cancer cells, due to the activation of membrane glucose transporters (GLUT1 and GLUT3) and of HK II, by HIF-1α, myc, ras activations and loss of p53 (Bellance, 2009; Feron, 2009; Grüning, 2010; Israël, 2004, 2005; Kim, 2006; Kroemer & Pouyssegur, 2008; Marin-Hernández, 2009; Olovnikov, 2009; Vander Heiden, 2009). F2,6P is considered as a key intracellular signal in cancer cells (Yalcin, 2009), enhancing glycolysis by activating PFK1, while inhibiting gluconeogenesis by inactivating fructose1,6-bisphosphatase (3-5). Therefore, citrate inhibits PKF2 and counteracts its effects on PFK1.

- Citrate also inhibits pyruvate kinase (PK), at least indirectly, because it decreases the powerful activation exerted by fructose 1-6 bisphosphate on PK, which in normal cells, allows an immediate adjustment of the activities of PFK and PK, thus closely adjusting flux at the entrance and at the exit of glycolysis (Campbell & Smith, 2000; Lehninger 1975; Stryer, 1981). Citrate regulates and adjusts also the flux of the tricarboxylic acids cycle (TCA cycle): it inhibits PDH (Taylor, 1973), the complex enzyme which produces acetyl-CoA from pyruvate, a step that allows the final product of glycolysis, to enter in the TCA cycle. Citrate inhibits at the end of the cycle, succinate dehydrogenase (SDH) (Hillar, 1975), which converts succinate to fumarate. SDH is part of complex II, located in the inner membrane, and is the sole enzyme that participates in both the TCA cycle and OXPHOS. Through SDH inhibition, citrate would reduce ATP production by OXPHOS.

Citrate stimulates fatty acid synthesis by providing acetyl-CoA which is required in abundance for this synthesis whereas it is an allosteric activator of the cytoplasmic Acetyl-Co Carboxylase (ACC), the main enzyme of this pathway consuming great amounts of ATP, and NADPH,H⁺ (Campbell & Smith, 2000; Lehninger 1975; Stryer, 1981). At the same time, citrate inhibits indirectly β-oxidation, because the first product of ACC, malonyl CoA, inhibits the carnitine acyl transferase I (CPTI), located on the outer mitochondrial membrane (Campbell & Smith, 2000; Lehninger 1975; Stryer, 1981).

Finally, the level of citrate is a main indicator of the energy inside cells, enabling cells to adjust their metabolism to their reserve and requirement. By regulating enzymes located at strategic places of the biochemical pathways, this molecule allows a close adjustment of the fluxes of glycolysis and of the TCA cycle. When the production of ATP is sufficient, citrate inhibits the ATP-producing catabolic pathways, blocking the catabolic pathways at their entrances (glycolysis, β-oxidation), whereas it stimulates biosynthetic pathways (neoglucogenesis and lipid synthesis). Consequently, if citrate is administered in excess to cancer cells that require a high production of ATP for their biosynthesis, it would fool the cell's energy level inside cells. While it would block all ATP-producing pathways, it would activate at the same time biosynthetic pathways consuming ATP, a situation that would quickly lead to a severe depletion of ATP, NADH,H^+ and NADPH,H^+, inside cells.

4.1 Other actions of citrate

The mechanism of action of citrate is not unique. In addition to the widely accepted biochemical effects of citrate (inhibition of PFK, activation of fructose1,6-bisphosphatase and of ACC) (Campbell & Smith, 2000; Lehninger 1975; Stryer, 1981), this molecule might have other actions, either on histone acetylation or on calcium homeostasis inside cells, that should have anti-cancer properties: - it could exert an action on the nuclear histone acetyltransferases (HATs), which use acetyl-CoA to acelytate the histones (Wellen, 2009). Indeed, citrate provides acetyl for HATs, after it is transformed by the ATP-citrate lyase (ACLY) in acetyl-CoA and OAA. Knowing that histone deacetylation plays a key role in the re-expression of genes (especially embryonic) and or in expression of oncogenes (Israël, 2004, 2005), citrate would favor the re-acetylation of histones, and might have an anticancer activity similar to that of the inhibitors of histone deacetylation (Mutze, 2010).

Citrate led also to an early inhibition of the antiapoptotic protein Mcl-1, which plays a key role with the protein Bcl- xL in chemoresistance of cancers (Burz, 2009; Warr, 2008; Willis, 2005; Yip, 2008), especially of mesothelioma cancers (Varin, 2010). Citrate could be usefully associated with Bcl-xL inhibitors, since inhibition of these two key anti-apoptotic protein is necessary to obtain a strong cytotoxic effect, as we showed for mesothelioma (Varin, 2010).

Interestingly, addition of citrate to Bcl-x_L-expressing cells leads to increase protein N-alpha-acetylation and sensitization of these cells to apoptosis(Yi, 2011). It has been suggested that cytosolic acetyl-CoA might influence the apoptotic threshold in multiple oncogenic contexts. In turn, Bcl-x_L would be able to control the levels of acetyl-CoA and protein-N-acetylation, this providing a clear example of a linkage between metabolism and apoptotic sensitivity.

Knowing that, there are few or any available specific inhibitors of Mcl-1 (Warr, 2008), whereas inhibitors of Bcl-x_L are currently under clinical evaluation (as BH3 mimetic compounds such antimycin A3 or the inhibitor of LDH, gossypol), this anti-Mcl-1 action of citrate reinforces the interest of this agent.

Citrate is also a known well known chelating agent of Ca^{2+}. Because it might reduce the pool of ATP required by Ca^{2+} ATPases, this inhibition might reduce or suppress the cell's ability to do work by increasing the cytosolic concentration of Ca^{2+}. When the increase of this concentration is beyond a threefold, it might lead to necrosis or to apoptosis in relation with calcium-dependent concentration. By diminishing also Mcl-1 at the outer membrane, which inhibits mitochondrial Ca^{2+} elevation, citrate would favor also mitochondrial apoptosis (Bergner, 2008).

4.2 Are 3-BrPA and citrate toxic?

3-BrPA should be not toxic for normal cells (Ihrlund, 2008), and none toxicity has been observed in animals *in vivo* studies reporting its anti-cancer action (Geschwind, 2004; Ko, 2004). To our knowledge, clinical studies should be currently performed at the John

Hopkins Hospital in Baltimore, to evaluate the beneficial effect of 3-BrPA in the treatment of human hepatocarcinoma.

Citrate is a physiological product, which does not seem toxic, except at very high dosages. Neither experimental studies nor literature data have reported toxicity, except the occurrence of hypocalcemia after massive blood transfusion (Diaz, 1994), which was reversed by intravenous infusion of calcium (Vagianos, 1990). No accidental ingestion of high doses of citrate has been reported to our knowledge. The LD 50 of 4 g per kg after ip injection we observed in mice was consistent with data reported in the literature, ie 4 g per kg for mice and 6 to 11 g per kg for rats (see, citric acid in International Chemical Safety Cards : ICSC 0704). We observed signs of clinical acute toxicity at doses > 500 mg / kg, with convulsions occurring within 3 to 8 minutes after the injection, which were reversed by ip calcium chloride injection at equimolar dose. Then, all animals survived. Therefore lethality and clinical signs observed in animals receiving lethal doses of citrate where interpreted as indirect evidence of severe hypocalcemia. Reversions of convulsions and of heart failure have been reported in animals treated with intra-vascular administration of calcium (Vagianos, 1990). Hypocalcemia after administration of citrate has also been documented after massive blood transfusions associated with liver failure following transplantation, the liver being responsible of the metabolism of citrate. In such cases the administration of calcium chloride restored normal calcium baseline levels and suppressed the cardiovascular toxicity that was related to this hypocalcemia (Vagianos, 1990). We did not find any sign of chronic toxicity in organs with the protocol we tested (ip doses ranged up to 500 mg per kg, administered either by peritoneal injections or by oral gavages for several weeks. By extrapolating, the daily dose in an adult male weighing 70 kg should be 28 g, a dose that could be administered through a peritoneal or pleural catheter.

Because citrate is a physiological molecule, it is likely there exist a range of elevated doses, where citrate might become cytostatic or toxic for proliferating cancer cells (as in our studies in vitro), without it would have no significant side effects for normal cells, which are most often in a quite steady state, and do not require an intense production of ATP for sustaining enhanced metabolism. Interestingly, an author has recently reported that a patient with primary peritoneal mesothelioma was improved after taking citric acid orally at a daily dose up to 45 gr per day (Halabé Bucay, 2011). However, because, as we have shown (Zhang, 2009a), there are clones of cells that can be only totally destroyed by the combination of citrate and cisplatin, we think future studies should focused more on testing citrate as a sensitizer of current chemotherapy.

Finally, association of these antiglycolytic agents with chemotherapy should be particularly considered for treating patients suffering advanced cancer disease, such as pleural or peritoneal carcinomatosis.

5. Conclusions

In conclusion, the understanding of the biochemical pathways involved in cancer cells helps to propose models of the reprogramming of the cell's metabolism and to imagine new strategies for counteracting cancer development. It can be easily understood that cancer cell death could be induced, at least experimentally, by molecules blocking glycolysis, glutaminolysis, the malate shuttle, β-oxidation, or by stimulating PDH. Because key regulator enzymes are generally located at the entrance of the metabolic pathways, strategies for blocking or activating such enzymes should be particularly investigated such as we showed using citrate, and combined together in "pluritherapies", since cancer cells may find new routes for escape any blockage. Citrate and 3-BrPA should be considered for clinical studies, and association of these agents with cisplatin should be tested as local therapy particularly in patients suffering pleural or peritoneal carcinomatosis.

6. Acknowledgements

This work was supported by the "Ligue Contre le Cancer" (Comité du Calvados).

7. References

Bellance, N.; Lestienne, P. & Rossignol, R. 2009. Mitochondria: from bioenergetics in the metabolic regulation of carcinogenesis. *Frontiers in Bioscience*, 14, 4015-4034.
Bergner, A. & Huber, R.M. 2008. Regulation of the endoplasmic reticulum C2+-store in cancer. *Anticancer Agents Med Chem.*, 8, 705-709.
Burz, C.; Berindan-Neagoe, I.; Balacescu, O. & Irimie A. 2009. Apoptosis in cancer: key molecular signaling pathways and therapy targets. *Acta Oncol.*, 48, 811-821.
Campbell, P.N. & Smith, A.D. 2000. *Biochemistry illustrated (fourth edition)*, Harcourt Publishers Limited, Churchill Livingstone.
Carretta, A.; Landoni, C.; Melloni, G.; Ceresoli,G.L.; Compierchio,A.; Fazio,F.& Zannini,P. 2000. 18-FDG positron emission tomography in the evaluation of malignant pleural diseases - a pilot study. *Eur J Cardiothorac Surg.*, 17, 377-383.
Chesney, J. 2006. 6-phosphofructo-2-kinase/fructose-2,6-bisphosphatase and tumor cell glycolysis. *Curr Opin Clin Nutr Metab Care.*, 9, 535-539.
Christofk, H.R.; Vander Heiden, M.G.; Harris, M.H.; Ramanathan, A.; Gerszten, R.E.; Wei,R.; Fleming, M.D.; Schreiber, S.L. & Cantley, L.C. 2008a The M2 splice isoform of pyruvate kinase is important for cancer metabolism and tumour growth. *Nature*, 13, 452, 230-233.
Christofk, H.R.; Vander Heiden, M.G.; Wu, N.; Asara, J.M.& Cantley, L.C. 2008b. Pyruvate kinase M2 is a phosphotyrosine-binding protein. *Nature*, 13, 452, 181-186.
Comerford, K.M.; Wallace, T.J.; Karhausen, J.; Louis, N.A.; Montalto, M.C. & Colgan, S.P. 2002. Hypoxia-inducible factor-1-dependent regulation of multidrug resistance (MDR1) gene. *Cancer res.*, 62, 3387-3394.
Danial, N.N.; Gramm, C.F.; Scorrano, L.; Zhang, C.Y.; Krauss, S.; Ranger, A.M.; Datta, S.R.; Greenberg, M.E.; Licklider, L.J.; Lowell, B.B.; Gygi, S.P. & Korsmeyer, S.J. 2003. BAD and glucokinase reside in a mitochondrial complex that integrates glycolysis and apoptosis. *Nature*, 424, 952-956.
DeBerardinis, R.J. & Cheng, T. 2010. Q's next: the diverse functions of glutamine in metabolism, cell biology and cancer. *Oncogene* , 29, 313-324.
DeBerardinis, R.J.; Sayed, N.; Ditsworth, D. et al. 2008. Brick by brick: metabolism and tumor cell growth. *Curr Opin genet Dev*, 18, 54-61.
Diaz, J.; Acosta, F.; Parrilla, P.; Sansano, T.; Bento, M.; Cura, S.; Contreras, R.F.; Belmonte, J.G.; Bueno, F.S.; Robles, R.; et al. 1994. Citrate intoxication and blood concentration of ionized calcium in liver transplantation.*Transplant Proc.*, 26, 3669-3670.

Eagle, H.; Oyama, V.I.; Levy,M.; et al. 1956. The growth response of mammalian cells in tissue culture to L-glutamine and L-glutamic acid. *J Biol Chem*, 218, 607-616.

Feron, O. 2009. Pyruvate into lactate and back: From the Warburg effect to symbiotic energy fuel exchange in cancer cells. *Radiotherapy and Oncology*, 92: 329-333.

Ganapathy-Kanniappan, S.; Vali, M.; Kunjithapatham, R.; Bujis, M.; Syed, L.H.; Rao, P.P.; Ota, S.; Kwak, B.K.; Loffroy, R. & Geschwind J.F. 2010. 3- Bromopyruvate: a new targeted antiglycolytic agent and a promise for cancer therapy. *Current Pharm. Biotech.*, 11, 510-517.

Geschwind, J.F.; Georgiades, C.S.; Ko, Y.H. & Pedersen,P.L.2004. Recently elucidated energy catabolism pathways provide opportunities for novel treatments in hepatocellular carcinoma. *Expert Rev Anticancer Ther.*, 4, 449-457.

Gogvadze, V.; Orrenius, S. & Zhivotovsky, B. 2009. Mitochondria as targets for chemotherapy. *Apoptosis*, 14, 624-640.

Green, D.R. & Kroemer, G. 2004. The pathophysiology of mitochondrial cell death. *Science*, 305, 626-629.

Grüning, N.M.; Lehrach, H. & Ralser, M. 2010. Regulatory crosstalk of the metabolic network. *Trends Biochem Sci*, 35, 220-227.

Halabe Bucay, A. 2011. Clinical report: A patient with primary peritoneal mesothelioma that has improved after taking citric acid orally (letter). *Clinics and Research in Hepatology and Gastroenterology*, 35, 241

Hatzivassiliou, G.; Zhao, F.; Bauer, D.E.; Andreadis, C.; Shaw, A.N.; Dhanak, D.; Hingorani,S.R.; Tuveson, D.A. & Thompson,C.B. 2005. ATP citrate lyase inhibition can suppress tumor cell growth. *Cancer Cell*, 8, 311-321.

Hillar, M.; Lott, V. & Lennox, B. 1975. Correlation of the effects of citric acid cycle metabolites on succinate oxidation by rat liver mitochondria and submitochondrial particles. *J Bioenerg.*, 7, 1-6.

Icard, P. & Lincet, H. The central role of citrate in the metabolism of cancer cells. 2012. *Biomedical Research.*, 2012;23 (1), in press.

Ihrlund, L.S.; Hernlund, E.; Khan, O. & Shoshan, M.C. 2008. 3-Bromopyruvate as inhibitor of tumour cell energy metabolism and chemopotentiator of platinum drugs. *Mol Oncol.*, 2, 94-101.

Israël, M. & Schwartz, L. 2005. *Cancer: a dysmethylation syndrome*, éd. John Libbey Eurotext,.

Israël, M. 2004. *Four hidden metamorphoses: a remark on blood, muscle, mental diseases and cancer.* éd. John Libbey Eurotext.

Kim, J.W.; Tchernyshyov, I.; Semenza, G.L. & Dang, C.V. 2006. HIF-1-mediated expression of pyruvate dehydrogenase kinase: a metabolic switch required for cellular adaptation to hypoxia. *Cell Metab.*, 3, 177-185.

Ko, Y.H.; Smith, B.L.; Wang, Y.; Pomper, M.G.; Rini, D.A.; Torbenson, M.S.; Hullihen, J. & Pedersen, P.L. 2004. Advanced cancers: eradication in all cases using 3-bromopyruvate therapy to deplete ATP. *Biochem.Biophys.Res.Commun.*, 324, 269-275.

Kroemer, G. & Pouyssegur, J. 2008. Tumor cell metabolism: cancer's Achilles' Heel, *Cancer cell*, 13, 472-482.

Lehninger, A.L. 1970, 1975. the molecular basis of cell structure and function. *Biochemistry*, Worth Publishers, Inc.

Leist, M.; Single, B.; Castoldi, A.F.; Kuhnle, S. & Nicotera P. 1997. Intracellular adenosine triphosphate (ATP) concentration: a switch in the decision between apoptosis and necrosis. *J Exp Med.*, 185, 1481-1486.

Lelli, J.L., Jr.; Becks, L.L.; Dabrowska, M.I. & Hinshaw D.B. 1998. ATP converts necrosis to apoptosis in oxidant-injured endothelial cells. *Free Radic Biol Med.*, 25, 694-702.

Lopez-Rios, F.; Sanchez-Arago, M.; Garcia-Garcia, E.; Ortega, A.D.; Berrendero, J.R.; Pozo-Rodriguez, F.; Lopez-Encuentra, A.; Ballestin, C. & Cuezva, J.M. 2007. Loss of the mitochondrial bioenergetic capacity underlies the glucose avidity of carcinomas. *Cancer Res.*, 67: 9013-9017.

Lu, Y.; Zhang, X.D.; Lan, J.; Huang, G.; Varin, E.; Lincet, H.; Poulain, L. & Icard P. 2011 : Citrate induces the apoptosis death of human carcinoma cells : an anti-cancer agent for gastric cancers ? *Anticancer Res.*, 31, 3, 797-805.

Marin-Hernandez, A.; Gallardo-Perez, J.C.; Ralph, S.J.; Rodriguez-Enriquez, S.& Moreno-Sanchez, R. 2009. HIF-1alpha modulates energy metabolism in cancer cells by inducing over-expression of specific glycolytic isoforms. *Mini Rev Med Chem.*, 9, 1084-1101, Review.

Mazurek, S.; Grimm, H.; Boschek, C.B.; Vaupel, P.& Eigenbrodt,E. 2002. Pyruvate kinase type M2: a crossroad in the tumor metabolome. *Br.J.Nutr.*, 87, Suppl 1:S23-S29.

Mutze, K.; Langer, R.; Becker, K.; Ott, K.; Novotny, A.; Luber, B.; Hapfelmeier, A.; Göttlicher, M.; Höfler, H. & Keller, G. 2010. Histone Deacetylase (HDAC) 1 and 2 Expression and Chemotherapy in Gastric Cancer. *Ann Surg Oncol.*, 17, 3336-3343.

Olovnikov, I.; Kravchenko, J.A. & Chumakov P.M. 2009. Homeostatic functions of the p53 suppressor: regulation of energy metabolism and antioxidant defense. *Seminars in Cancer Biology*, 19, 32-41.

Pastorino, J.G. & Hoek, J.B. 2008. Regulation of hexokinase binding to VDAC. *J Bioenerg Biomembr.*, 40, 171-1 82. Review.

Paumen, M.B.; Ishida, Y.; Muramatsu, M.; Yamamoto, M. & Honjo,T. 1997. Inhibition of carnitine palmitoyltransferase I augments sphingolipid synthesis and palmitate-induced apoptosis. *J Biol Chem.*, 272, 3324-3329.

Pedersen, P.L.; Mathupala, S.; Rempel, A.; Geschwind, J.F. & Ko, Y.H. 2002. Mitochondrial bound type II hexokinase: a key player in the growth and survival of many cancers and an ideal prospect for therapeutic intervention. *Biochim Biophys Acta.*, 1555, 14-20.

Quin, J.Z. & Nickoloff, B.J. 2010. Targeting glutaminase metabolism sensitizes melanoma cells to TRAIL-induced death. *Biochem Biophys Res Commun.*, 398, 146-152.

Reitzer, L.J.; Wice, B.M. & Kennell, D. 1979. Evidence that glutamine, not sugar, is the major energy source for cultured Hela cells. *J Biol Chem*, 254, 2669-2676.

Samudio, I.; Fiegl, M. & Andreeff M. 2009. Mitochondrial uncoupling and the Warburg effect: molecular basis for the reprogramming of cancer cell metabolism. *Cancer Res.*, 69, 2163-2166.

Simonnet, H.; Demont, J.; Pfeiffer, K.; Guenaneche,L.; Bouvier,R.; Brandt,U.; Schagger, H., & Godinot,C. 2003. Mitochondrial complex I is deficient in renal oncocytomas. *Carcinogenesis*, 24, 1461-1666.

Stryer, L. 1975. 1981. *Biochemistry*, W.H. Freeman and Compagny, San Franscisco.

Taylor, W.M. & Halperin, M.L. 1973. Regulation of pyruvate deshydrogenase in muscle. Inhibition by citrate. *J Bio Chem.*, 248, 6080-6083.

Vagianos, C.; Steen, S.; Masson, P.; Fåhraeus, T.; Sjöberg, T.; Kugelberg, J. & Solem, JO. 1990. Reversal of lethal citrate intoxication by intravenous infusion of calcium. An experimental study in pigs. *Acta Chir Scand.*, 156, 671-675.

Vander Heiden, M.G.; Cantley, L.C. & Thompson, C.B. 2009. Understanding the Warburg effect: the metabolic requirements of cell proliferation. *Science*, 324, 1029-1033.

Varin, E.; Denoyelle, C.; Brotin, E.; Meryet-Figuiere, M.; Giffard, F.; Abeilard, E.; Goux, D.; Gauduchon, P.; Icard,P. & Poulain, L. 2010. Down-regulation of Bcl-xL and Mcl-1 is sufficient to induce cell death in mesothelioma cells highly refractory to conventional chemotherapy. *Carcinogenesis*, 31, 984-93.

Wang, J.B.; Erickson, J.W.; Fuji, R.; Ramachandran, S.; Gao, P.; Dinavahi, R.; Wilson, K.F.; Ambrosio, A.L.; Dias, S.M.; Dang, C.V. & Cerione,R.A. 2010. Targeting mitochondrial glutaminase activity inhibits oncogenic transformation. *Cancer cell*, 18, 207-209.

Warburg, O. 1930. The Metabolism of Tumors. Constable and Company, Ltd. London, 327.

Warburg, O. 1956. On the origin of cancer cells. *Science*, 123, 309-314.

Warr, M. & Shore, G.C. 2008. Unique biology of Mcl-1: Therapeutic opportunities in cancer. *Current Mol Med.*, 8, 138-147.

Wellen, K.E.; Hatzivassiliou, G.; Sachdeva, U.M.; Bui, T.V.; Cross, J.R. & Thompson, C.B. 2009. ATP-citrate lyase links cellular metabolism to histone acetylation. *Science*, 324, 1076-1080.

Willis, S.N.; Chen, L.; Dewson, G.; Wei, A.; Naik, E.; Fletcher, J.I.; Adams, J.M. & Huang, D.C. 2005. Proapoptotic Bak is sequestered by Mcl-1 and Bcl-xL, but not Bcl-2, until displaced by BH3-only proteins. *Genes Dev.*, 19, 1294-1305.

Xu, R.H.; Pelicano, H.; Zhou, Y.; Carew, J.S.; Feng, L.; Bhalla, K.N.; Keating, M.J. & Huang,P. 2005. Inhibition of glycolysis in cancer cells: a novel strategy to overcome drug resistance associated with mitochondrial respiratory defect and hypoxia. *Cancer Res.*, 65, 613-621.

Yalcin, A.; Telang, S.; Clem, B. & Chesney,J. 2009. Regulation of glucose metabolism by 6-phosphofructo-2-kinase/fructose-2,6-bisphosphatases in cancer. *Exp Mol Pathol.*, 86, 174-179.

Yi, C.H.; Pan, H.; Seebacher, J.; Jang, I.H.; Hyberts, S.G.; Heffron, G.J.; Vander Heiden, M.G.; Yang, R.; Li, F.; Locasale, J.W.; Sharfi H.; Zhai, B.; Rodriguez-Mias, R.; Luithardt, H. & Cantley, L.C. 2011. Metabolic Regulation of Protein N-Alpha-Acetylation by Bcl-xL Promotes Cell Survival. *Cell*, 146, 607-620.

Yip, K.W. & Reed, J.C. 2008. Bcl-2 family proteins and cancer. *Oncogene*, 27, 6398-6406.

Zhang, X.; Varin, E.; Allouche, S.; Lu, Y.; Poulain, L. & Icard P. 2009a. Effect of citrate on malignant pleural mesothelioma cells: a synergistic effect with cisplatin. *Anticancer Res.*, 29, 1249-1254.

Zhang, X.; Varin, E.; Briand, M.; Allouche, S.; Heutte, N.; Schwartz, L.; Poulain, L. & Icard, P. 2009b. Novel therapy for malignant pleural mesothelioma based on anti-energetic effect: an experimental study using 3-Bromopyruvate on nude mice. *Anticancer Res.*, 29, 1443-1448.

Zhang, X.D.; Deslandes, E.; Villedieu, M.; Poulain, L.; Duval, M.; Gauduchon, P.; Schwartz, L. & Icard, P. 2006. Effect of 2-deoxy-D-glucose on various malignant cell lines in vitro. *Anticancer Res.*, 26, 3561-3566.

Permissions

The contributors of this book come from diverse backgrounds, making this book a truly international effort. This book will bring forth new frontiers with its revolutionizing research information and detailed analysis of the nascent developments around the world.

We would like to thank Alexander Zubritsky MD, PhD, for lending his expertise to make the book truly unique. He has played a crucial role in the development of this book. Without his invaluable contribution this book wouldn't have been possible. He has made vital efforts to compile up to date information on the varied aspects of this subject to make this book a valuable addition to the collection of many professionals and students.

This book was conceptualized with the vision of imparting up-to-date information and advanced data in this field. To ensure the same, a matchless editorial board was set up. Every individual on the board went through rigorous rounds of assessment to prove their worth. After which they invested a large part of their time researching and compiling the most relevant data for our readers. Conferences and sessions were held from time to time between the editorial board and the contributing authors to present the data in the most comprehensible form. The editorial team has worked tirelessly to provide valuable and valid information to help people across the globe.

Every chapter published in this book has been scrutinized by our experts. Their significance has been extensively debated. The topics covered herein carry significant findings which will fuel the growth of the discipline. They may even be implemented as practical applications or may be referred to as a beginning point for another development. Chapters in this book were first published by InTech; hereby published with permission under the Creative Commons Attribution License or equivalent.

The editorial board has been involved in producing this book since its inception. They have spent rigorous hours researching and exploring the diverse topics which have resulted in the successful publishing of this book. They have passed on their knowledge of decades through this book. To expedite this challenging task, the publisher supported the team at every step. A small team of assistant editors was also appointed to further simplify the editing procedure and attain best results for the readers.

Our editorial team has been hand-picked from every corner of the world. Their multi-ethnicity adds dynamic inputs to the discussions which result in innovative outcomes. These outcomes are then further discussed with the researchers and contributors who give their valuable feedback and opinion regarding the same. The feedback is then collaborated with the researches and they are edited in a comprehensive manner to aid the understanding of the subject.

Apart from the editorial board, the designing team has also invested a significant amount of their time in understanding the subject and creating the most relevant covers. They scrutinized every image to scout for the most suitable representation of the subject and create an appropriate cover for the book.

The publishing team has been involved in this book since its early stages. They were actively engaged in every process, be it collecting the data, connecting with the contributors or procuring relevant information. The team has been an ardent support to the editorial, designing and production team. Their endless efforts to recruit the best for this project, has resulted in the accomplishment of this book. They are a veteran in the field of academics and their pool of knowledge is as vast as their experience in printing. Their expertise and guidance has proved useful at every step. Their uncompromising quality standards have made this book an exceptional effort. Their encouragement from time to time has been an inspiration for everyone.

The publisher and the editorial board hope that this book will prove to be a valuable piece of knowledge for researchers, students, practitioners and scholars across the globe.

List of Contributors

Philip A. Rascoe, Xiaobo X. Cao and W. Roy Smythe
Texas A&M Health Science Center College of Medicine, Scott & White Memorial Hospital & Clinic, Olin E. Teague Veterans' Medical Center, USA

Jesus Montesinos, Sílvia Catot, Francesc Sant and Montserrat Domenech
Althaia, Xarxa Assistencial de Manresa, Fundació Privada, Barcelona, Spain

Zachary Klaassen, Kristopher R. Carlson and Martha K. Terris
Department of Urology, Georgia Health Sciences University, United States of America

Jeffrey R. Lee and Sravan Kuvari
Department of Pathology, Georgia Health Sciences University, United States of America

Alexander N. Zubritsky
Moscow, Russian Federation

Bonnie W. Lau
Brown University, USA

Elif Aktas, Kemal Arda and Nazan Çiledağ and Bilgin Kadri Aribas
Ankara Abdurrahman Yurtaslan Oncology Education and Research Hospital, Turkey

Bora Aktas and Sahin Coban
Ankara Yildirim Beyazit Diskapi Education and Research Hospital, Turkey

Winnie A. Merlo and Adriana S. Rosciani
Servicio Diagnóstico Histopatológico y Citológico, Facultad Ciencias Veterinarias Universidad Nacional del Nordeste, Argentina

R. Cornelissen, J.G.J.V. Aerts and J.P.J.J. Hegmans
Erasmus Medical Centre, Rotterdam, The Netherlands

Hiromi Sato and Koichi Ueno
Graduate School of Pharmaceutical Sciences, Chiba University, Japan

Saly Al-Taei, Jason F. Lester and Zsuzsanna Tabi
Department of Oncology, School of Medicine, Cardiff University and Velindre NHS Trust, Cardiff, United Kingdom

Parviz Behnam-Motlagh, Andreas Tyler, Thomas Brännström, Terese Karlsson, Anders Johansson and Kjell Grankvist
Umeå University, Umeå, Sweden

Julija Hmeljak and Andrej Cör
University of Primorska, Faculty of Health Sciences, Izola, Slovenia

T. Fukamachi, H. Saito and H. Kobayashi
Chiba University, Japan

M. Tagawa
Chiba Cancer Center Research Institute, Japan

Philippe Icard
Department of Thoracic Surgery, University Hospital of Caen Basse-Normandie, France
Groupe Régional d'Etudes sur le Cancer (EA 1772), IFR 146 ICORE, University of Caen
Basse-Normandie, France

Xiao-Dong Zhang, Emilie Varin, Pascal Gauduchon, Hubert Lincet and Laurent Poulain
Groupe Régional d'Etudes sur le Cancer (EA 1772), IFR 146 ICORE, University of Caen
Basse-Normandie, France

Stéphane Allouche
Department of Biochemistry, University Hospital of Caen Basse-Normandie, France

Antoine Coquerel
Department of Pharmacology, University Hospital of Caen Basse-Normandie, France

Maria Paciencia
Department of Pathology, University Hospital of Caen Basse-Normandie, Unité "Biologie
et Thérapies Innovantes des Cancers Localement Agressifs" and Centre de Lutte Contre le
Cancer François Baclesse, Caen, France

Luc Joyeux
Department of Thoracic Surgery, University Hospital of Caen Basse-Normandie, France